Praise for
*The Art of Plant-based Cheesemaking*

I knew the moment I walked into Karen McAthy's cheese shop a few years ago that this lady knew what she was doing. Karen has spent the last few years honing her craft and understanding the new science of making cheese from plants, and demonstrates it for us here in her beautiful new book, which elevates vegan cheese to a whole new level. Brava, Karen—I only wish I lived closer to your shop!

—Miyoko Schinner, founder and CEO, Miyoko's Creamery, author, *Artisan Vegan cheese*

For years, Karen has been a source of inspiration and guidance to many who are delving into the world of great vegan cheese. Her expertise, matched with her generosity in sharing her knowledge and skill, makes this volume a must-have in the collection of any culinary aficionado!

—Margaret Coons, founder/CEO, Nuts for Cheese

If you don't use dairy products, or are vegan, here is a true culinary prize for you! *The Art of Plant-based Cheesemaking* delivers the real goods like no other. You'll enjoy cheese and other cultured, dairy-free products with the richness of texture, the depth of flavor, and the myriad health benefits of a plant-based diet.

—Vesanto Melina, MS, Registered Dietitian, author, *Becoming Vegan* and *Kick Diabetes Cookbook*, lead author, Academy of Nutrition and Dietetics' Position Paper on Vegetarian Diets

Karen is a food magician! I've been a fan of her plant-based cheeses for years, and none other compare. She reveals the careful food science behind her art on these pages, so we can all try creating delectable vegan cheeses in our own homes. Let's eat!

—Em Von Euw, cookbook author, creator, *This Rawsome Vegan Life*

Karen McAthy has been at the forefront of artisanal plant-based cheese since the beginning. Her influence is felt everywhere as she strides to bring traditional cheesemaking techniques to vegan cheese. *The Art of Plant-based Cheesemaking* is the best resource for home chefs seeking to delve into the world of real cheesemaking with plant-based ingredients. If vegan cheese analogs have left you wanting, Chef Karen's cheeses will leave you wanting for more.

—Aaron Adams, owner and chef, Farm Spirit and Fermenter

I'm not sure if I've ever met someone who has so much passion, drive, and knowledge for one specific field. Karen has all of these attributes coming out of her cheesy pores. Coming from me, I don't think I can give a bigger compliment actually. She blew my mind with her amazing plant-based dairy products. I've tasted thousands of cheeses, but trying her products opened up a new world to me. This book is incredibly informative. It's technical and fun at the same time. It's a must-read for anyone who loves plant-based dairy products or anyone who likes cheese. Karen is an icon and artist in her field and this book may just be her Sistine Chapel. BUY THIS BOOK.

—Afrim Pristine, owner, Cheese Boutique

# THE ART OF PLANT-BASED CHEESEMAKING

**REVISED & EXPANDED SECOND EDITION**

HOW TO CRAFT REAL, CULTURED, NON-DAIRY CHEESE

**KAREN McATHY**

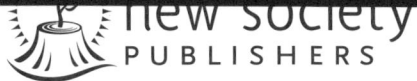

The Westport Library
Westport, Connecticut
203-291-4800

Copyright © 2021 by Karen McAthy
All rights reserved.

Cover design by Diane McIntosh. Main cover image: © Catherine Downes; Background: seal elements, marble plinth ©iStock.
Back cover photo © Andre Shepperd, Dremond Studio.
All interior photos by Karen McAthy, unless otherwise noted.

Printed in Canada. First printing April 2021.

This book is intended to be educational and informative. It is not intended to serve as a guide. The author and publisher disclaim all responsibility for any liability, loss or risk that may be associated with the application of any of the contents of this book.

Inquiries regarding requests to reprint all or part of *The Art of Plant-based Cheesemaking* should be addressed to New Society Publishers at the address below. To order directly from the publishers, please call toll-free (North America) 1-800-567-6772, or order online at www.newsociety.com

Any other inquiries can be directed by mail to:
New Society Publishers
P.O. Box 189, Gabriola Island, BC V0R 1X0, Canada
(250) 247-9737

**LIBRARY AND ARCHIVES CANADA CATALOGUING IN PUBLICATION**

Title: The art of plant-based cheesemaking : how to craft real, cultured, non-dairy cheese / Karen McAthy.

Names: McAthy, Karen, author.

Description: Revised & expanded second edition. | Includes index.

Identifiers: Canadiana (print) 20210124024 | Canadiana (ebook) 20210124032 | ISBN 9780865719620 (hardcover) | ISBN 9781550927559 (PDF) | ISBN 9781771423519 (EPUB)

Subjects: LCSH: Cheesemaking. | LCSH: Cheese. | LCSH: Vegan cooking. | LCSH: Cooking (Cheese) | LCSH: Dairy substitutes. | LCSH: Milk-free diet.

Classification: LCC TX837 .M4152 2021 | DDC 641.5/63971—dc23

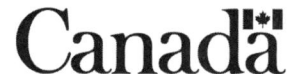

New Society Publishers' mission is to publish books that contribute in fundamental ways to building an ecologically sustainable and just society, and to do so with the least possible impact on the environment, in a manner that models this vision.

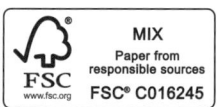 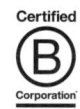 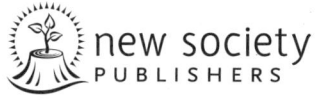

# Contents

Foreword  ix

Preface  xi

Introduction  1

### Chapter 1: On History and Definitions  7
    Cheese, a Product and a Process  13
    Terminology: Cheese Versus Cheeze  16
    Cheeze, Cheese, Crossover Methods: Definitions and Boundaries  17

### Chapter 2: Equipment, Sanitization, and Food Safety  21
    Food Safety and Sanitization  22
    Tools and Equipment  26
    Ingredients  27

### Chapter 3: Making Quick Non-Cultured Cheeze  29
    Non-Cultured Soft Cheeze  31
        Soaking nuts, seeds, and legumes  32
    Non-cultured Semi-firm or Set Cheezes  39
        Starches  39
        Gelling agents  41

### Chapter 4: Fermentation and Culturing: Role in Cheesemaking  57
    Lactic Acid Fermentation  59
    LAB Acidification  60

Rejuvelac 61
    Making rejuvelac 63
Kefir: Water Kefir Versus Dairy Kefir 68
    Experimentation 68
    Water kefir as bulk starter 69
    Making water kefir 72
    Making coconut kefir using water kefir 74
    Back slopping 77
Other Starter Cultures 77
    Probiotic capsules 77
    Miso 78
    Sauerkraut brine 78
    Tempeh culture 79
    Mesophilic direct-set culture 79

## Chapter 5: Fresh Cultured Cheeses 81

Forming and Aging for Short-Term Aging 94
Coconut Kefir-based Cheeses 96
Lactic Acid (cultured) Almond Curd 107
    Feta-style cheeses 111
Longer-Aged Cheeses 118
    Cashew and coconut havarti/gouda-style cheeses 123
    Cheddar-style cheeses 129

## Chapter 6: Mold Ripened Cheeses and Affinaging 135

Before You Start 137
White Mold Ripened Cheese 137
Blue Cheese Method 146
Affinaging 159
    Salt: dry salting, brining (soaking), washing 159
    Oil curing/leaf wrapping/bandaging 164
    Cold smoking 166

## Chapter 7: Recipes: Putting Your Cheeses to Work 167

More Cultured Foods (that are not cheese) 169
Something Sweet 177
Something Savory 191

## Appendix 1: Resources 211

Ingredients 212
Tools and Equipment 215

**Appendix 2: Record-keeping** 217
    Cheesemaking Culturing Log 217
    Cheesemaking Observation Log 220

**Appendix 3: Common Issues for Starter Cultures** 221

**Appendix 4: Choosing a Base** 225

**Appendix 5: Preparing Dry Beans** 229

**Index** 231

**About the Author** 239

**A Note about the Publisher** 240

# Foreword

The story of how I ended up as Karen McAthy's business partner starts on a beautiful autumn evening in 2014. I was out with Eden, my wife at the time, at our favorite dinner spot, Graze Vegetarian. I remember our evening started with a short walk and enjoying the ethereal painter's sky as we made our way to the restaurant. We had been longtime fans of the culinary artistry that Karen had been pioneering as executive chef at this lovely restaurant in East Vancouver.

Being a creature of habit, I ordered the same thing every single time I was lucky enough to eat Karen's food (to this day I still crave that phyllo lentil dish). So my only opportunity to try new offerings was either the appetizer we'd share or the odd taste from Eden's plate.

This night was a special one, in particular as it was the first time we had ordered the antipasto tasting plate that included a variety of different cultured and aged dairy-free cheeses that Karen had been experimenting with. At that time, I was teaching plant-based cooking and nutrition classes alongside Eden, who was a nutritionist and culinary artist at our business, Feed Life. As someone who had tried almost every single plant-based cheese on the market in Vancouver and Seattle at the time, I was very inquisitive about Karen's cheeses.

I had always found that most dairy-free cheeses tasted synthetic and starchy. You could tell they were mass-produced and aimed at emulating the outward appearance of cheese. They failed to capture the complexity of flavor and enzymatic nature of a cultured and aged dairy-based cheese.

The moment I tried some of Karen's cheese is one I will always remember. The initial taste literally froze me in pure palate pleasure. I was speechless for a dozen seconds, then muttered a simple, "wow!" The entire plate was the craft of someone who not only captured the pleasing visual of a well-designed board but wove a complex symphony of flavor and texture with each component. We were regulars at Graze throughout its tenure and thoroughly enjoyed the cuisine that Karen created during her three years as executive chef. Little did I know it would be that very cheesemaking method that I was tasting that would change my life in the years to come.

Fast-forward to early 2016 and I was giving a talk at a community movie night hosted by the Juice Truck. We had co-hosted a few of these nights where we would watch a captivating documentary on plant-based eating and environmental impact and lead a discussion afterward. When I showed up to the evening, there was Karen sampling some of her delightful cumin cultured cashew cheese. She shared with me that after Graze closed the demand for her cheeses followed her and that she had decided to create a plant-based cheese company called Blue Heron. In the months that followed, I was grateful to be involved with the creation of Blue Heron, and after a year and a half of R&D, Karen asked me to be her business partner.

Creating Blue Heron with Karen has been some of the most rewarding and challenging work of my life. We have had the blessing of being in the spotlight and the forefront of what is a completely new emerging food sector. That comes with a host of unique challenges, but the journey of entrepreneurship is demanding and exciting.

*The Art of Plant-based Cheesemaking* is an edifying text that defines dairy-free cheese and explores the craft of culturing non-dairy mediums. Karen's important writing will take you on a journey that will expand your understanding of the transformative process of culturing and how you too can explore working with microbes and the magic they create.

Colin Medhurst

# Preface

Since *The Art of Plant-based Cheesemaking* was first published in 2017, much has transpired in the plant-based cheese world both globally and for my company, Blue Heron. At the time, my business partner, Colin Medhurst, and I were preparing to open the Blue Heron plant-based cheese shop in Vancouver, BC, the first fully stand-alone plant-based cheese shop in Canada, selling our hand-crafted, cultured, vegan cheeses. We hosted a pre-opening event on a cold, rainy, February evening, and because in the lead-up to opening we had considerable local media attention, we were met with unexpectedly large lineups a block long consistently for several hours. On the day of our grand opening, we sold out in less than three hours, and the large lineups and sell-outs persisted for several weeks before stabilizing. We knew there was demand, we already had a small but dedicated local following, and we knew and know that this sector is really only in its infancy.

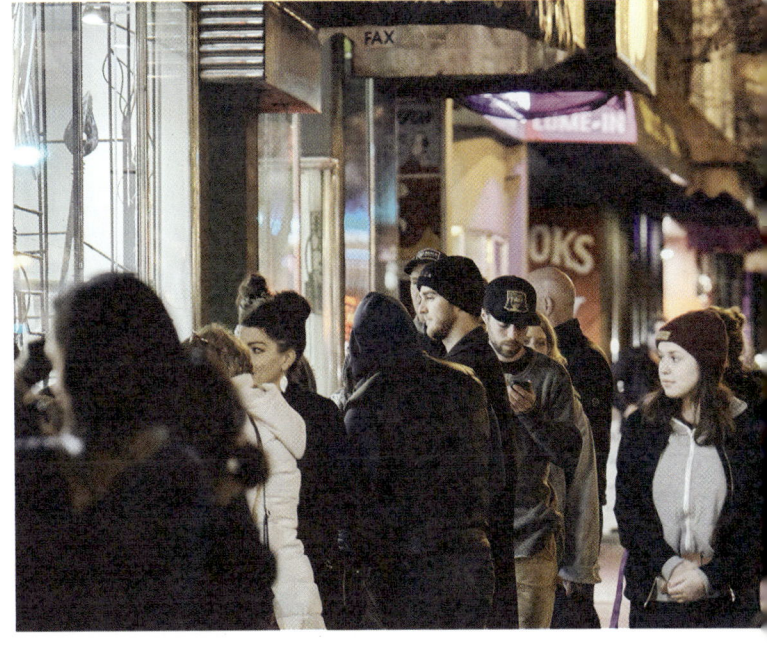

*Opening night, Blue Heron Cheese Shop, Vancouver, February 2018.*
CREDIT: ANDRE SHEPPERD, DREMOND STUDIO

Since the opening of the shop, we've had steady and increasing demand for our products from shops, individuals, restaurants, and large grocery brands and are working to meet this demand. We've attended dozens of events, participated in numerous fundraisers

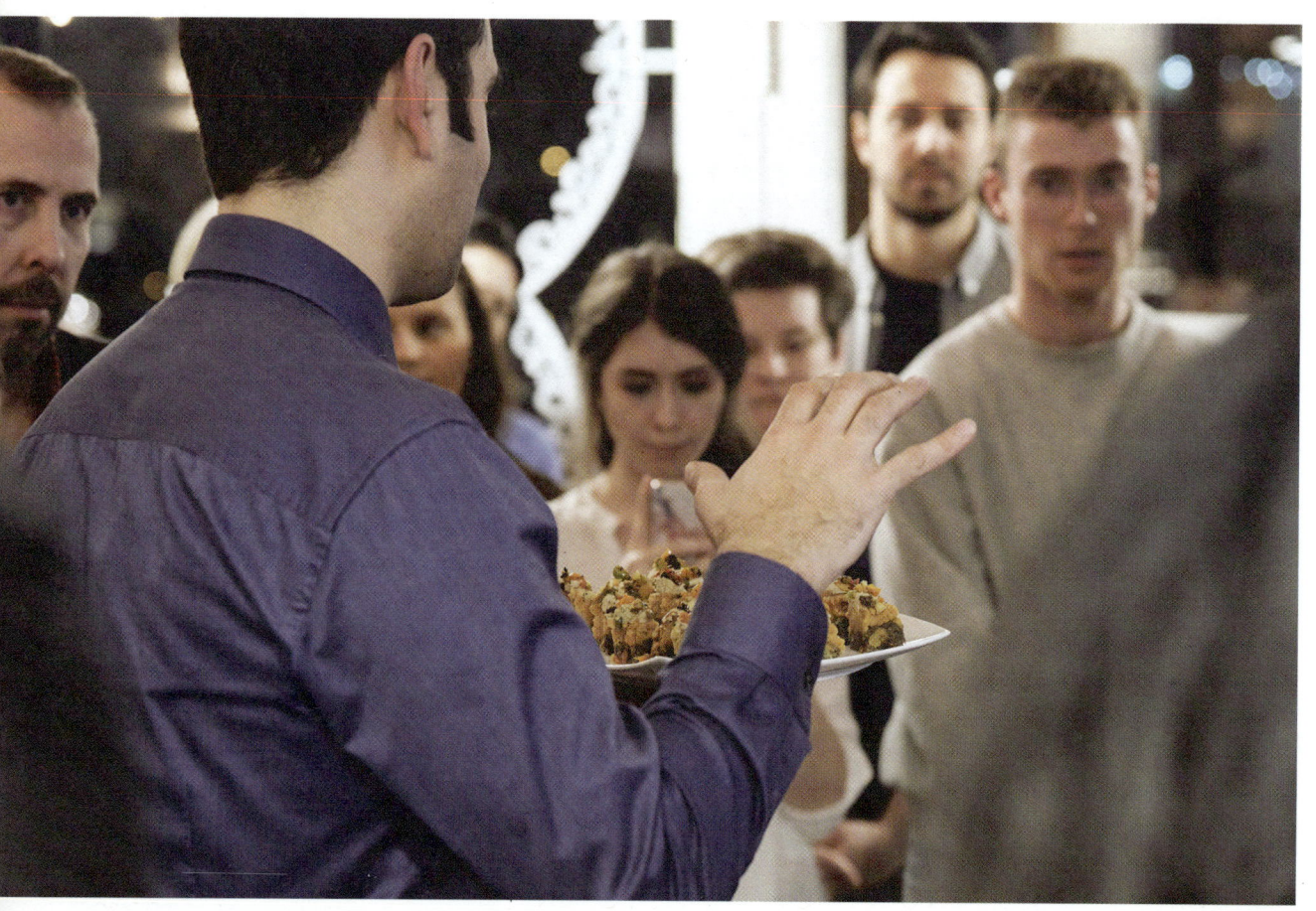

*Colin Medhurst educating guests, Blue Heron opening party, Vancouver, February 2018.* CREDIT: ANDRE SHEPPERD, DREMOND STUDIO

for other organizations; my first version of this book won its category, Vegan, at the 2018 Gourmand World Cookbook Awards; our company, Blue Heron, was nominated for and was a finalist for the Innovation Award in the BC Food Processors Awards in 2018; we opened a restaurant, SOIL, closed the restaurant; Colin, my business partner, got married; I broke my wrist; all of this amidst large scale global challenges, including a pandemic, an economic slowdown, and necessary calls for social and environmental changes. It has been busy.

As we continue to refine our processes and prepare for larger scale manufacturing, there has been an explosion around the globe of new commercial vegan cheesemakers and demand for education on the science and art of vegan cheesemaking. I hear from many new and aspiring vegan cheesemakers, both commercial and home DIYers, frequently. Fellow Canadian brands The Cultured Nut and Nuts For Cheese are growing and thriving in British Columbia and Ontario respectively. New Roots (Switzerland), Happy Cheeze (Germany),

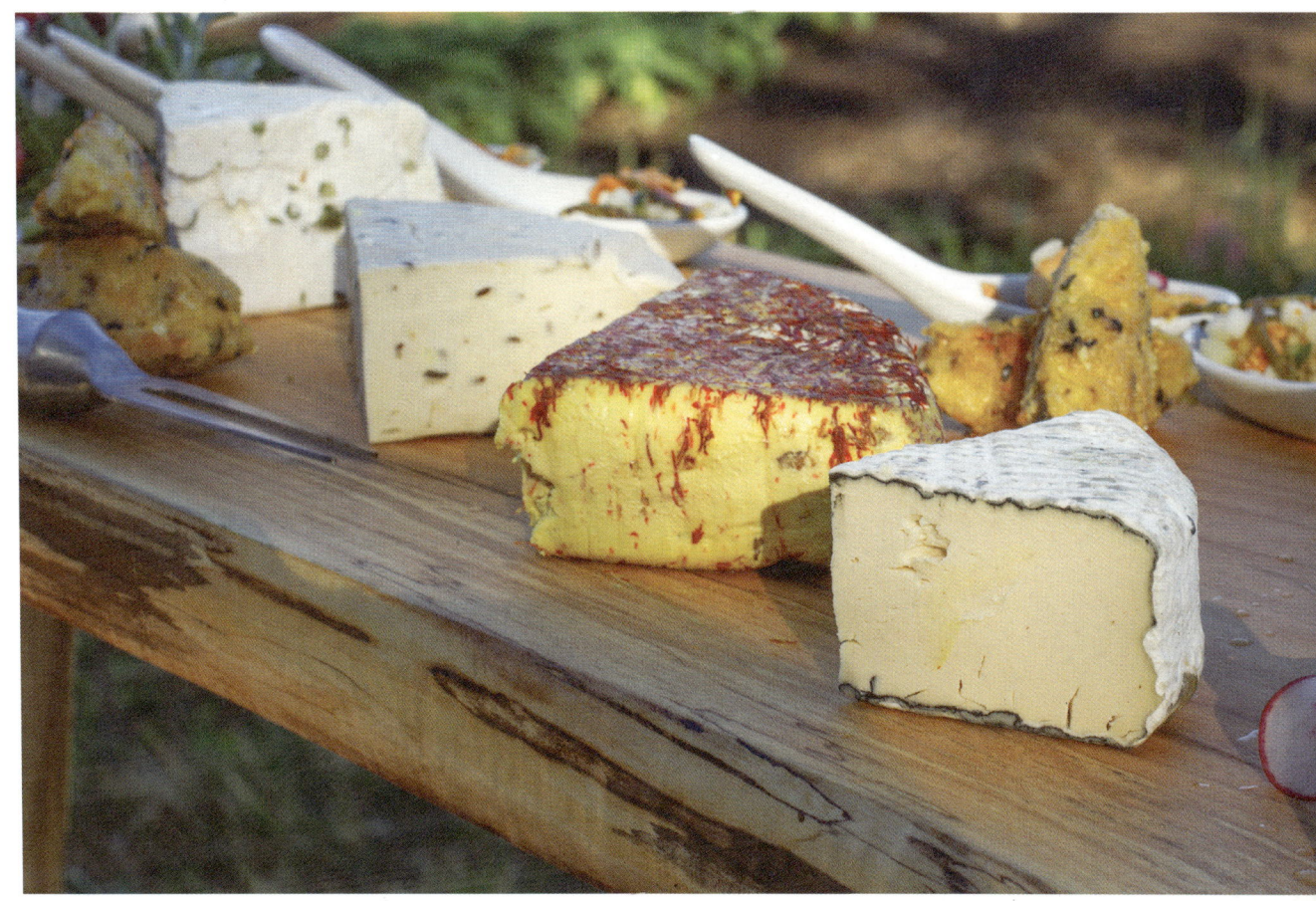

*Blue Heron Cheeses.*
CREDIT: COLIN MEDHURST

Kinda Co. and Palace Culture (United Kingdom), and dozens of others are expanding rapidly in Europe. Artisa in Tasmania is excelling and winning awards in Australia, and brands are popping up in Central and South America, India, and parts of Southeast Asia. Vegan cheese shops offering cheeses from a range of vegan brands are a natural development in the arena like Riverdel in New York (which has been around for several years now), La Fauxmagerie, a fairly new vegan cheese shop in London, United Kingdom, and Rebel Cheese in Austin, Texas (opened 2019, and also makes its own cheeses in addition to selling other brands).

This former niche market has begun to have an impact on the global dairy market, and in late winter of 2019, Blue Heron, my company, was met with an industry driven complaint filed with the CFIA (Canadian Food Inspection Agency) regarding the use of the word "cheese." This complaint stimulated a rapid and intense response after food writer Alexandra Gill published a story in the *Globe and Mail*.[1]

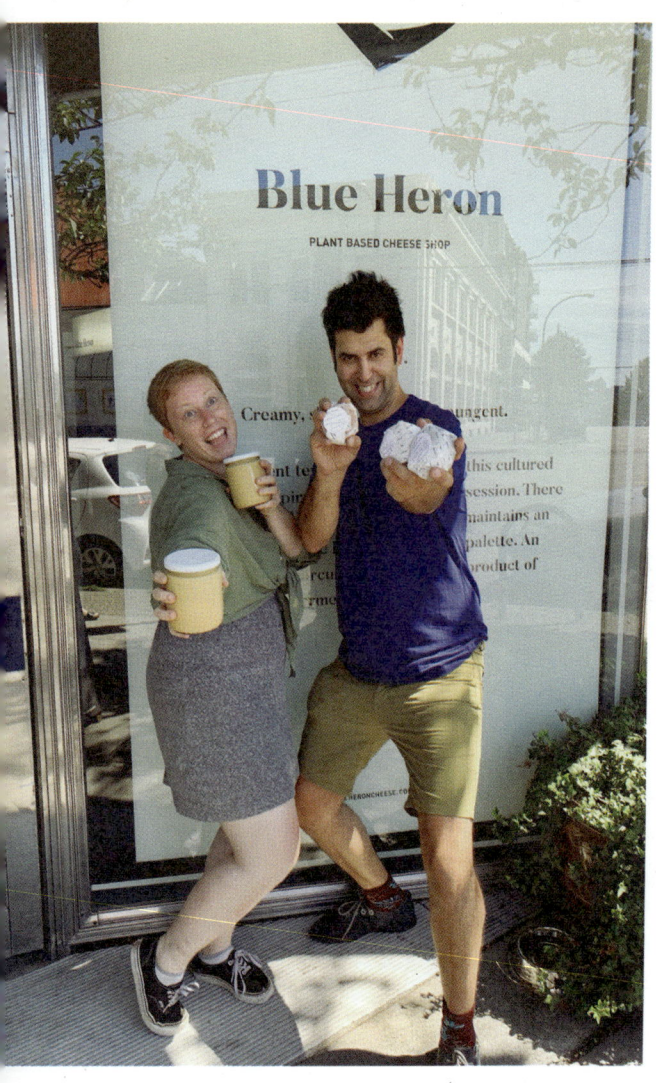

*Jolene & Colin, Cheesy Greetings in front of the Blue Heron Shop door, 2019.*

Critics were vitriolic and prolific in their insistence that cheese can be made only from animal milk. Supporters were so many more and from many more places than we could have anticipated, and they were active, writing letters to the CFIA, commenting publicly, writing articles or other responses. The result, we were given approval to use the term "cheese" in our language provided we precede it with "100% dairy-free" and "plant-based," which we were already doing.

In many ways this complaint, the public response, and the CFIA response highlight the inherent tensions attendant on a shift within the population regarding the ethics of consumption. Younger people (eighteen to forty) in many jurisdictions around the world are adopting plant-based or vegan lifestyles. Those over forty are more hesitant. As people desire and seek animal-free protein, their consumption choices are impacting traditional animal agriculture products and the industries in that sector, and those consumers committed to the sector exercise their objections when vegan, plant-based companies challenge the established line.

It is my sense that this indicates that this is not simply a food trend that will pass, but rather, an ethical, perhaps moral shift, as people begin to consider the impact of their food choices on the environment, their personal health, and finally, to actually consider more seriously the impact on the animals used in large scale animal agriculture.

The CFIA complaint showed that the vegan cheese sector has much work to do to develop shared knowledge, identify common practices, methods, and standards of identity to facilitate better engagement with regulators and expand the creative and scientific boundaries of what is possible as cheesemakers, and this seems increasingly possible now.

I have found the adage it takes a village to raise a child to be true in my work establishing Blue Heron, teaching classes, and writing both the first book and this second edition. One can have an idea, a talent, a skill set, and the drive to do something with them, but without people who believe in you, support you in terms of your personal well-being as well as your concept or business, you exist in an echo-chamber of your own imaginings. Despite the long hours and the creeping self-doubt that inevitably comes when one is exhausted and things do not feel as though they are going as I might wish, I am fortunate and deeply grateful for the people I know: students, readers, clients and guests, friends, fellow food business owners, fellow commercial vegan cheesemakers, food writers, fellow chefs. Many are people I have met; some are people I have only conversed with via the internet; some have known me for years; some are new and now very dear.

Their tangible support in words and actions has given me the exceptional privilege (albeit hard won and not the least bit luxurious) of being able to pursue a set of ideas that adds new knowledge to the plant-based food sector and continues to deepen my knowledge and craft. Without all of them, I would not have been able to write a book.

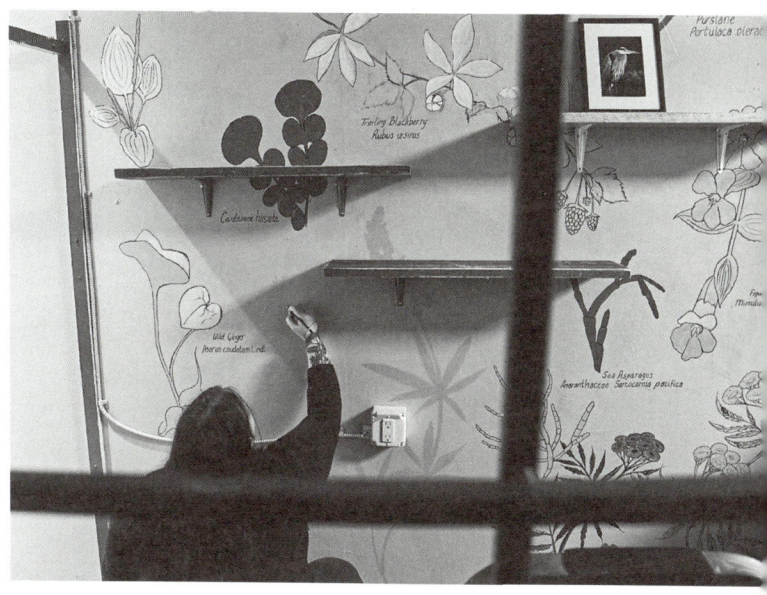

*The author illustrating Blue Heron cheese shop wall before opening, January 2017.* CREDIT: ANDRE SHEPPERD, DREMOND STUDIO

This list of individualized thanks will undoubtedly be incomplete, but my gratitude goes to all who have been part of my life these past few years.

Colin Medhurst: business partner, friend, brother. Our journey has really only begun, and now, as we prepare for new challenges, I am glad we are in it together.

Emily Davies: my most recent sous chef, who, determined to work with me, persisted until it was realized. Your presence in my life and your friendship mean well more than you know. Your belief in me astounds me, and I only hope that I can be half the mentor you hope for. Go Be Great!

Brad Hendrickson: for your friendship, collaborations, hours of fermentation talk, and beer. Here's to always learning. Thank you, Chef!

Naomi Arnaut: colleague, collaborator, and friend in this food industry. I am eternally grateful for you and for rescued groceries.

Jill Aiken: a friendship enduring past our introduction through the food game, you bring such warmth and wonderful energy to everything you do, including the quality of your friendship.

Jolene Vasallo: for hanging in there through every kind of ridiculousness that is me. How am I and how is Blue Heron so fortunate? I hope we can help you realize some dreams.

Natalie Swatez: for all the commiseration, the wine, the friendship, and your discerning palate for all the tasting. Here's to more.

Blue Heron 2018/19 team: Joel, Jaroslav, Gwendolyn, Maria, Christine: gratitude for your general good natures, your willingness, your effort.

Lucia Valenzuela: your joining the team is one of the best things of 2019. I am truly grateful, and I look forward to conducting further research with you.

Kassandra Linklater: how lucky am I to have you as a confidante, cheerleader, and friend. I will always seek to return the generosity.

Ryan Lanji: because you know me, and because always, and because you know.

A final note of thanks to my dear colleagues and friends who shared recipes or took photos for this book. I believe it is worth knowing more about them and discovering their talents for yourself, so here is the list of folks and their respective Instagram handles:

Chef Emily Davies: wholesomeslice@gmail.com
Chef Lucia Valenzuela: @giardino_kitchen
Chef Karima Cellouf: @heyhaveyoueatenx
Chef Kaide Tighe: @vegankraftdinner
Jolene Vasallo: @traderjo_lene

Photographers:
Catherine Downes: @catherinedownes
Colin Medhurst, Blue Heron co-founder: @feedurlife
Andre Shepperd, Dremond Studios: @expirydateunknown

---

[1] Gill, Alexandra. "Vegan food producer ordered to drop the word 'cheese' from its marketing." *Globe and Mail*. February 17, 2019. https://www.theglobeandmail.com/business/small-business/marketing/article-vegan-food-producer-ordered-to-drop-the-word-cheese-from-its/.

# Introduction

In the spring of 2013, I accepted the post as executive chef of Graze Vegetarian, a new, plant-based restaurant opening in Vancouver, British Columbia. Creation of a solely plant-based menu that would have broad appeal and yet be creatively interesting was our primary goal. As part of that, we decided plant-based, dairy-free cheese, or cheese analog, would have a place on the menu. Not satisfied by what was available in the market at the time, I began searching for compelling recipes or methods on the internet.

Much of what I found were recipes that involved a nut or seed component blended with nutritional yeast, water, salt, and some sort of acid, usually lemon juice or apple cider vinegar. Some included miso, others onion and garlic powder, an attempt to capture an umami sensation. These cheesy spreads were tasty but more relevant as dips than cheese. Other recipes involved cooking similar-type mixtures with agar agar or kappa carrageenan and sometimes incorporating a starch. These methods ostensibly create firm cheeses, as agar agar and kappa carrageenan are strong binders that yield a semi-firm set in the final product.

Then there were the recipes including some level of fermentation using a rejuvelac. Rejuvelac is a fermented liquid made from sprouted grains, very often wheat berries. This fluid is rich in microbes (bacteria and some yeasts) and works effectively as a culturing agent. A mixture of blended nuts or seeds is fermented with the addition of some rejuvelac and then drained and shaped and "aged" or, in some cases, then cooked with agar agar or kappa carrageenan and sometimes mixed with coconut oil to create a cultured semi-firm cheese of sorts. What these particular recipes often demonstrated was an incomplete understanding of what role the fermentation component was playing, and in some recipes that I found, the culturing agent was added when the mixture was at too high a temperature. Nonetheless, I began my own experiments informed by this background.

My initial cultured cheeses were primarily in either the ricotta or chèvre style (meaning fresh, young, soft) and employed rejuvelac, sauerkraut brine, kombucha, or probiotic capsules. The results, while interesting and able to create tasty cheese-like results, always seemed limited to one note with respect to acidity and flavor, and in the case of using probiotic capsules, highly inconsistent. As I began to think more about what cheesemaking itself is, I was fortunate to have a young chef, Katie Luebke, apply to stage with me at Graze.

Katie, already working full-time as a cook at another restaurant, had heard that I was doing a lot of fermentation and culturing and making plant-based cheeses. She had a serious interest in culturing processes herself, and spent two days a week for nearly six months in the Graze kitchen helping me carry out a variety of experiments testing mediums, cultures, aging processes, archiving the cheese and taking notes—so many notes.

We explored the recipes and methods available to us from the plant-based realm and found that most recipes had insufficient method and explanation for

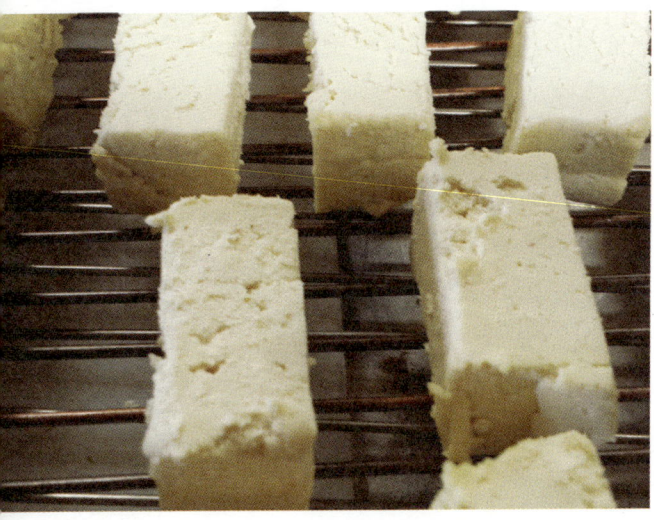

Above: *Almond Feta Test, Graze, 2014.*

Right: *Almond, cashew, and Brazil nut/coconut milk cheeses on aging boards, ready for inspection at Graze.*

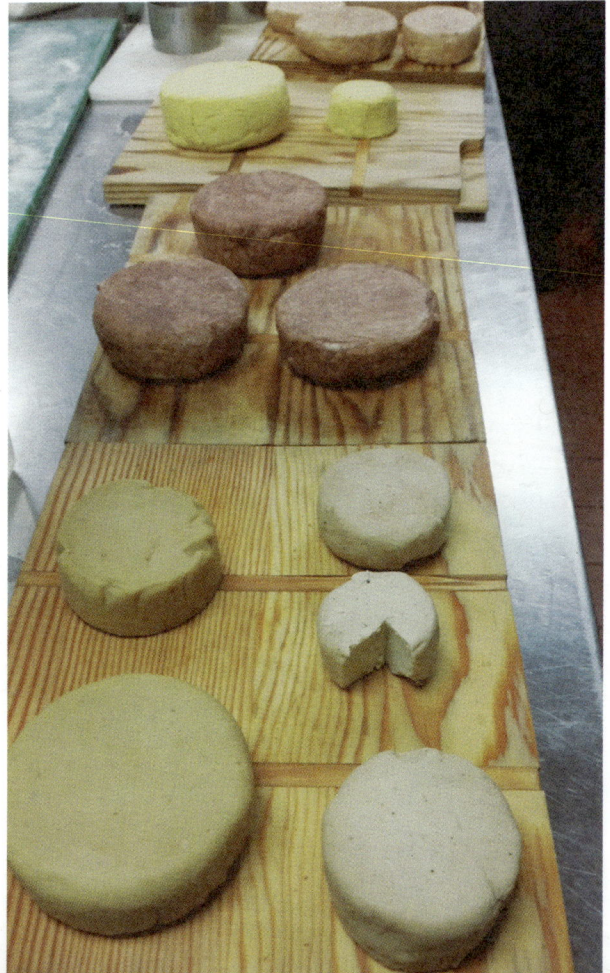

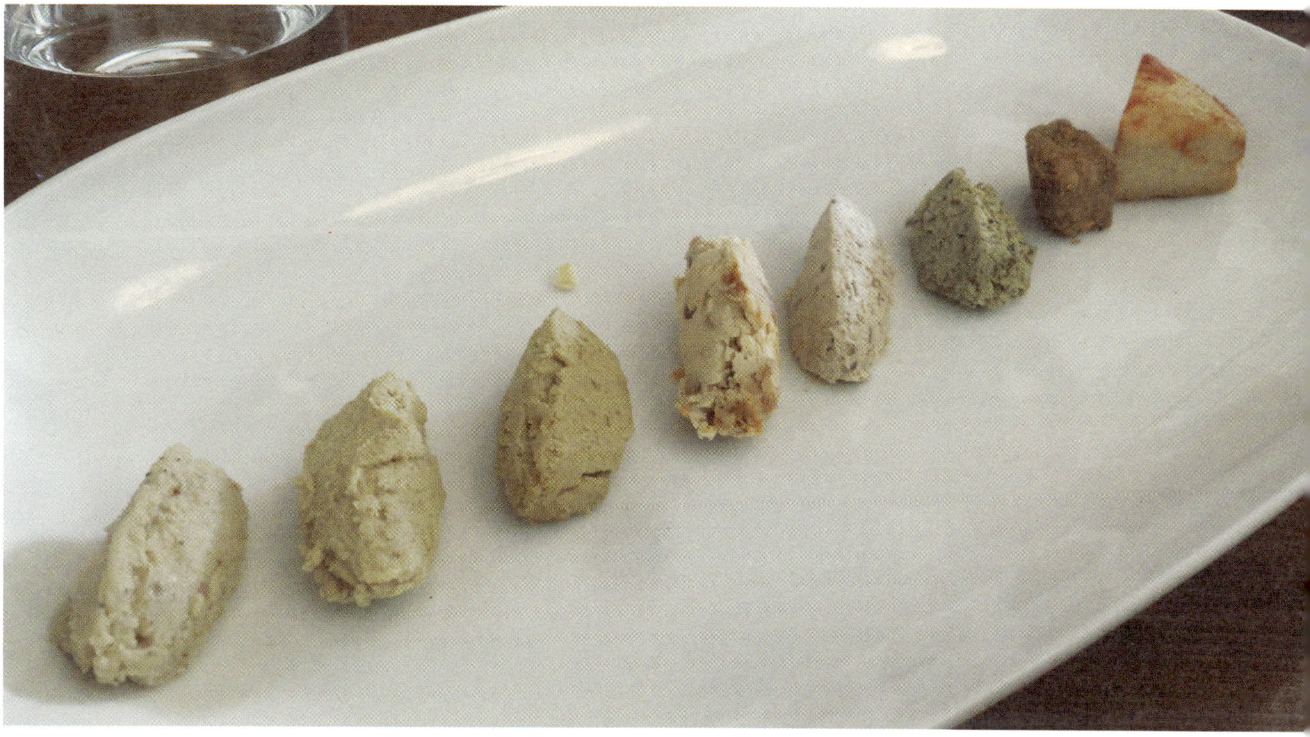

*Curd tests, Graze, 2014.*

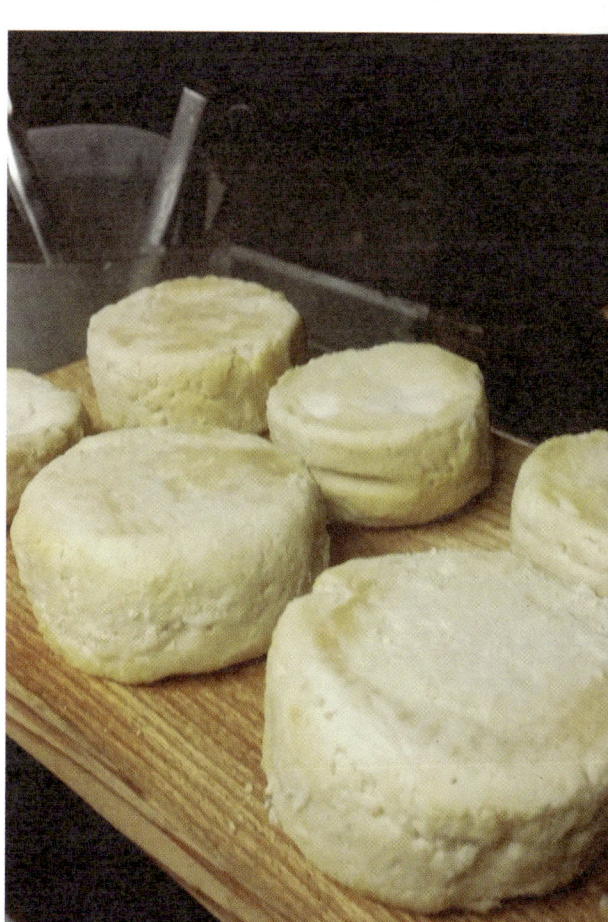

how and why particular ingredients were selected. In our naïve experiments, we were able to identify aspects we wanted to understand better, and we had some interesting and sometimes unintentional outcomes (accidents) that demonstrated there was so much more to know. What was abundantly clear was that fermentation and culturing were going to be integral to what I wanted to do.

I wanted a deeper understanding of the role of fermentation within cheesemaking, and I wanted to make products that could feel satisfying from both flavor and textural perspectives. Thus, I turned to studying traditional dairy cheesemaking methods. Developed over centuries, dairy methods reveal the evolution of a craft from accident to scientific and intentional.

In the course of reading and researching, I began thinking of cheese as a concept. Any particular cheese within the traditional, dairy cheesemaking (and here I am

*Cheeses at Graze, 2015.*

focused on the craft of cheesemaking and not the dairy industry as a whole) context is an end product, the result of several processes, beginning with the use of microbes and or digestive enzymes that begin the transformational process. Although all foods that begin with raw materials become the end product through a series of processes, there is something essential about the act of fermentation, the use of microbes, in relation to desired outcomes in cheesemaking.

For instance, you cannot simply mimic a blue cheese by adding color or sharp flavor. The recognizable aroma and flavor of blue cheese is inherently a result of the metabolic action of the *P. roqueforti* mold on the dairy medium along with other microbes. Similarly, to make a hard cheese, simply adding agar agar or kappa carrageenan or other setting agents is not sufficient. They retain moisture, whereas in true hard cheeses, there is low moisture content, a result of the time and processes required to remove moisture from a cheese, which then leads to a densification of the cheese curd.

Understanding cheese this way, as a concept, invigorated my desire to test and refine my own approach to cultured plant-based cheesemaking. It also made me really want to comprehend what the various microbes do and why what they do is important. I wanted to understand the microbes as living agents, not as "probiotics" or some other blanket term that renders their agency invisible or, at best, neutralizes them as being just another ingredient.

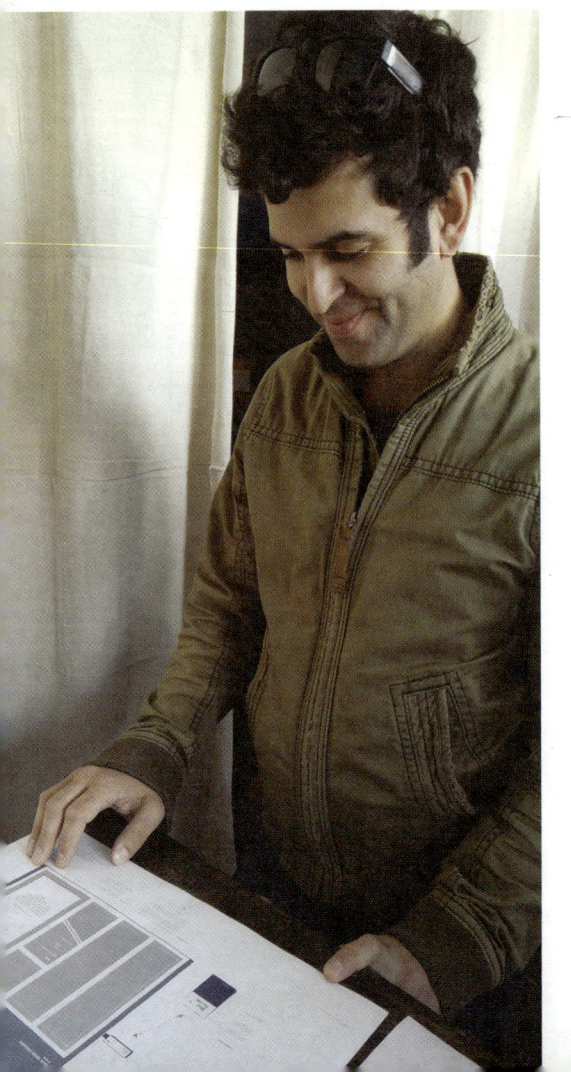

*Colin viewing Blue Heron storefront design plans, 2018.*

After Katie and I began pursuing this understanding through further tests, we had a number of happy surprises, a few unexpected results, and, of course, some things that didn't quite work out as desired. And I developed an appreciation for a type of food that I had never had much attachment to previously. Our effort resulted in production of a few consistent "types" of plant-based cheese that Graze then sold at the Vancouver Farmers Market in 2015.

With the closure of Graze Vegetarian in November of 2015, I continued pursuit of my research and interest in making cultured plant-based cheese, deciding that I would eventually launch my own plant-based, vegan cheese brand. I landed on the name Blue Heron, which represents my love of the British Columbia west coast (unceded lands), and my long-standing admiration of the great blue heron. In early 2016, I reconnected with a former Graze guest, Colin Medhurst, at an event at which I was sampling some of my cheeses. From there, it quickly turned into a business partnership, and I have discovered a brother in Colin.

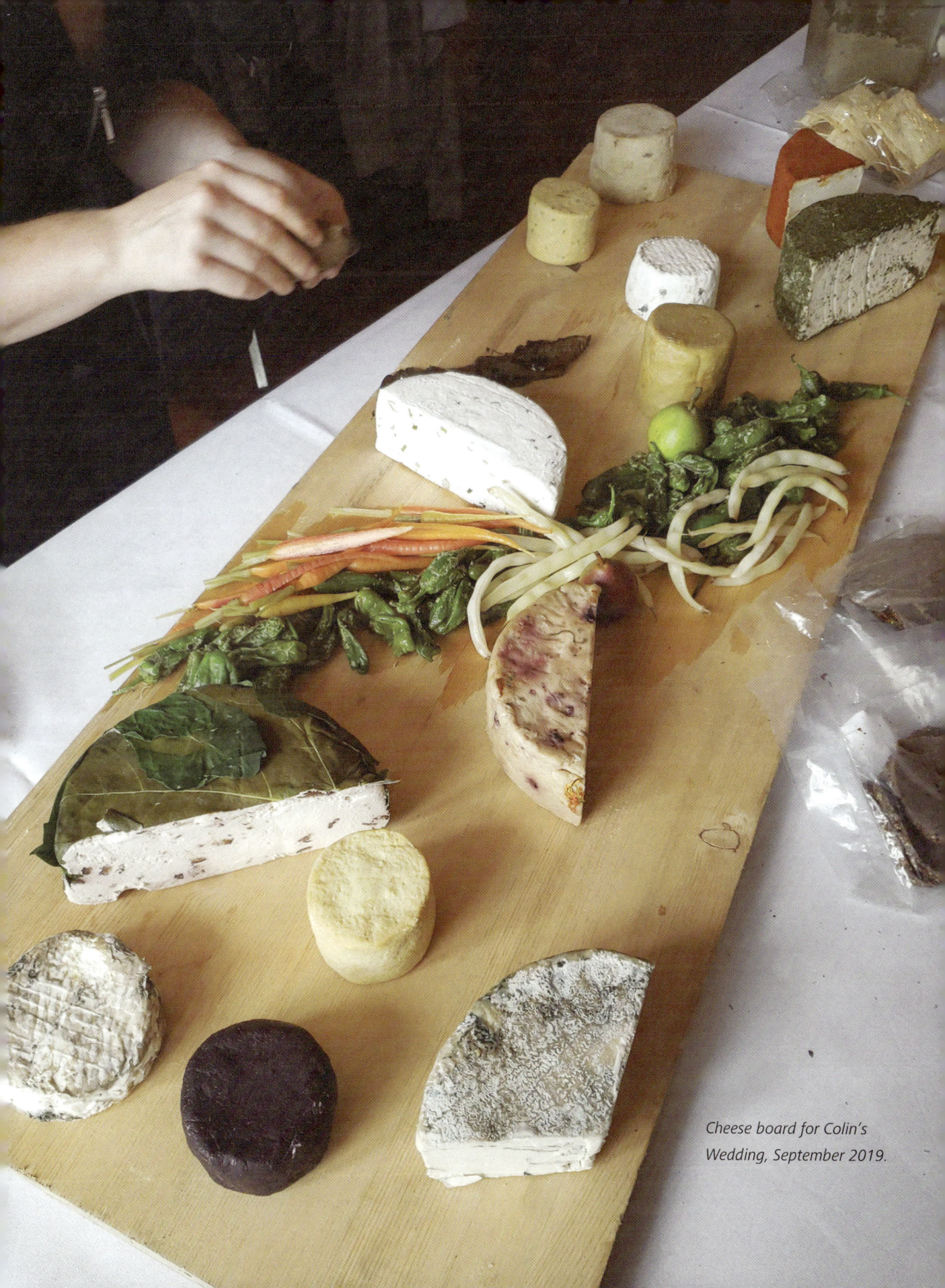

*Cheese board for Colin's Wedding, September 2019.*

I have learned many things over the past few years. The most significant are that this is an exploration driven by endless curiosity and that I remain a novice with an insatiable desire to learn. Things that I have written or taught or thought or practiced have changed, evolved. Making cheese and working with cultures means committing to learning constantly, practicing patience, and studying the smallest details. This is something I hope to be doing for a very long time.

This book is an invitation to the seriously interested and actively curious in cheesemaking, hopeful to participate with me in an exploration and development of cheese, to participate with the now many others seeking to expand the idea of cheesemaking itself, to choose patience, observation, and time over speed and instant gratification. It is an invitation to deeper understanding and, therefore, more care. More care about making food. More care about where food comes from. More care about how we feed ourselves and share with others. More care about our impact on this planet. Making food, and cheese, is ultimately the way I choose to express love.

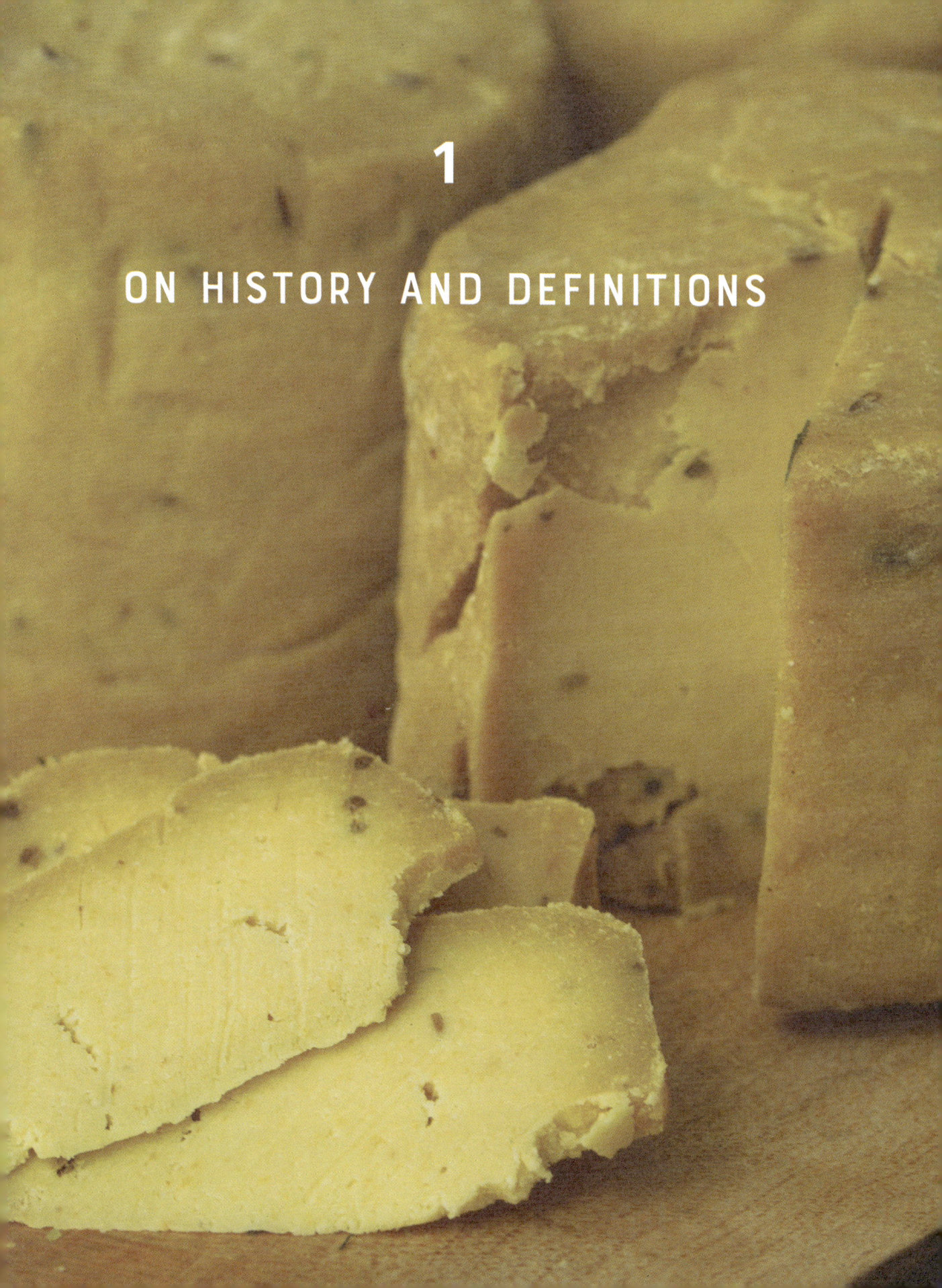

# 1
## ON HISTORY AND DEFINITIONS

Cheese. Creamy, sharp, firm, tangy, pungent, mild, aromatic—the sensory adjectives are plentiful. The textures and redolent aromas of this cultured food have inspired a romantic obsession. There are thousands of varieties of cheese, all cultured from goat's milk, cow's milk, sheep's milk, buffalo milk. In principle it is a simple food. Rarely made up of more than ingredients—a medium (historically, animal milk of some kind), salt, enzymes, microbial cultures—cheese maintains an almost primitive hold on the human palate.

Cheese is one of the oldest of modern foods. Humans across nearly every culture have developed some form of animal milk into this cultured and (sometimes) aged foodstuff. Cheese craft has thousands of years of history behind it, with some estimates that cheesemaking with animal milk has been happening for about 4,000 years. Cheese is the outcome of an accident of circumstance (lack of refrigeration for preserving milk) and organisms (bacteria and molds). Cheese is a by-product of fermentation, culturing, and time (aging). Early versions of cheese would have been soured curd, loose, soft, not shaped, and eaten as a subsistence food by nomadic peoples. Evolving from this early product of accident, thousands of varieties of cheese have been created and hundreds of localized, artisan practices. There is not one dairy cheese that defines all dairy cheeses.

Like all forms of fermentation and culturing, cheesemaking evolved as a means of preserving food for the long months after the harvest when food was sparse. Now, along with many fermented and cultured food practices such as sauerkraut, kimchi, tempeh, beer, and wine, cheesemaking has become one of a growing number of do-it-yourself pursuits of ardent foodies. In recent years, a number of books have been written with this pursuit in mind, including *The Cheesemaker's Apprentice* by Sasha Davies and *Basic Cheesemaking* by Gianaclis Caldwell. Cheesemaking kits for the home user are readily available online and in boutique food shops, allowing folks to explore making their own ricotta, cream cheese, burrata, mozzarella, and others.

Cheese and cheesemaking are continually evolving, and the latest area of development is plant-based, dairy-free alternatives. Understanding why this pursuit has gained traction is relevant. As plant-based and vegan eating and lifestyle choices in general have moved from the periphery of most cultures to the mainstream of many—especially in some of North America and Western Europe—and is growing rapidly in other places, forsaking cheese is often seen as the last barrier to overcome. Three primary areas of concern inform this dietary shift to embracing plant-based/plant-forward eating and lifestyle choices, particularly in the West: environmental, personal health, and animal welfare/animal rights. As evidence mounts for the benefits of, at the very least, minimizing as much as possible our consumption of animal products for both personal health, environmental, and ethical reasons, a growing market is seeking alternatives to favorite items. This has included a surge in alternatives to cheese and other dairy foods such as butter and yogurt.

In many ways, Miyoko Schinner's book *Artisan Vegan Cheese* set the stage for the direction of the evolution, advancing the idea of plant-based, dairy-free cheese beyond cheesy flavored pâtés and spreads, which have primarily filled the void for those avoiding dairy cheese. Putting forward recipes that involve some degree of culturing (probiotic or rejuvelac application) and flavor outcomes that are at least somewhat familiar, this book has inspired many home foodie and prospective artisan plant-based cheesemakers alike.

*Blue Heron Herbed Coconut Kefir cheese.*
CREDIT: CATHERINE DOWNES

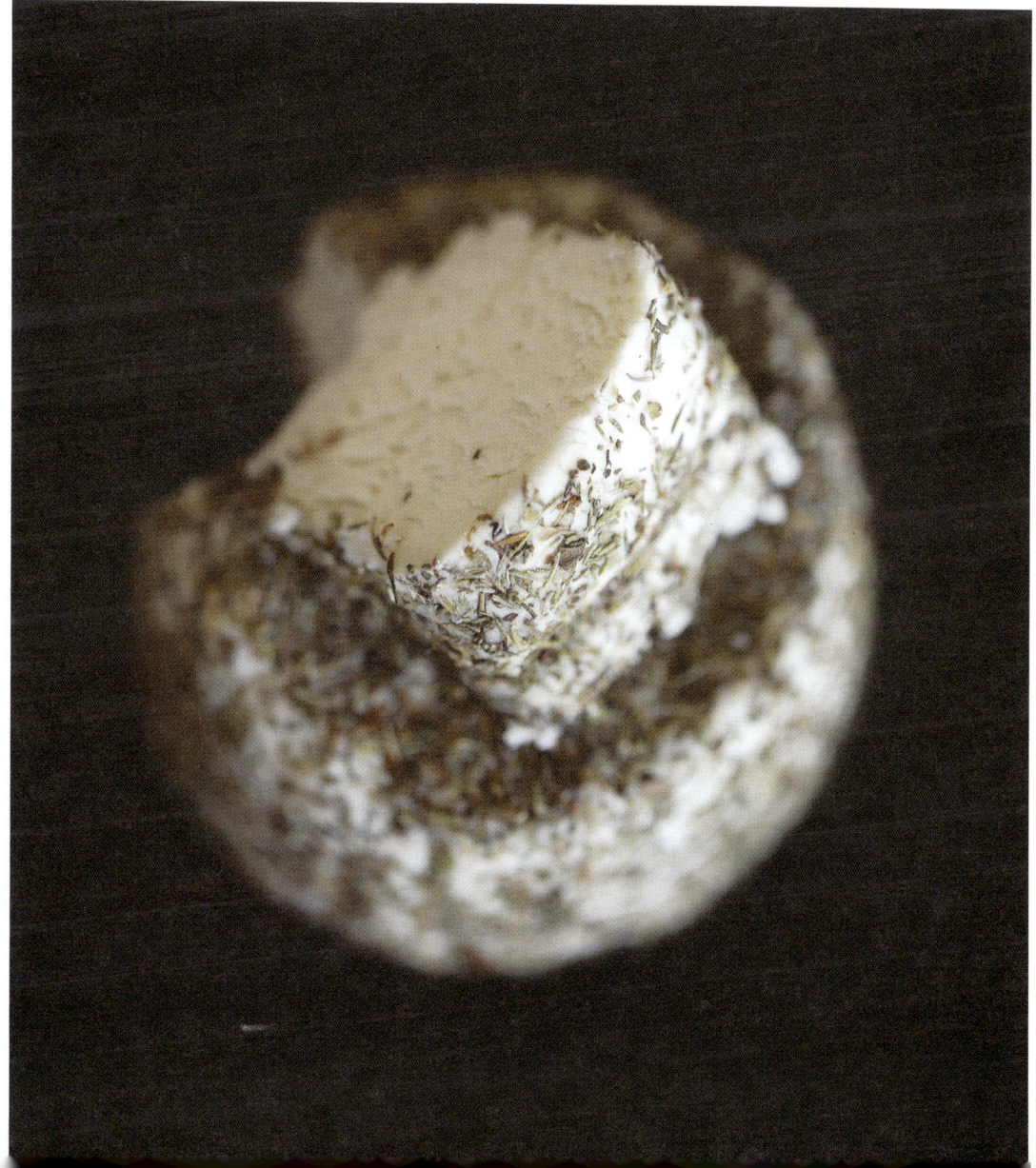

A claim that processes such as these produce some form of cheese is seen as controversial, particularly by ardent dairy cheese lovers and many in the dairy cheesemaking industry. This controversy is not necessarily unfounded or even irrelevant. To understand a little of why there is controversy around the growing vegan, dairy-free cheesemaking sector using the beloved word "cheese," and even around the premise underlying this book, it is important to know how the traditional sector understands what constitutes cheese.

The Codex Alimentarius of the Food and Agriculture Organization of the United Nations is a set of standards regarding different foods that is accepted internationally. These standards assist producers and trading nations alike in terms of providing definitions and guidelines that allow a common understanding to form. The Codex, then, is a set of "international food standards, guidelines and codes of practice that contribute to the safety, quality, and fairness of (the) international food trade." According to the Codex:

> Cheese is the ripened or unripened soft, semi-hard, hard, or extra-hard product, which may be coated, and in which the whey protein/casein ratio does not exceed that of milk, obtained by: (a) coagulating wholly or partly the protein of milk, skimmed milk, partly skimmed milk, cream, whey cream or buttermilk, or any combination of these materials, through the action of rennet or other suitable coagulating agents, and by partially draining the whey resulting from the coagulation, while respecting the principle that cheese-making results in a concentration of milk protein (in particular, the casein portion), and that consequently, the protein content of the cheese will be distinctly higher than the protein level of the blend of the above milk materials from which the cheese was made; and/or (b) processing techniques involving coagulation of the protein of milk and/or products obtained from milk which give an end-product with similar physical, chemical and organoleptic characteristics as the product defined under (a).[2]

For a complete list of the cheese standards outlined by the Codex, visit fao.org. Even without this formal definition, many ardent cheese lovers and makers alike do balk at the notion that a plant-based dairy-free cheese could be made and be legitimately understood as cheese.

Indeed, my company, Blue Heron, received an industry stimulated complaint from the Canadian Food Inspection Agency in January of 2019, and in

2015, Zengarry, another Canadian vegan cheesemaking company, also met with regulatory challenge regarding the use of the word "cheese." The underlying basis for regulatory complaints about the use of the word "cheese," aside from the political, is that there are complex standards of identity for each type of dairy cheese and that the processes employed in non-dairy cheesemaking do not meet these standards. Underpinning all of it is the notion that animal milk alone can become cheese, regardless of process employed.

In contrast to clearly established standards of identity for (commercial) dairy cheesemakers, the vegan dairy-free sector lacks any coherent standards of identity, lacks ubiquitous practices and methods, and even an understanding of just what vegan cheese is. At best, the term "vegan cheese" refers, colloquially, to a product that is simply dairy-free, animal-product-free, and is generally made to physically resemble, either in form or via packaging, dairy-cheese products.

It is expected that as the methodology and practices in the plant-based cheese sector continue to evolve, the sector will develop its own standards of identity, and possibly even push the boundaries of dairy cheesemaking within a regulatory context.

To that end, after considerable and loud pushback by our supporters and efforts on our part to ensure that we would be compliant with the current regulatory framework, Blue Heron received approval from the CFIA to use the word "cheese" provided we precede it with "100% dairy-free, plant-based." While not a ruling that can be ubiquitously applied to others in our sector, it serves as evidence that despite emotional attachments to the notion, the boundaries of what constitutes cheese are shifting, albeit slowly.

Although the majority of mass produced plant-based cheeses are of the non-cultured variety, (for instance, Daiya, Chao, Earth Island, Violife, Parmela), the number of companies focusing on cultured vegan cheeses is growing rapidly. Miyoko's Creamery is the largest and most recognizable brand in this arena, but notable participants such as New Roots (Switzerland), Happy Cheeze (Germany), Cashewbert (Germany), Artisa (Tasmania, Australia), Blue Heron (Canada), Nuts for Cheese (Canada), The Cultured Nut (Canada), La Fauxmagerie (Canada), Zengarry (Canada), Wandering Deli (Canada), Reine (USA), Blöde Ku (USA), Rebel Cheese (USA), Cheezehound (USA), Conscious Cultures (USA), Living Food BCN (Spain) are a cross-section of companies from the very small to medium-sized companies applying various aspects of fermentation and culturing processes in an effort to create products that have more depth, flavor, and cheese-like qualities than the analogs, which are primarily combinations of starches, proteins, and seasoning or flavoring.

Certainly, these efforts open the door for those advancing the culturing of non-dairy mediums, and other companies or projects such as Perfect Day and Impossible Foods are poised on the horizon to disrupt the dairy industry further with the production of non-animal derived casein and whey proteins for use in making non-dairy cheeses. What cheese is and what vegan cheese is will continue to be volubly and actively challenged in the coming years. It is my intention with this book to offer up on a small and practical scale insight into what informs some of this discourse, allowing the user-reader to understand and to participate in the development of cultured plant-based cheesemaking as a legitimate evolution of cheesemaking itself.

Exploring a small sampling of approaches to making plant-based cheeses from non-cultured processes to more involved culturing and aging processes, this book intends to help the user recognize and understand the differences between non-cultured and cultured cheeses via hands-on exercises. This is primarily a methodology book, with recipes intended to highlight core principles and processes. Since the first edition of this book was published, I have had the opportunity to re-evaluate some of the original processes and methods based on reader feedback, the content in the classes I teach, and my own ongoing research. Subsequently, I have made amendments to several processes and methods, added new information, more photos, and, significantly, there are three new chapters.

There are many fascinating things about culturing and fermentation, and the principles learned in this book do not apply only to cultured vegan cheesemaking, so I have also included easy, basic methods for making live cultured vegan yogurt and cultured butter.

I have added a chapter on using molds in vegan cheesemaking. While not as comprehensive or as robust as a parallel section in a dairy cheesemaking book, this chapter is a good introduction to how molds work in cheesemaking and why they are used. Additionally, I provide a couple of relatively simple methods for making a vegan blue cheese and a vegan white mold or bloomy rind cheese. The objective of the chapter is to help the reader become familiar with and understand what molds are, why they are used in cheesemaking, and how to work with them toward a successful outcome.

Finally, with all the focus on methodology in the early chapters of this book and given how often I am asked by Blue Heron clients, readers, and students, "what can I do with this?" I have also added a recipe chapter. This includes recipes demonstrating easy ways to use cultured and non-cultured cheeses. Recipes such as Artichoke and Spinach Dip, Pear Tarte Tatin, Herb, Potato, Mushroom, and Asparagus Galette will give you a framework for building out your own creativity.

This book invites the curious reader to try their hand at a few of their own plant-based cheesemaking experiments and to find ways of expanding their personal understanding of what cheese is. As readers explore making and using cultures, they have an opportunity to experiment with creating cheeses to suit their own preferences, to understand how the culturing process works (and sometimes fails), and to become familiar with a practice that has its roots in thousands of years of human history and food preservation.

## Cheese, a Product and a Process

Traditional cheese or "true cheese" as the New England Cheese Making Supply company calls it, is generally defined by the consolidation of milk proteins

*Selection of Blue Heron Creamery cheeses. Vegan cheesemaking is rapidly evolving both in homes and commercially. Advances in knowledge and technology will see this sector expand further into the mainstream.*
CREDIT: YUSHIIN LABO

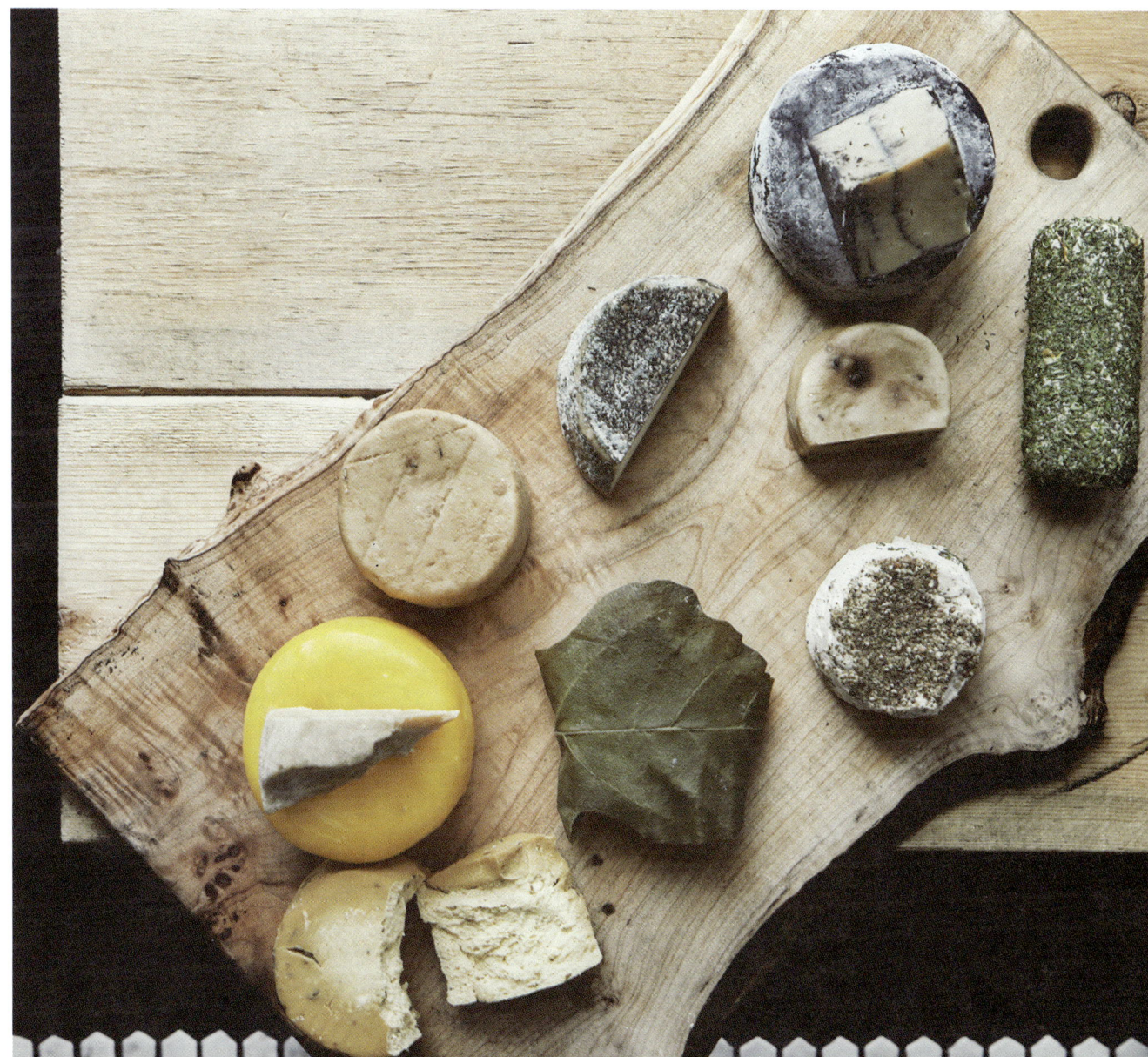

(caseins) with calcium and enzymes (rennet), followed by the development of acidity using lactic acid forming bacteria, which converts the sugars of the dairy to lactic acid, followed by the modification of protein during the aging process, resulting in different textures and flavors.

Earlier, I referred to the United Nations Codex Alimentarius definition, or, rather, standard for identifying cheese. When articulating how I understand cheese and therefore how I perceive the differences between cultured vegan cheese and non-cultured cheese-like products, I turn to this definition that emphasizes the process employed in making cheese, not the end product, in determining what cheese is.

It may seem difficult to see how I find my definition of plant-based cheese within these strict confines, but in opening up the traditional and official definition of cheese, I am choosing to understand and evaluate cheese as a concept. That is, I have elected to pull apart the Codex definition and focus on process components: coagulation of a protein rich medium (in my case nut, seed, and other bases), acidification of the medium with a lactic acid forming bacterial culture, and the use of aging methods to develop different characteristics.

As with "true cheese" in the Codex definition, I do not consider the use of thickening agents, oils, emulsifying agents, or umami rich ingredients such as nutritional yeast, in a recipe-based process to make something that is cheese. These products I understand to be "cheeze" or cheese analogs, and though entirely tasty results are found with this approach, the approach itself is devoid of what is integral to the "true cheese" process, which relies on flavor and texture evolving from microbes metabolizing. I do include some recipes in this vein because they are easy to make, yield tasty results, and serve as a good way to compare the difference in flavor and texture between cultured and non-cultured cheeses.

My approach with respect to the cultured vegan cheeses mirrors the "true cheese" definition insofar as I focus on the use of microbes (and their subsequent enzymes) to metabolize carbohydrates (sugars) and coagulate proteins to create flavor and texture. In conjunction, I employ a variety of aging (affinaging) techniques that help develop different characteristics for my cheeses. Central to my focus in this realm is the use of minimal ingredients and the avoidance of unnecessary fats, starches, proteins. The methods I highlight in this book allow the reader to develop a very intimate relationship with their own culturing experiments at home and thus an opportunity to witness up close the amazing things that microbes can do in the creation of food.

However, there is a middle area of vegan cheesemaking that has been developing for some time, a crossover between strict culturing and aging processes only (this takes more time) and the quicker cheeze/analog processes. In this undefined realm, many makers use some combination of a fermented or cultured base (e.g., cultured cashew), which is then combined with other ingredients such as carrageenan, agar agar, miso, coconut oil, sometimes starches, and other seasoning or flavoring elements. These products are often aged for a short duration, usually two to four weeks. A potential complication of this crossover approach is that because the microbes are not metabolizing all of the components at the same time, you will not achieve the same kind of textural changes as with a culturing only process. Additionally, if oils are used, they risk trapping microbes and inhibiting their metabolic processes. Aside from a maker's comfort with this crossover process, there is the fact that products made in this manner take less time to make than their cultured only cousins and usually have more depth of flavor and texture than the non-cultured products.

I do not expect to unravel all of the necessary scientific elements of this claim within this book, but I do hope that the boundaries of definition I provide are helpful for the reader in understanding how I define cheese, the approach I am taking, and that it is possible and likely that a more comprehensive, formal definition of vegan plant-based cheese will eventually be developed. I invite the home-based reader-user to reconsider the possibilities of cheese, to think outside the confines of formal definition, and to allow the progress of recipes and methods to reveal the possibility that advanced plant-based cheesemaking could indeed be an evolution of the cheesemaking process itself.

Further, in presenting the three approaches to vegan cheesemaking (non-cultured, cultured, and crossover), I also seek to provide an overview of plant-based cheese methods and styles. While not exhaustive, it will give you a sense of how vegan cheesemaking has been and is evolving and offer you many options to choose from for the fun of your own home-based experimenting!

*Art of Plant-based Cheesemaking course student cheese tasting, 2018, at Bluhouse Market & Cafe, Deep Cove, North Vancouver.*

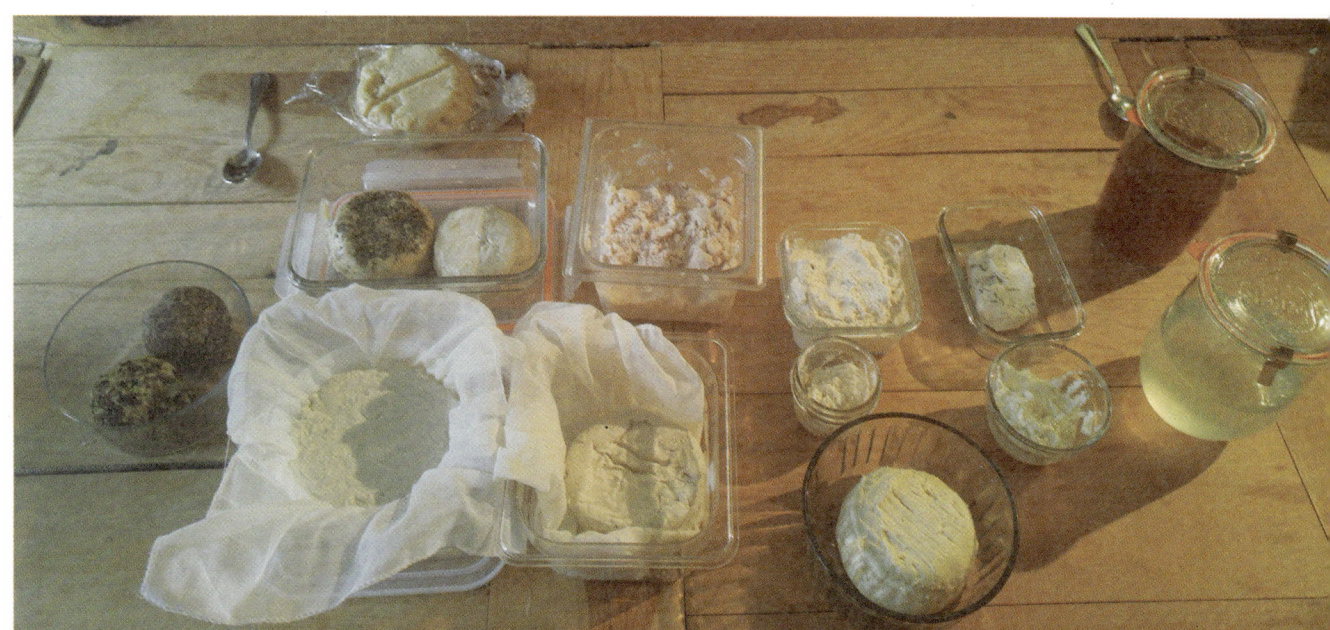

In contrast to the long history of dairy-based cheesemaking, which like so many of humankind's food preserving methods started out as a bit of an accident, plant-based cheesemaking began with intention. As cheese is often the last hurdle for those desiring to pursue a fully plant-based lifestyle, it comes as no surprise that many, many people have set about to explore a variety of means of creating the flavor and texture that so many people miss.

Until relatively recently (thirty years), there has been very little available in the way of formal culinary education in this realm and even less so with respect to culturing and fermentation. In the absence of formal culinary education with a vegan plant-based focus, community and homes have been the source of the development of plant-based cuisine knowledge and early recipe developments. People seeking solutions not offered on the market have brought about a robust DIY culture in vegan communities.

Vegan plant-based cheese has evolved through the commitment to do-it-yourself practices in the vegan community. This embrace of DIY in vegan circles, inherent to the culture, is a result in part of there being limited access to so many different types of food (processed/prepared) and lack of good quality options in restaurants. Vegans and plant-based folks from around the world have become adept at finding solutions and becoming creative in their experimental pursuit of plant-derived foods. This essentially empirical approach has led to increased intentional development of vegan cheese methods and to the widespread sharing of knowledge developed at the individual level.

## Terminology: Cheese Versus Cheeze

Dairy cheesemaking has its own nomenclature and classification system largely defined by the process and culture used to make the cheese. Surface ripened, washed rind, cave aged, cheddaring, et cetera, are all related to processes that affect specific outcomes. Soft, semi-soft, and hard cheeses are descriptors that imply specific characteristics, which are applied to identify cheese styles. In many cases, multiple categories apply to one kind of cheese.

Currently there is no official or formal classification system or common nomenclature for identifying plant-based cheeses by either style or method. For the purposes of guiding you through this book I will use an informal classification system organized, first, according to whether the cheese is cultured or not, and second, according to either texture or process. These are very loose and broad categories that have no formal standing.

The basic categories I put forward are non-cultured cheezes, cultured cheeses, and crossover cheeses. When I use the word "cheeze," I am referring to recipes that do not use cultures or aging processes. When I use the traditional term "cheese," I am referring to recipes that are cultured, aged, or otherwise mirror some elements of traditional cheesemaking. The cultured and aged cheeses range from simple fresh cheeses to more advanced cheeses and processes that bring us closer to bridging the gap between dairy and plant-based cheesemaking. When I use "crossover," I am referring to cheeses that employ some culturing method along with added ingredients such as coconut oil, miso, starches, and emulsifiers.

## Cheeze, Cheese, Crossover Methods: Definitions and Boundaries

Cheese analogs, or cheeze, are not cultured. These products generally aim to capture something familiar or nostalgic for folks missing dairy cheese. Whether it be a cheesy flavor, a stretchy or meltable consistency, or a sharp density, these characteristics are achieved (or attempted) through the use of multiple ingredients without engaging in culturing or aging processes that do the primary work in the creation of dairy cheeses (after the milk production by the animals themselves, of course). The terms "cashew cheeze" or "nut cheeze" arose a few years ago in relation to this style of product, and these terms have become nearly synonymous with the (mainstream) idea of vegan plant-based cheese, meaning many people now assume that vegan cheese is always or almost always cashew or nut based because cashews were one of the first and most widely used ingredients for this purpose.

However, this style of cheese can be and often is made with a combination of many ingredients other than cashews. Ingredients common in these types of analogs are agar agar, kappa carrageenan, modified tapioca starch, tapioca starch, potato starch, pea protein, other plant proteins, nutritional yeast, miso, apple cider vinegar, lemon juice, lactic acid powder, coconut or other oil, proteins for structure, starches for stretchiness/meltability, acids for tanginess/sharpness, umami rich compounds for that cheesy flavor, and a fat for a creamy mouthfeel. Another feature of this style of cheeze (and even cultured vegan cheese) is the tendency to add distinctive flavors through the addition of herbs, spices, fruits, something that is less common in the traditional dairy cheesemaking realm.

With dozens if not hundreds of recipes existing on the internet for a quick cheeze-like substance to be used in ravioli, lasagne, salads, and so on, cashew cheeze/nut cheeze has almost become comfortably mainstream. Chefs at non-plant-based restaurants are increasingly trying some version or other, increasing the quality and range of vegan plant-based options on restaurant menus.

While non-cultured cheeze recipes tend to focus heavily on the use of cashews, the use, in either a creamy paste or milk form, of sunflower and pumpkin seeds, chickpeas, tofu, and white beans have become more prominent as a starting base. Depending on the style of the cheeze being made, you can use varying amounts of the different components (the base, oils, proteins, starches, umami, acid) to make a product that is firmer, softer, creamier, and so forth. In this manner, this method is much more in line with cooking and using traditional style recipes, though it is still important to understand the individual ingredients with respect to what they do and how they work.

These cheezes can be heated and then shaped or made as uncooked preparations (without the agar agar or other thickening agent). To a small extent they can be air dried to remove moisture but generally have a shorter shelf life due to the fact that non-cultured cheeses lack the acidity and protective enzymes produced through the microbial metabolizing of carbohydrate by lactic acid forming bacteria that occurs during fermenting and culturing processes.

This user-friendly analog is highly adaptable and relatively low risk for the home user. It allows for broad experimentation and multiple applications, from sauces to thicker preparations, and without additional ingredients, aside from cashews (or other nut/seed/legume of choice) and filtered water, also serves as a base medium for culturing processes that can be used in some cultured cheeses. I think of these as the gateway plant-based cheezes, and with its generally broad appeal, cashew cheeze/nut cheeze at least allows the skeptic to consider the possibility of non-dairy cheese. Recipes detailing different versions, soft, semi-soft, semi-firm, are provided further on.

With cultured cheese we begin to explore in greater depth the realm and effect of microbes in culturing and fermentation. In traditional cheesemaking, a variety of bacteria, yeasts, and molds are employed to create different flavors, aromas, and textures. In many dairy cheese processes, different species of lactic acid forming bacteria (LAB) are added in early stages. The bacteria then metabolize the sugars, producing lactic acid and other enzymes, which then break down the proteins, causing coagulation into a curd. In dairy cheesemaking, this coagulation process is often aided by the addition of other digestive enzymes (calf rennet or microbial rennet), and flavor enhancing enzymes (lipases).

Other bacteria are or can be added later on in addition to the initial culture for ripening or developing flavor and texture in different directions. Yeasts and molds are employed for their metabolic activity as well, though they do not produce lactic acid. They have significant impact on flavor and texture outcomes and are very obviously present in cheeses such as brie, camembert, cambazola, gorgonzola, stilton, morbier, and many others. The knowledge within this sector of what these microbes do is considerable, and it is a valuable place to seek information. Essentially, much of the craft of traditional cheesemaking is microbiology.

Cultured vegan cheesemaking is very much in its infancy. Miyoko's book *Artisan Vegan Cheese* popularized the concept by introducing the application of rejuvelac, a microbially rich solution made from sprouted grain (most often wheat berries), to a plant-based medium.

The first edition of my book furthered work in this arena in its discussions of rejuvelac, water kefir, coconut kefir, and probiotics, and others such as Thomas's blog *Full of Plants* and Cashewbert with their e-book *A Guide to Vegan Cheese* continue to broaden the scope of publicly available, user friendly information out there for the vegan cheesemaker.

However, that said, the diversity of culture types, their limited availability (inconsistent availability in different countries), and the lack of in-depth research by food scientists and others with respect to how traditional cultures behave on the diversity of plant mediums means that the complexity of flavors, textures, aromas, and styles of vegan cheeses are still largely underexplored. Hopefully, as companies such as Dupont, which makes Danisco cheese cultures, finally begin to turn their attention to making culture sets specifically for plant-based culturing, there will be an increase in the number and diversity of microbes and in the understanding of their behavior on plant-mediums and it will result in an expansion of what is possible in vegan cheesemaking.

I knew from the beginning of my engagement with vegan cheesemaking that the use of microbes was essential, but over the last few years, it has become apparent to me that what may be possible in vegan cheesemaking is only just beginning to be understood. In my research, development, and production work for Blue Heron and in the courses I teach, increasingly my emphasis is on understanding the behavior of the microbes we use in order to find conditions for them that lead to best outcomes. These microbes, after all, are living organisms and not simply another ingredient.

Unofficially, that is, not within the confines of a formal food science laboratory, I have tested the use of several traditional starter cultures and discovered so much more depth of flavor and textural changes than rejuvelac alone can offer and, without question, substantially better outcomes than from probiotic capsules. It is also clear to me that much more research needs to be done in terms of identifying enzymes that will break down a wide range of plant proteins, because in plant-based cheeesemaking we are working with a larger number of types of proteins than in dairy cheesemaking.

So, knowing that research in this area of cultured vegan cheese is active, ongoing, and changing, my intention in this book is to offer information that is understandable and relatively easy for the home user and small scale experimenter to work with. This book in no way provides the depth of knowledge required by a commercial producer, and those reading it with that in mind should be prepared to do considerably more work of their own. It is a measure of my knowledge and experience to date and is not all encompassing or the final stop in this evolution of a new craft and is specifically designed for folks who wish to enhance their home-based food adventures.

In order to be fully plant-based, I focus on the use of rejuvelac, water kefir, coconut kefir, and some other lactic acid microbial starters that can be grown at home or easily found. Importantly, I no longer recommend the use of probiotic capsules for culturing. Probiotics are primarily a product of the wellness industry and are not a classification of bacteria. Capsules, powders, and other probiotic products are designed for human consumption, and the microbes they contain are related to the kinds of microbes that are found within the human gut biome. While some of these products are related to the same microbes that do optimal culturing of food, they are often inconsistent in their performance, and outcomes can vary from low acidity to too much acidity, and flavor-wise they usually produce flat flavor because not all of the species of bacteria in these products are lactic acid forming, which is necessary for a lactic acid culturing process. The other starter cultures produce better flavor and texture results and provide the user a more direct understanding of the relationship of microbes and variables (conditions) to cheesemaking outcomes.

New in this second edition is the introduction of blue mold, *P. roqueforti*, and white molds, a couple of types, for use in making a blue cheese and a brie- or camembert-type cheese. Molds are more complex to work with and do require more diligence with respect to maintaining food safety conditions and inhibition or prevention of jumping of spores as they grow, but it is possible to make blue and white mold ripened vegan cheeses at home. Blue mold is the mold responsible for the sharp piquancy, pungency, and creaminess of dairy cheeses like stilton, gorgonzola, cambazola. White molds are those that create the mushroomy, earthy qualities associated with camembert and brie and form the white mold rind that grows on them.

It is worth reiterating that the focus of this book is methodology. Instead of dozens of vegan cheese recipes, this book gives you an understanding of how the materials we use work, how microbes behave, and some key principles and concepts that allow us to make vegan cheese, and this will result in your being able to be more creative at home.

---

2. Joint FAO/WHO Codex Alimentarius Commission. "Codex General Standard For Cheese, Codex Standard 283–1978." *Codex Alimentarius*. Food and Agriculture Organization of the United Nations.

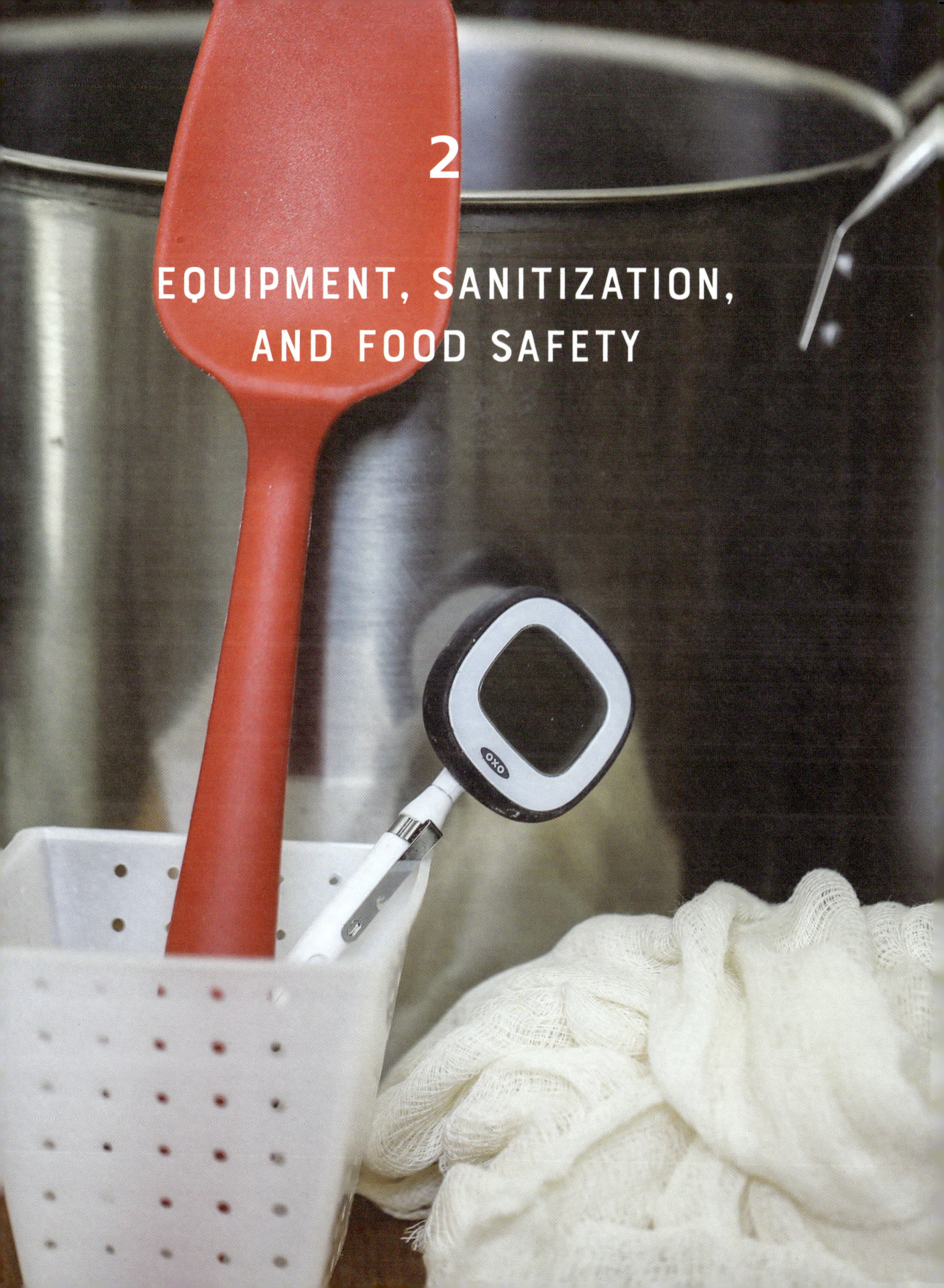

# 2
# EQUIPMENT, SANITIZATION, AND FOOD SAFETY

In this chapter, I discuss food safety and sanitization practices and I provide an overview of the key equipment you will find useful in your home experiments. Prior to undertaking any of these experiments and recipes, make sure you are well equipped and aware of how to prepare food in a safe manner for yourself and those you love.

## Food Safety and Sanitization

Regardless of whether one is working with fermentation processes, preparing any kind of food for consumption should be done with a view to doing so safely. Food borne illness is one of the most common forms of illness and is easily preventable with good preparation, cleanup, and storage practices. Yes, many of us will have consumed a bite of something that has dropped to the floor, crying out "three second rule, three second rule!" and yes, the vast majority of those who do consume that bite will be just fine (after all, we have hydrochloric acid in our stomachs, and with 7.5 billion people on this planet and counting, it's guaranteed more than one person has been less than hyper-cautious about food preparation). However, there is no such thing as a "three second rule," and it is not just the floor or ground that can be a source of contamination. I often tell students in my classes that it is not as though microbes are waiting to contaminate or move onto a surface. If they are there, they are there. There is no microbial bouncer telling the other microbes "wait; she has three seconds before we move in!"

Wild yeast, bacteria, and molds exist everywhere, the presence of which enables wild fermentation processes. It is the pathogenic (unwelcome) microbes that present concern. *Listeria, E.coli,* and *Salmonella* are among the familiar pathogenic bacteria that we want to ward against. *Listeria, E. coli* and *Salmonella* can come into an environment through opportunistic channels, for example, being present on another food, and can thrive in the right conditions of food, moisture, and warmth.

Although it is not possible to ensure a sterile environment (nor is that even a desirable objective), it is essential to ensure that all of the equipment you will be working with and all the surfaces you will be working on are clean and sanitized and that you have a safe, clean working and storage environment. Though all of this may seem obvious, there are some optimal ways to prepare your food preparation environment. Here is a recommended approach for preparing your tools and surfaces.

## Step 1: Wash

You can't sanitize a dirty or contaminated surface or item. The first step in preparing your space is to make sure your tools, equipment, and surfaces are clean.

# Equipment, Sanitization, and Food Safety

Use hot water and soap. Hot means not tepid, not lukewarm, but *hot*. Hot water and soap and a little elbow grease will remove any grime and unwanted debris from your utensils, the stovetop, and working counter. Any household soap will work for this purpose, including dish soap.

## Step 2: Rinse/Dry

After washing the surface with hot soapy water, use a clean, unused towel to wipe up any excess soapy water residue. The towel is for picking up excess moisture, not for drying off the surface. Leave the surface to air dry. After washing utensils and tools, rinse them in hot water and leave to air dry fully. If you do not have a dishwasher, air drying is the best way to ensure that all moisture has evaporated. Unwanted bacteria and microbes thrive in moist environments, and towel drying, rather than removing all moisture, actually can create a thin layer of pervasive moisture that can last for a long time, in addition to contributing unwanted fibers and potentially spreading microbes if you are not using a clean towel.

## Step 3: Sanitize

Only after the cleaning process is completed can sanitization occur. Four sanitizing options are outlined here.

### Acid based

I use an acid based sanitizer, Star San, which is available in self-brew shops (do-it-yourself wine or beer shops), or online. Star San is commonly used by commercial beer brewers and other fermenters. It is made from food grade phosphoric acid and is considered safe for both the environment and people. When used in the correct dilution, 1 fluid ounce Star San to 5 gallons of water, and with only 1 to 2 minutes of contact time, it does not require post application rinsing. It has good shelf stability, and in a covered container, a pre-mixed solution can last up to 3 to 4 weeks. It is effective at pH 3 or lower, and can be used in a spray bottle. Please ensure you follow the manufacturer's instructions for mixing and storing all chemicals. Store all chemicals in clean, previously unused containers to avoid chemical reactions.

### Alkaline (ammonium chloride) based

A quaternary sanitizer, or quaternary ammonium chloride, is also effective. Quaternary sanitizer (sometimes referred to as hard surface sanitizer) is the generic name for quaternary ammonium chloride based sanitizers. These sanitizers are low in toxicity and corrosiveness,

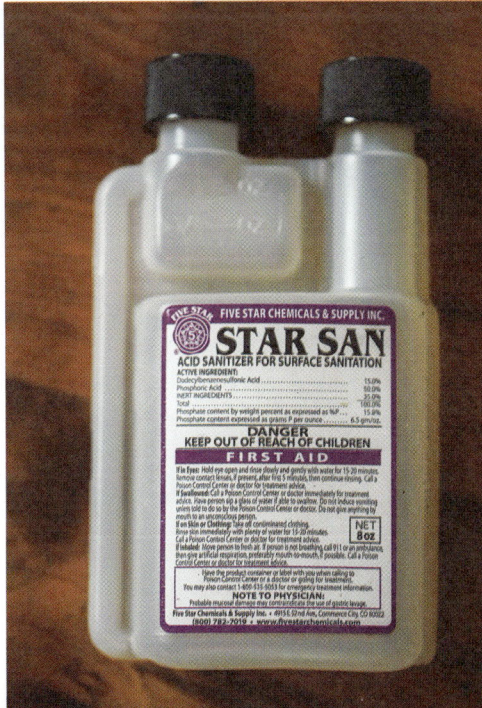

*Sanitizer.*
CREDIT: CATHERINE DOWNES

and because of this they are commonly used in restaurant and food service kitchens and on guest-related surfaces. Quaternary ammonium chloride has a wide-spectrum antimicrobial function, low or no odor, a good shelf life, and is effective across a range of pH levels, making it easy to use. Quat sani also contains surfactants (a compound that lowers surface tension between two liquids and is a common compound in detergents), so they do have some cleaning efficacy. However, even if you choose to use a quat sani, precede its use with a proper hot water and soapy water cleaning. Quaternary sanitizer products can be found online and at restaurant supply and janitorial supply stores. Follow the manufacturer's directions for mixing the solution and store the solution in a new, not previously used, spray bottle.

**Alkaline (bleach and water) based**

Those who do not want to order sanitizer online or have difficulty finding either an acid based sanitizer or quat sani, may use a bleach and water solution.

I mix this at 1 fluid ounce to 1.04 gallon (30 milliliters to 3.8 liters) of water. Bleach is a sodium chlorite and water compound, and is readily available. Household bleach (sold in most grocery stores, pharmacies, and many other places) contains a 5% sodium chlorite solution. It is a highly effective disinfectant and has high alkalinity, but there are some things to be mindful of when using bleach.

- It is highly corrosive and oxidative, and even household solutions can cause damage to a variety of materials (bleach stains anyone?).
- It has strong fumes that can be irritating to eyes and lungs.
- It can form toxic gasses if accidentally combined with other chemicals.
- It dissipates quickly, meaning that you cannot store a pre-made bleach/water solution for prolonged periods of time but must make it just before use each time you need it.

After the washing process, use the sanitizing solution to wipe down utensils, all related tools, and surfaces on which you will handle any of the cheese-related ingredients. If you are using the bleach solution, allow the tools to rest and allow the chlorine to evaporate, or rinse the tools in clean water and allow them to air dry.

**6 % Distilled White Vinegar (acetic acid)**

For folks looking to use a natural sanitizer, (I avoid saying "chemical," even though acetic acid is indeed a chemical) 6% acetic acid distilled white vinegar (or cleaning vinegar) can be effective. It is also very inexpensive. Most distilled white vinegar in grocery stores is 5%, so you may have to do a little searching to find a 6% solution. According to the David Suzuki Foundation's *Queen of Green* website, 5% distilled white vinegar will kill up to 80% of microbes, so for increased effectiveness, do be sure to seek out the 6% solution. At a strength of 6%, distilled white vinegar can effectively kill gram-negative bacteria such as *E.coli* and *Salmonella*, and in a clinical study, with prolonged time exposure it was found to be effective at killing tuberculosis.

At 6% strength white vinegar can be used in a 50/50 (vinegar to water) ratio applied directly to the washed and dried surface and tools and should be left on for at least 30 minutes. This time requirement does mean a little bit more planning. Shortening the exposure time of the vinegar lowers its effectiveness as a sanitizing agent. Acetic acid permeates the cell membranes of bacteria, causing them to explode, and this requires some time to work.

If you do use white vinegar as a sanitizing agent, be mindful that some aroma residue will remain.

## Step 4: Hand-washing

Hand-washing as a means of controlling contamination spread cannot be overemphasized. It is one of the most effective means we have of preventing movement of unwanted microbes from one place to another. Though your hands will be quite clean after cleaning and sanitizing tools and surfaces, washing your hands before you begin working directly with ingredients is still important and a good habit to develop.

Hand-washing is often done hastily and without deep attention. However, as you are about to handle cultures and apply them to food ingredients, making sure your hands are as clean as possible is helpful.

- Under warm running water rinse your hands; then add 3–5 milliliters of soap (if liquid). If you are using bar soap, make sure you lather it up quite well.
- Rub your hands together well, making sure to wash your fingers, backs and palms of hands, and up to your wrists. Use a nail brush to scrub your nails, making sure to remove foreign debris. Take your time, sing a song to prolong the time you spend scrubbing your hands.
- According to food safety guidelines from several nations, states, and provinces, 15 to 30 seconds of vigorous handwashing under warm water with soap will be effective.
- After washing with soap, rinse your hands well and dry them completely with a paper towel or on a clean towel.

## Tools and Equipment

Just before you get started on your project, you should make sure that you have all of the equipment you will need. It is not a lot, and you do not need to have anything specialized to get started, but it will be less frustrating if you make sure you have the equipment assembled beforehand.

The following lists the equipment you will need. Keep in mind that you may not need all of the equipment listed here for each method or recipe you choose to explore.

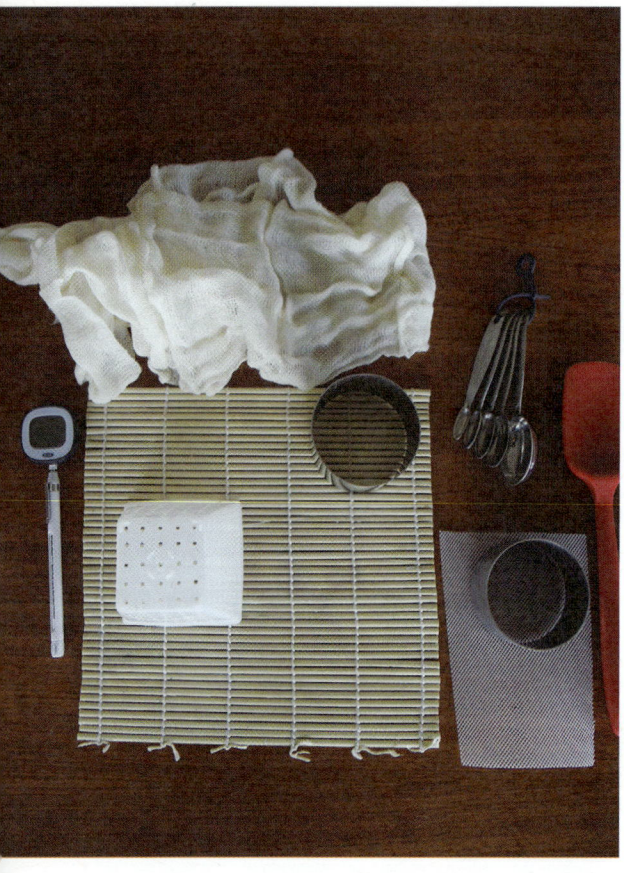

*Useful tools to have on hand: bamboo mat, probe thermometer, cheesecloth, cheese mold, stainless steel rings, silicone spatula, measuring spoons.*
PHOTO CREDIT: CATHERINE DOWNES.

### Key Tools

High-speed blender

Wooden/silicone spoon and spatula

Stainless steel stock pot with thick cast bottom, medium-sized pot, 3–5 L, depending on the size of the batch you wish to make

Glass or food grade plastic bowl (medium-sized, enough room to stir and mix if necessary)

Probe thermometer

pH meter

Cheesecloth or butter muslin (Butter muslin has a tighter weave than most cheesecloth and is easily reusable with washing.)

Measuring cups

Measuring spoons

Mason jars, 500 mL to 1 L for making rejuvelac and kefir (again, depending on the size of batch you make)

Cheese molds or food grade stainless steel ring molds, for cheese shaping

Wooden boards

Colander or fine mesh sieve

Bamboo sushi mats/cheese aging mats

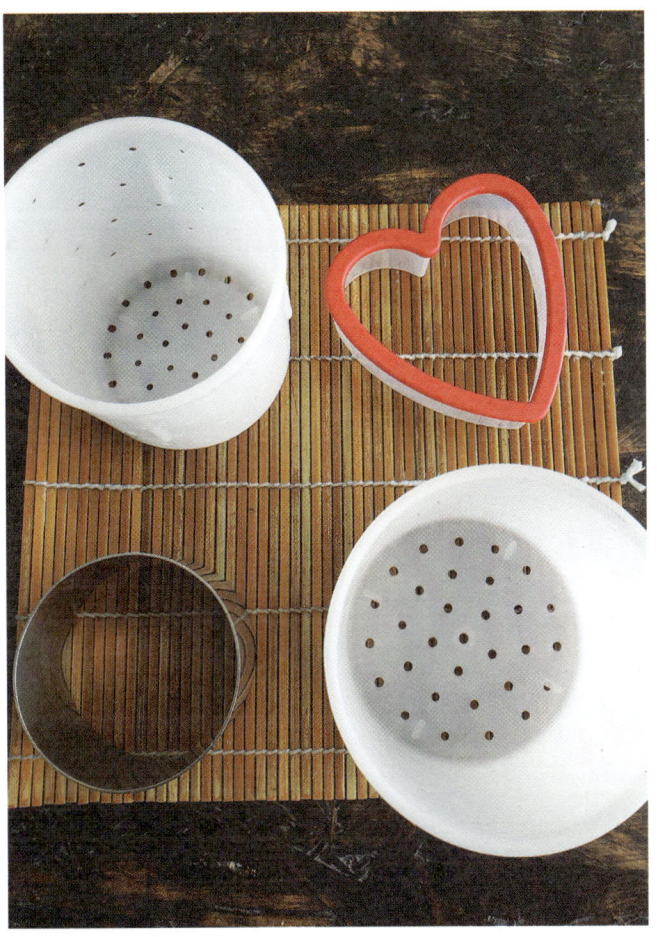

*A variety of cheese molds for forming cheese shapes.*

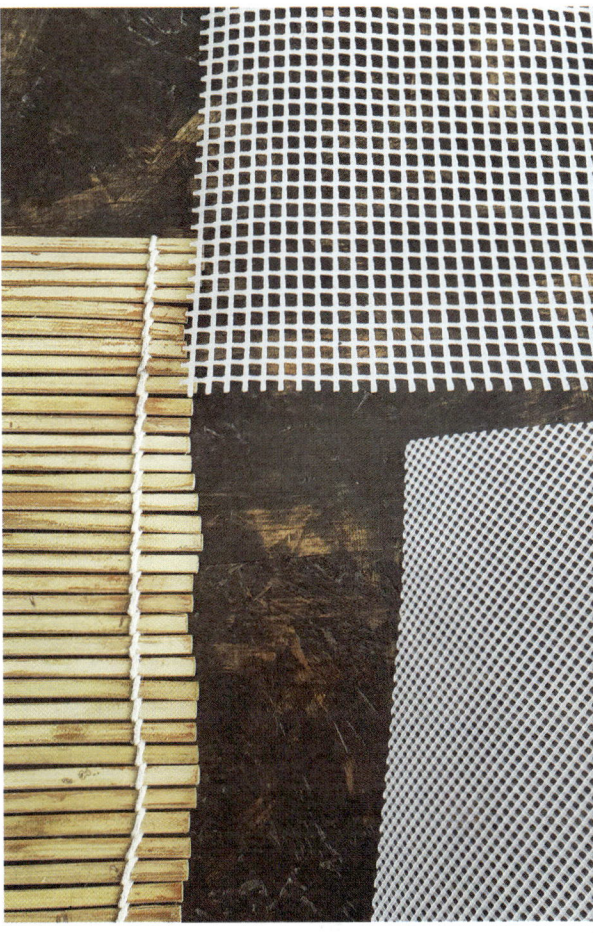

*A selection of aging mats, including bamboo, food grade plastic wide mesh, and fine mesh cheese mats.*
CREDIT: CATHERINE DOWNES

## Ingredients

Given that any vegan cheese (cultured or non-cultured) is trying to replace something in the way of flavor and texture, it makes sense to give some consideration to what ingredients will yield the most satisfying results. There is room for a lot of creativity and experimentation, but I do think that understanding the ingredients always helps me make choices that lead to the kind of outcomes I am seeking.

So, how do you choose the base material for your process? I am often asked this question in the classes I teach and in messages from readers. Cashews have become nearly synonymous with vegan cheese. They offer a good balance of sweetness, creaminess (fatty), and density. However, there are other ingredients and combinations of ingredients that can produce favorable, even preferable results.

When I am considering what ingredients I want to work with, I think about their protein, fat, and carbohydrate content, not what this means with regard to nutrition (that is a secondary thought), but what they mean for the kind of product that will result. Fat content provides a sense of creaminess, carbohydrates, an element of sweetness, and protein gives structure or supports texture. If an ingredient has too much protein (to use on its own), I will combine it with another or other ingredients that provide more fattiness and sweetness, particularly in non-cultured cheeze processes. For instance, if I use lentils in a quick cheeze process, I may combine them with some cashews or oats and maybe some coconut cream. Other considerations for building flavor in soft, non-cultured vegan cheeze and even in cultured cheeses include creating sharpness (acidity), creaminess/fattiness, and depth of flavor (umami).

Sharpness or tanginess in a non-cultured cheese comes from the use of acidity. Commonly, lemon juice and apple cider vinegar are used, but you may also use other vinegars as well as citric acid powder or lactic acid powder (vegan source). Creamy or fatty mouthfeel comes from fat content, and you may want to increase this component in your cheeze by blending nuts, seeds, and/or legumes with oat milk, coconut milk, a high quality cashew or almond milk, or by adding coconut oil or cacao butter.

Finally, and likely the most important element of flavor with regard to cheeze or cheese, is umami. Umami is one of the five primary taste components: sweet, sour, bitter, and salty. It is often described as a deep, savory or meaty flavor. Often this depth of flavor is lacking, especially in non-cultured vegan cheezes, but there are ways to address this through the addition of particular ingredients.

"Umami" is a term initiated by the Japanese scientist Kikunae Ikeda, who first identified umami in 1908. It was recognized officially in 1985 as a scientific term referring to the flavor and its sensation in the human mouth. Umami, then, refers to the taste of glutamates and nucleotides GMP and IMP (guanosine monophosphate and inosine monophosphate). Glutamate or its precursor, glutamic acid, is found in a number of foods, and while many people assume that it is mostly animal products that possess this important flavor compound, there are plenty of sources to be found in the plant world. Plants particularly noted for their umami include mushrooms, tomatoes, and potatoes, and fermented foods in general are high in umami compounds.

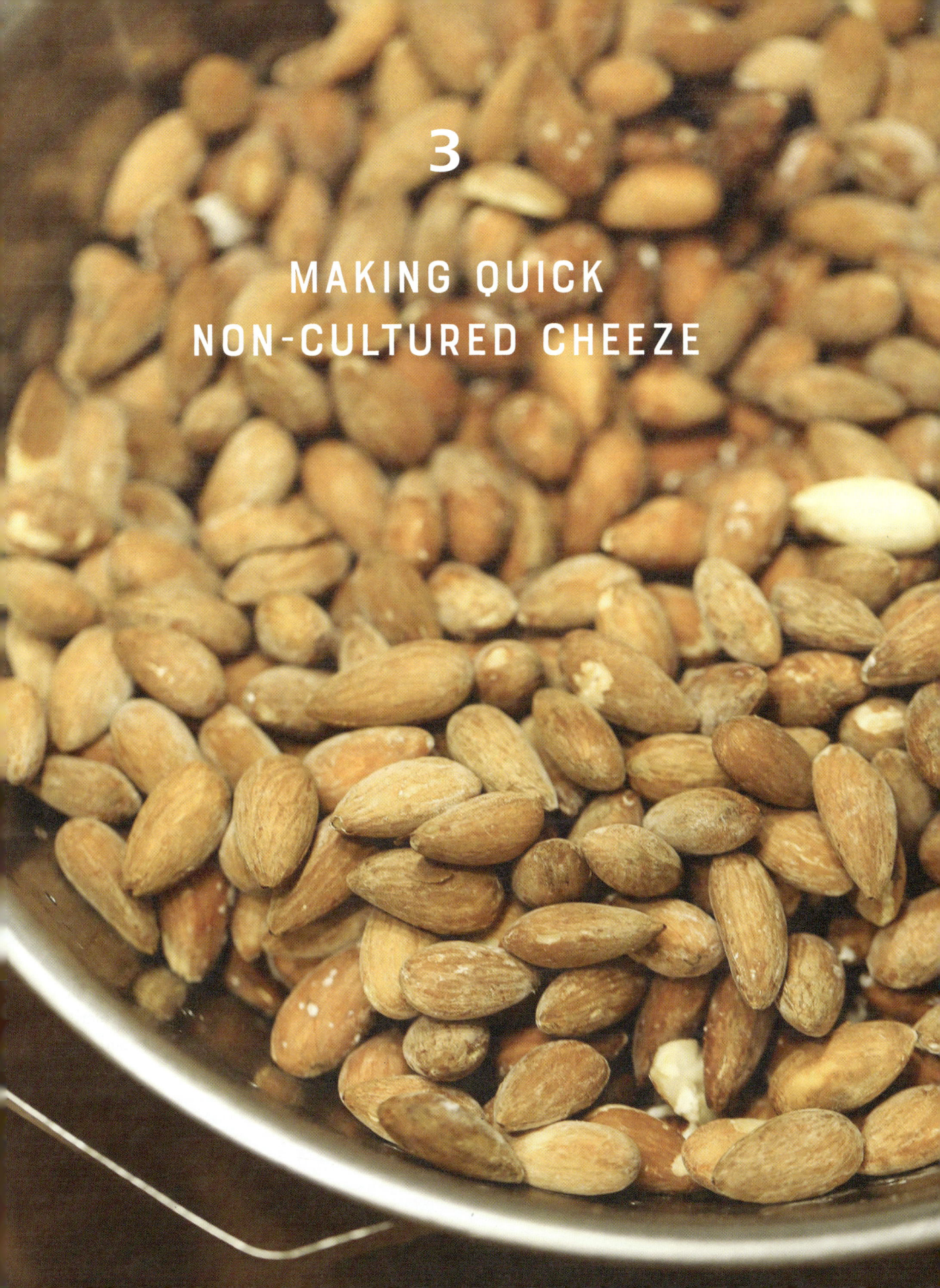

# 3
# MAKING QUICK NON-CULTURED CHEEZE

This chapter provides a brief overview of some easy base recipes for creating do-it-yourself quick cheeze. Although some of these can be adapted and altered for a culturing approach, typically, these types of cheezes are meant to be produced quickly and to evoke a sense of cheese through the use of added ingredients to create familiar flavor and/or texture rather than relying on the application of a culture and aging time to produce taste and texture. The recipes highlighted in this section are examples of what you can do and of how to work with different ingredients (e.g., legumes versus seeds and nuts) and are a great way to practice blending with emulsification in mind and to play with building flavor profiles you enjoy.

Dairy cheeses, for those who still choose to eat them or for those who have a sense memory from when they once did, possess characteristics that are often cited by their fans as being essential, never mind that not all dairy cheeses share the same traits. Texture is often identified as important, particularly for lovers of hard cheese, who lament the dearth of similar options in the vegan cheese sector. Aroma is missed by those who enjoy strong, pungent cheeses. Finally, there is flavor. There is something about the combination of tangy, salty, and fatty that causes some people to virtually swoon when eating cheese and to lament the prospect of giving it up.

Then there is the fact that dairy cheese, which contains casein proteins that when metabolized (digested) break down into casein peptides (casomorphins), some of which interact with our dopamine receptors, pulls the cheese lover back for more with each pleasure-releasing bite. A study published in the US National Library of Medicine discusses this and the results of the Yale Food Addiction Scale. You can read more about this in the study itself, "Which foods may be addictive? The roles of processing, fat content, and glycemic load," by Schulte et al.[3] With this in mind, quick vegan cheezes aim to capture some combination of these characteristics, often aiming at the most popular or most widely recognized realm of dairy-based cheeses, like cheddar, monterey jack, nacho cheese, or even brie. The idea with these cheezes is to create something that is flavorful and creamy and texturally fulfilling so that the substance can be used to replace dairy in items such as lasagne, ravioli, pizza, nachos, and really for whatever one wishes. There is very much a comfort food connection to these items.

The general approach I take in this section is intended to be easily modifiable by the user. I focus on concept and principles first and use recipes as guidelines. It is a dominant trend these days for people to seek quickly accessible information and fast ways of doing things, and often, in my opinion, this leads to unsuccessful results, especially with food. Making food, and cheese, is a way of reconnecting to process, to understanding through observation and patience. It is an opportunity to create some time for you, to slow life down a little, and to enjoy the act of doing something. Thus, I've chosen to write these recipes in a manner that allows room for experimentation based on key information about the use of particular ingredients.

I have found this is a useful approach, if mildly provocative, as I find when people rely solely on recipes, they are not paying close attention to the food and the process itself. It is the marriage of recipe and user that yields the best results, and once you are using the culturing recipes, observation, patience, and deeper involvement are necessary to good outcomes. The approaches to quick vegan cheezes that follow begin with soft cheeze, which is essentially a cheesy dip or pâté. This approach is followed by methods for making quick, non-cultured mozzarella- and feta-type cheezes, which use, in addition to some of the ingredients in the spreadable cheezes, ingredients such as starches and gelling agents, or tofu. Last in the non-cultured cheeze section are a few recipes for semi-firm cheezes. These rely on different combinations of gelling agents and emulsifiers and sometimes added oils to create a cheese that holds its shape and is a bit firmer and drier than the soft cheezes.

## Non-Cultured Soft Cheeze

This simple flowchart outlines the core processes, in order, required to make soft spreadable cheezes. You can use this as a quick reference guide, but I recommend that you closely review the specific recipes first.

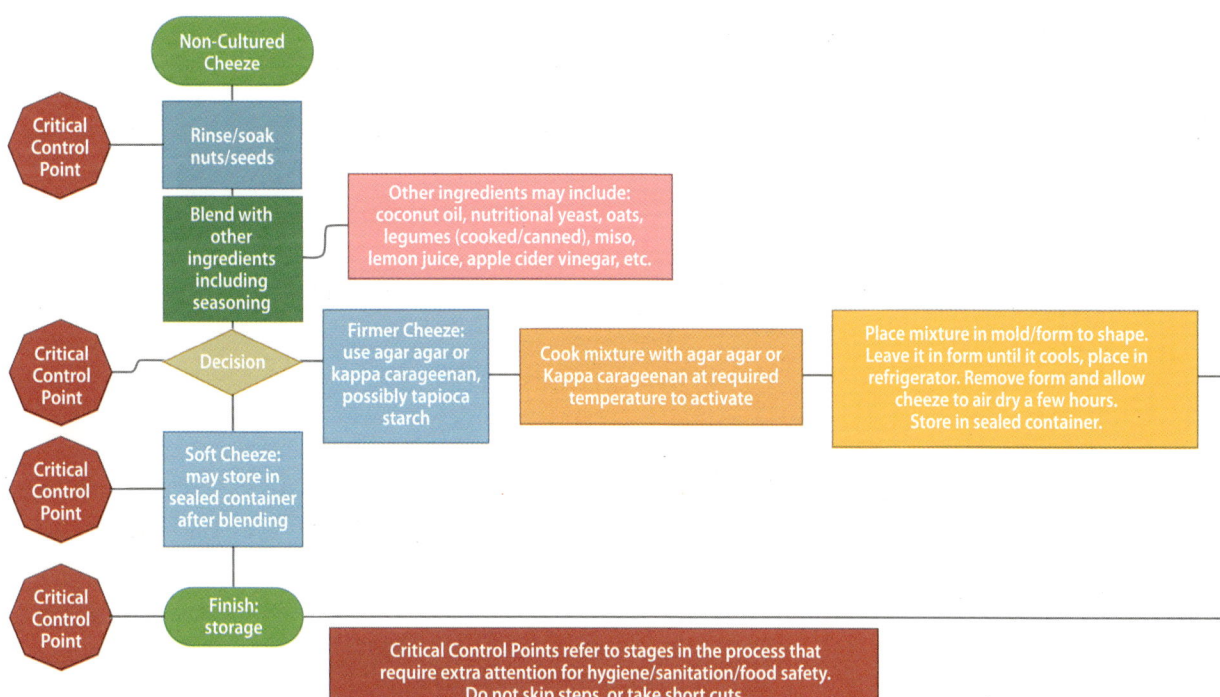

Although plant-based cheesemaking is still in its infancy and there is no formal nomenclature, soft cheezes are non-cultured and on the spectrum of spreads, dips, and pâtés in consistency.

When working with nuts, seeds, and dry legumes, it is generally advisable to soak them first, even if you are not going to be making fermented or cultured cheese, although there are some exceptions.

### *Soaking nuts, seeds, and legumes*

Soaking nuts, seeds, and legumes in advance of using them removes inhibiting enzymes such as phytic acid, saponins, and trypsins, and this makes them easier for us to digest. These inhibiting enzymes (or anti-nutrients, as they are referred to in the wellness industry) serve an evolutionary purpose for these containers of new plant life. They ensure that these nuts and seeds can pass through digestive tracts and come out the other end, so to speak, and fulfill their evolutionary purpose of growing into new members of their respective species. These enzymes also protect the seeds and nuts from decomposing and allow them to survive a wide variety of conditions.

Moreover, soaking them in advance protects delicate oils (particularly in the case of nuts and seeds) when toasting them, because the water absorbed will heat up and that heated moisture will heat the oil in the nuts and seeds, preventing them from burning.

Cashews are an exception to the soaking rule because they are already removed from their protective casing and most of the acid has been removed through the curing process cashews need to go through prior to being packaged. I rinse cashews under cold running water to remove remnant materials, and I do a short soak, approximately 1 hour at room temperature, just to make it easy for blending.

It is important to note that soaking should be done with care to prevent pathogen growth or contamination. Follow this protocol for safe soaking.

1. Ensure the container you soak the nuts or seeds in is clean and sanitized.
2. Rinse the nuts or seeds under cold running water.
3. Use cold water for soaking. Warm water can be a good growing ground for pathogens.
4. Make sure that the nuts or seeds are fully covered by the water and that the container is covered with an impermeable cover such as a fitted lid.
5. Soaking of nuts and seeds can be done for as short a duration as 2 hours at room temperature provided the ambient temperature is not above 72°F (22°C). Soaking time may vary based on how fresh the seeds or nuts are, and you should make careful observations about this prior to soaking.

6. If the room is above 72°F (22°C) or you are soaking overnight, soak the nuts or seeds in a covered container in the refrigerator.
7. Nuts such as walnuts, hazelnuts, and almonds (nuts with skins) should be soaked longer than other nuts because the skins contain not only phytic acid, but also tannic acid.
8. After soaking, discard the soaking water and rinse the nuts or seeds under cold running water to remove residual debris.

There is much and varied information about how long to soak what types of nuts and seeds. This table provides recommendations. Most soaking recommendations are intended for nuts and seeds that are being used in non-fermented food-making processes. As such, I recommend using longer soaking times when you make non-cultured cheezes and using reduced soaking times when you make fermented/cultured vegan cheese.

## Soaking Guidelines

| | Soaking Time Non-cultured Process | Soaking Time Cultured Process | Soaking with Salt | Soaking with Baking Soda |
|---|---|---|---|---|
| Almond, Pumpkin Seed, Hazelnut, Pecan/Walnut | 7–8 hours | Minimum 4 hours refrigerated | 1 tsp/1 gal (3.78 L) | Pinch baking soda with pumpkin seed |
| Cashew, Sunflower Seed, Hemp | 4 hours | 1 hour (at room temperature) 2–4 hours refrigerated | 1 tsp/1 gal (3.78 L) | Pinch baking soda with sunflower seed |
| Pistachio, Brazil | 4–6 hours | Minimum 4 hours refrigerated | 1 tsp/1 gal (3.78 L) | N/A |
| Macadamia | 6–7 hours | Minimum 6 hours refrigerated | 1 tsp/1 gal (3.78 L) | N/A |

Note: Be mindful that the amount of moisture in the nuts and seeds before and after soaking will impact how much moisture you add during blending. Because you don't know what the pre and post soak moisture amount is, add moisture during blending a little at a time and focus on achieving the texture you want, rather than rushing the blending process.

# Walnut Ricotta

This cheeze is obviously not truly a ricotta, but it does have a ricotta-type texture and, more importantly, is a great replacement for ricotta in salads, pasta dishes, on sandwiches, and if blended until very creamy, is a good base for a pâté. This is a soft-style cheeze. When working with walnuts I recommend looking for walnuts that are plump and do not taste sour or bitter, which indicates that they are rancid. I suggest soaking walnuts before use, not just to remove tannin and inhibiting enzymes, but also to protect the delicate walnut oil in applications using heat, such as toasting them. Soak walnuts for a minimum of 1 hour following the soaking guidelines given in this chapter.

## Tools and Equipment

Jar or bowl for soaking
High-speed blender (or food processor and less fancy blender)
Spatula
Measuring spoons
Bowl
Colander or fine mesh sieve
Cheesecloth or butter muslin or nut milk bag
Container for storage

## Ingredients

2 cups walnuts, soaked and rinsed
½–1 tsp salt (Add a little at a time, and adjust to your taste.)
1 tsp lemon juice
2 tsp apple cider vinegar
2 Tbsp nutritional yeast (You may add more if you like.)
½ cup water (or almond milk, oat milk, coconut milk, etc. for more richness)
Optional: 1 Tbsp softened coconut oil or cacao butter for mouthfeel

## Method

1. Rinse the walnuts under cold running water.
2. Soak the walnuts from 1 hour to overnight in cold water. If soaking overnight, do so in the refrigerator. Walnuts have quite a bit of tannin in the skin, giving them a slight bitterness. Soaking them longer helps to remove much of this bitter flavor. You may also try adding 1 tsp of baking soda to the soaking water.
3. Drain the walnuts, and rinse under cold running water. At this point, you may toast the walnuts in the oven at 275°F (135°C) for 15 minutes.
4. Add the water (or your choice of plant-based milk), lemon juice, apple cider vinegar, salt, and nutritional yeast to the blender, add the walnuts, and start blending on low speed. Pulse a few times to allow the ingredients to break into smaller pieces.
5. Increase the speed only moderately. You are not aiming to achieve a creamy texture but rather a cottage cheese-style texture. If you have elected to add the coconut oil or cacao butter, this is when you add it.
6. Scrape the mixture out of the pitcher and into a cheesecloth-lined sieve or a nut milk bag and allow it to drain for 1 to 2 hours. Overdraining will result in a mixture that is too dry and crumbly.

7. Place the drained mixture in a sealed container. You may add garlic, parsley, or other herbs.

**Storage**

Keeps refrigerated up to 1 week.

*Walnut ricotta, non-cultured, is a quick and easy cheeze that works well on its own and used in recipes such as stuffed pasta.*

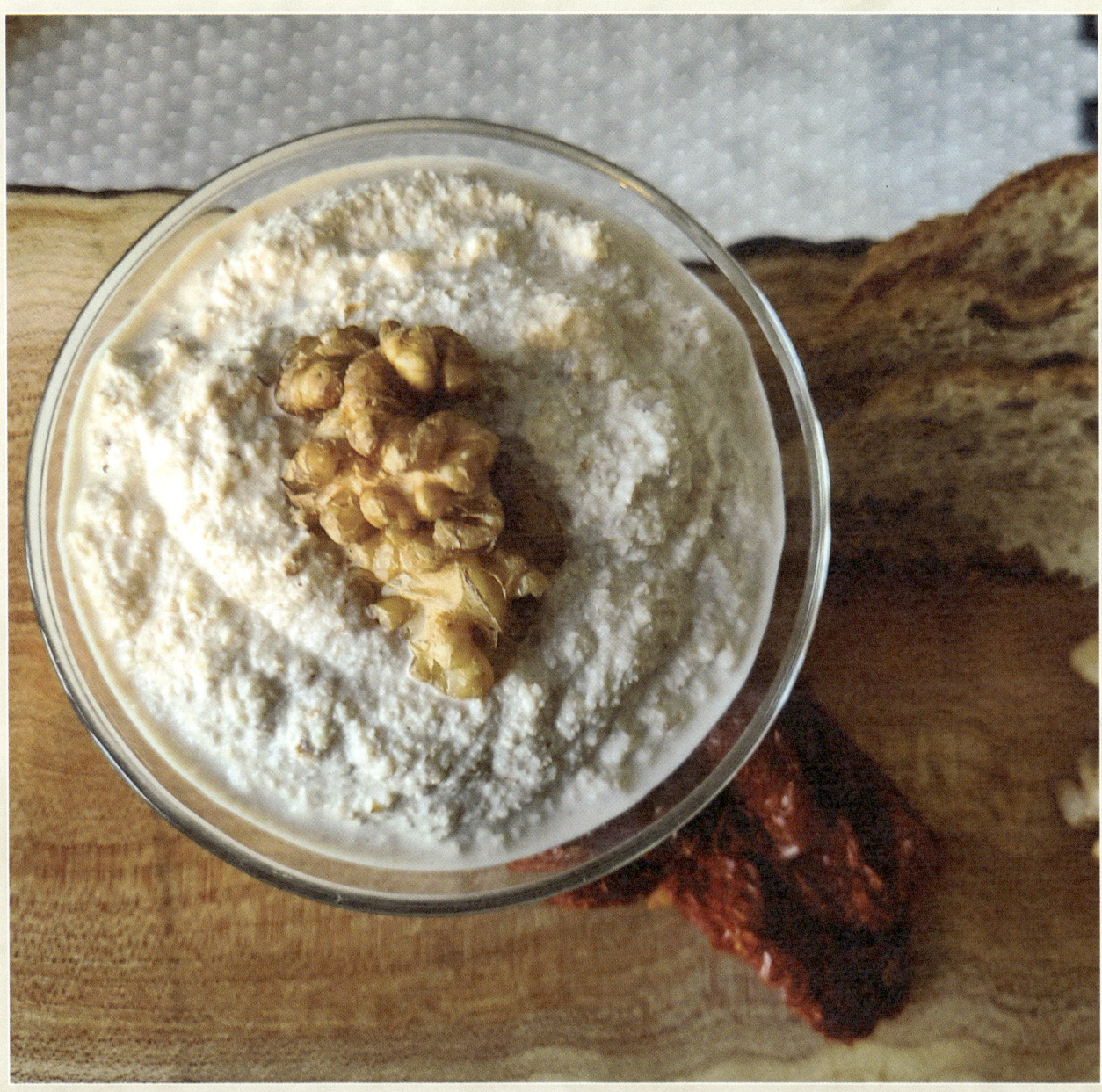

# Cashew, Sunflower Seed or Macadamia Cream Cheeze

**Tools and Equipment**

Jar or bowl for soaking
High-speed blender (or food processor and less fancy blender)
Spatula
Measuring spoons
Measuring cups
Bowl
Colander or fine mesh sieve
Cheesecloth or butter muslin
Container for storage

As suggested, you can use cashews, sunflower seeds, or macadamia nuts in this process. You may also elect to use a combination. I suggest ⅓ sunflower seeds to ⅔ cashew or macadamia nuts.

If you avoid adding cooked ingredients to this core recipe, it is suitable for raw food diets.

## Ingredients

2 cups cashews, sunflower seeds, or macadamia nuts
2 tsp salt (Use a good quality non-iodized salt. Kosher salt is non-iodized and does not contain anti-caking agents.)
2–3 Tbsp nutritional yeast (or 1 Tbsp miso)
1 Tbsp lemon juice (Fresh squeezed is best, but not necessary.)
2 tsp apple cider vinegar
1½ cups of water (Add more or use less depending on how much moisture the nuts and/or seeds absorbed during soaking.)

## Method

1. Rinse the nuts and or seeds under cold running water, or you may boil them for 5 minutes.
2. Soak the cashews, macadamia nuts, or the sunflower seeds in a clean, sanitized container with filtered water and a tiny pinch of salt (about 1 tsp for 1 gal, see Soaking Guidelines in this chapter). If you are using a combination of nuts and seeds, soak them separately and combine them only at time of blending.
3. After soaking, rinse under cold running water.
4. Blend until smooth, adding small amounts of filtered water a little at a time. Take time to interrupt the blending process. Use a spatula to clear the sides and then add water. Avoid turning the blender to the highest speed immediately (an instinct many have). It is best to start at lower speeds to allow the blender blades to catch the material and then gradually turn the speed up, combining this with spatula scraping and small additions of water. Blending at too high a speed can lead to poor emulsification of the ingredients and liquefaction. Blend until you reach the desired consistency. As you blend, check the seasoning to see if you need to adjust any of the elements, particularly the salty and acidic ones. If needed, add more salt, vinegar, or lemon juice.

Don't add too much water at once or you may end up with more of a sauce than a cheeze, though this may not be a terrible outcome.

5. Once you have reached the texture you desire, scrape the mixture out of the blender and place it inside a cheesecloth bag, (nut milk bags or synthetic porous produce bags are suitable alternatives). Hang the bag over a bowl and allow it to drain for up to 4 hours.
   a. Add any spices, herbs, dried fruit, olives, or other ingredient you want to the mixture before placing it into the cheesecloth.
   b. You may want to blend the mixture with ingredients like dried figs or apricots until smooth and then add chunks of these back in for texture.
6. After the cheeze has drained excess fluid, store it in a container as is, covered and refrigerated. If you wish to dress it up for presentation at a party or just for fun, you can place the cheeze mixture in a shaping mold or hand shape the mixture and then cover it in herbs, spices, dried fruit, or whatever pleases you.

## Flavoring Options

Herbs, spices, dried fruit, or peppers: If you add fresh herbs or garlic, the shelf life of the cheeze is reduced.

Fig, tarragon, and balsamic: Add ⅓ cup chopped figs, dried, and 1 Tbsp balsamic vinegar in place of the apple cider vinegar.

Roasted garlic, cracked pepper, and rosemary: Add ½ bulb of roasted garlic, ½ Tbsp coarse cracked black pepper, and as much chopped fresh rosemary as you like.

Dill, mint, and lemon: Add 4 Tbsp chopped fresh dill, 2 Tbsp chopped fresh mint, and zest of 1 lemon.

## Adjusting the recipe

This is a great base recipe to try with your own flavor combinations. When amending this recipe, you may want to consider using a white bean such as lima to add a thicker, creamier texture.

When using sunflower seeds in this recipe, if you do not wish to toast them, I recommend using them (as suggested in the main recipe) in combination with another nut, one with more carbohydrate or fat. Sunflower seeds, when raw, can become bitter after a few days. This can be minimized by soaking them for the maximum amount of time recommended in the Soaking Guidelines in this chapter.

## Storage

Storage time for this cheeze is up to 10 days, properly covered or wrapped, if you use dried herbs and spices, and up to 5 days if you use fresh herbs and spices. Even in the absence of a culture, the cashew may want to ferment on its own; don't be alarmed. If you find your batch getting a bit sharp tasting, it may be that the cashew paste has begun fermenting. So long as you have kept the container clean, not used your fingers to taste, or cross-contaminated the mixture in some way, you can continue to use the cheeze if you like the evolving flavor profile.

### Ways to use this cheeze

Sandwiches and toast

In raw lasagne

In baked vegan lasagne

In ravioli or any pasta dish

Scooped into small balls and used in vegan caprese salads, or salads in general

On flatbreads

In cheesecakes or dessert tarts if sweetness is added

## Non-cultured Semi-firm or Set Cheezes

It is possible in the non-cultured cheeze realm to make replacements for cheeses such as mozzarella, feta, cheddar (especially for grilled cheese type functionality) that take less time than their fermented counterparts. Added starches and gelling agents, or emulsifiers, are key ingredients for these types of cheeze, and it is useful to learn some tips for working with them. Tofu is also a useful ingredient in these types of recipes and is especially popular as a replacement for feta, but note that it can be blended with other ingredients and can provide a protein rich addition to a mixture that contains coconut milk and cashews, for instance.

In these methods that do not rely on culturing and aging time to remove moisture, starches and gelling agents create firmness by trapping moisture inside a matrix of other molecules (ingredients). Firmness achieved through moisture evaporation (aging) results in a very different texture as well as a greater depth of flavor.

Starches in these recipes are used for a couple of reasons: one, they absorb moisture, which means the mixture you make will set up more firmly, and two, some of them can provide some degree of stretchiness or pull, often considered a desirable trait for cheezes used on foods like pizza or in grilled cheese sandwiches. Tapioca starch or modified tapioca starch offer the greatest amount of stretch or pull, but potato starch and arrowroot starch may also be used, more for the density they give a cheeze than for stretchiness or give.

Emulsifiers are ingredients that help bind ingredients that might otherwise not combine well. Soy or sunflower lecithin is commonly used in raw vegan food applications to help stabilize and give hold to a recipe. Emulsifiers can also, in conjunction with other ingredients, provide a sense of stretchiness similar to what starches do. This depends on which emulsifier you use. They do not all behave the same way. Gelling agents behave somewhat like emulsifiers, pulling all the other ingredients into a matrix, but while they generally set firmer, they do not force molecules to bind with one another in the same way an emulsifier does, and they do require heating to become active. The most common gelling agents used in vegan cheezemaking, especially home based, are agar agar, kappa carrageenan, and pectin. All three offer very different characteristics when set, and all three respond differently to any acid used such as lemon juice, citric acid, or vinegars.

## *Starches*

Starches are polymeric carbohydrates, meaning that they are large molecules composed of many smaller units, and they represent the most common carbohydrate in the human diet. Potato, rice, corn/maize, cassava, taro, all root vegetables contain this ubiquitous energy. In vegan cheesemaking, especially in non-cultured cheezes, starch plays an important role in many commercial brands as well as in many DIY recipes. Not all starches behave the same way, and you cannot always substitute one starch for another at a 1:1 ratio, or, sometimes even at all.

In DIY recipes, tapioca starch is the most commonly used, but arrowroot, rice flour, and potato starch can also be used, although each will yield a different outcome. Tapioca starch is derived from the cassava root, a tropical root originating in Brazil and now grown in a number of tropical nations. It is a common thickening agent in many types of recipes and in sauces provides a clingy texture when used in small amounts and a stretchier consistency when used in more significant amounts. It is this latter characteristic that has made tapioca popular for cheeze recipes. Readily available, tapioca starch can be found in nearly any grocery store.

Modified tapioca starch is more common in commercial applications. It can also be used by the home user but is more difficult to find. Modified tapioca starch (as with all modified starches) has been treated in some manner (physically, enzymatically, or chemically) to change its properties in some particular way in order to enhance or amplify certain aspects of its behavior in recipes. How the modified starch behaves depends on what treatment it received. Modified tapioca starch product Expandex, for instance, is used in baking recipes to help with lift or expansion. Modified starches such as this typically need to be ordered from an online source.

In my first edition of this book, I mentioned that tapioca starch could not be replaced with another starch in a recipe, but this is not completely accurate. Arrowroot starch behaves similarly to tapioca and can be used as a replacement at a 1:1 ratio. Arrowroot does provide less stretchiness than tapioca, but for recipes that are not designed to amplify that characteristic, arrowroot does a capable job of absorbing moisture and providing textural stability to semi-firm vegan cheeze.

Potato starch and rice flour or rice starch cannot replace tapioca starch in a recipe, but you can use them in recipes for diffcrent purposes. Be mindful, however, that potato starch can be quite gummy and set heavy. I recommend potato starch for use in cheesy sauces or combined with tapioca, arrowroot, or rice flour.

**Adding Starches to Cheeze Recipes**

There are a few ways to add starches to your cheeze recipes.

1. Add the measured amount of tapioca (or other starch) directly to the recipe mixture at the time of blending. This will ensure full inclusion but will not

eliminate the need to whisk continuously once the mixture is on heat. As you heat the mixture up, it will tend to thicken very quickly, so keep the heat low to start and whisk continuously to ensure even absorption of moisture before gradually increasing heat.

2. Make a slurry. A slurry is a mixture of starch and water and is a very helpful way of including starches in soups, stews, and other cooked or heated recipes that you want to thicken. A slurry will work well for recipes you heat up, and mixing the starch with water first helps the starch combine with the rest of the mixture with greater ease. You will need to reduce the mixture a little longer to ensure evaporation of excess moisture, but keeping the heat low to low-medium and monitoring while whisking occasionally will ensure success. Use ⅓ cup water, preferably warm–hot, to 1 Tbsp starch, whisk together well, and then add to the gently warming mixture. As you pour the slurry into the mixture, whisk frequently but not too vigorously. The amount of slurry you make will depend on the amount of starch you need to add to your recipe. These two approaches work best for adding any starch to a vegan cheeze recipe.

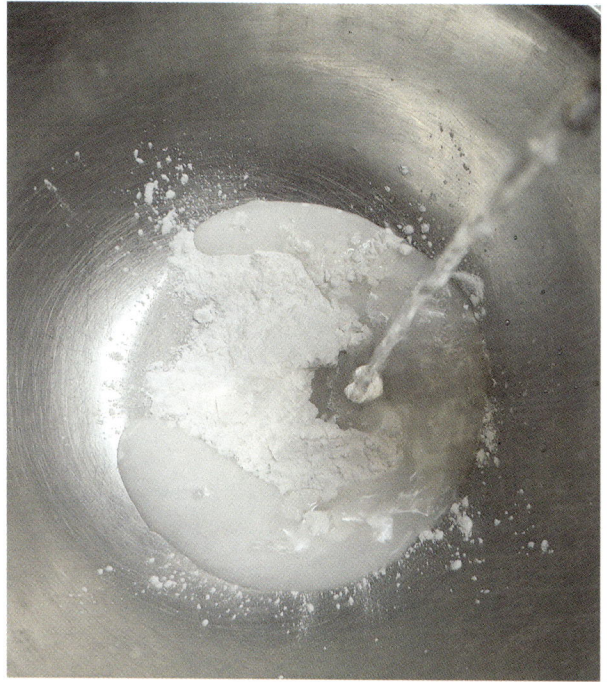

*Tapioca starch slurry.*

## Gelling agents

The most commonly used gelling agents are agar agar, kappa carrageenan, and pectin.

### Understanding agar agar

Agar agar is an agarose agaropectin (hence its common name is agar agar) compound derived from a particular kind of red seaweed. Agarose is a long chain carbohydrate (polysaccharide), and agaropectin forms the cell walls of the seaweed from which it is derived. Agar agar is a popular ingredient in many Asian desserts and in Japan is referred to as Kanten. It is also used in microbiological settings for growing cultures

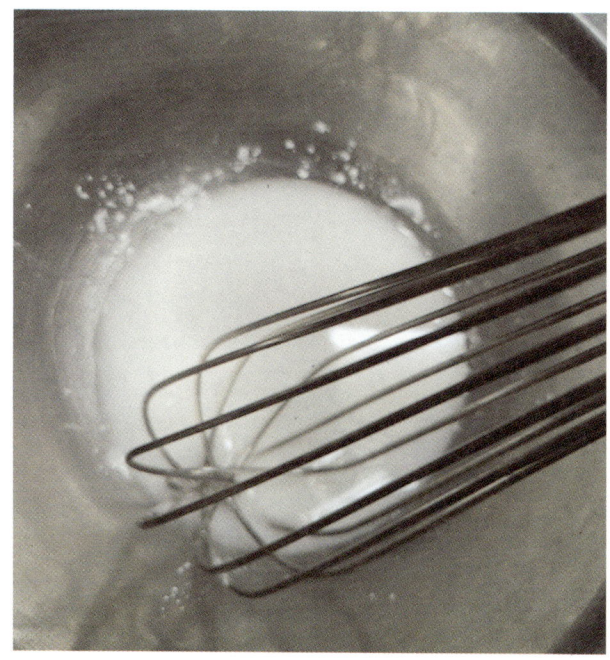

*Whisking the slurry to prevent lumps forming.*

because it is nutrient dense and forms a gel which does not liquefy under low to moderate temperatures. Additionally, it finds use as a clarifying agent in brewing processes. It is a high fiber ingredient and is considered to be helpful in digestion and may also act as (fun fact) a mild laxative. In commercial food, it is a highly effective binder or gelling agent, often replacing gelatin in vegan and plant-based recipes, and can also be used in place of pectin in making jams, jellies, and other preserves, particularly if you want a slightly firmer set. Agar agar comes in several forms, most commonly found are flake or powder. I recommend using the powder rather than the flake because it combines better with other ingredients and forms a better setting vegan cheeze. If you have not used agar agar before, I recommend playing with it first, just to get comfortable with the material. Agar agar needs to be activated in order to work. It becomes activated at 185°F (85°C), and you must keep it at that temperature for at least 5 minutes for it to be truly effective. It solidifies or gels at (89.6°F–104° F (32°C–40°C). At lower temperatures there will still be some flexibility and softness to the set, while at higher temperatures it will tend to set very firm. Once gelled it can be reheated and cooled multiple times without degrading. This applies primarily to agar agar/water solutions, not to complete recipes that it is used in, though some of them may be reheated more than once.

In high acid recipes, agar agar does not set well, so in desserts that use a large amount of acidic fruit, you will need to add more agar agar if you are seeking a very firm set. If you are looking for a soft set with good cling/viscosity, then agar agar will serve this purpose well.

**Preparing agar agar**

1. Place 1 cup of water in a saucepan, add 2 tsp of agar agar powder, and bring to a boil. Agar agar, as mentioned earlier, requires exposure to heat (up to 185°F/85°C) for a minimum of 5 minutes, before it will bloom, or become activated.

2. You will need to stir or whisk it as it comes to a boil, and this is a great opportunity to observe it as it changes. The mixture will start to become slightly more opaque and will start to cling to the whisk. You will notice that any mixture that ends up on the sides of the pan will start to set. Slide this off the side and back into the wet mixture. When working with such a small amount, stop after 5 to 10 minutes or you will lose too much moisture to evaporation.

3. To test how firmly the agar agar will set, use a trick from jelly and jam making, the cold plate test. Put a plate in the freezer or refrigerator for 30 minutes, and allow it to become quite cold. After you have heated the agar

agar and maintained it at the right temperature for the right amount of time, take a spoonful and drop it onto the cold plate. It should cling to the plate almost immediately rather than running like a loose fluid. This tells you that as it cools it will become firm or set.

**Adding agar agar to cheeze recipes**

1. As mixture: Add the measured amount of agar agar to ½–⅔ cup water. Bring the solution to a boil while stirring, and allow it to cook for 5 minutes at a sustained temperature of 185°F (85°C). Pour the solution into the heated cheeze mixture and stir frequently. Continue heating the cheeze mixture and stirring for several minutes to ensure that the agar agar solution is fully integrated into the cheeze mixture. If it is clumping or feels too thick, add small amounts of filtered water to loosen the mixture. On occasion, I have blended the mixture after heating to achieve a completely smooth texture. This is my preferred method for adding agar agar.
2. Directly: You can add powdered agar agar directly to the recipe mixture before heating up the mixture. As with the tapioca starch addition, you will need to stir frequently and monitor the temperature. Use a thermometer and do not raise the heat too quickly. With this method you can end up with clumps of agar agar forming on the bottom of the pot if it is not well whisked into the rest of the mixture. The caution with this approach is that the mixture will begin to thicken too quickly before other ingredients have had an opportunity to fully integrate (e.g., nutritional yeast, if it is being used, needs some time to break down). Continuous whisking and gradual increase of heat are recommended. This approach can work very well for non-cultured mozza-style recipes.

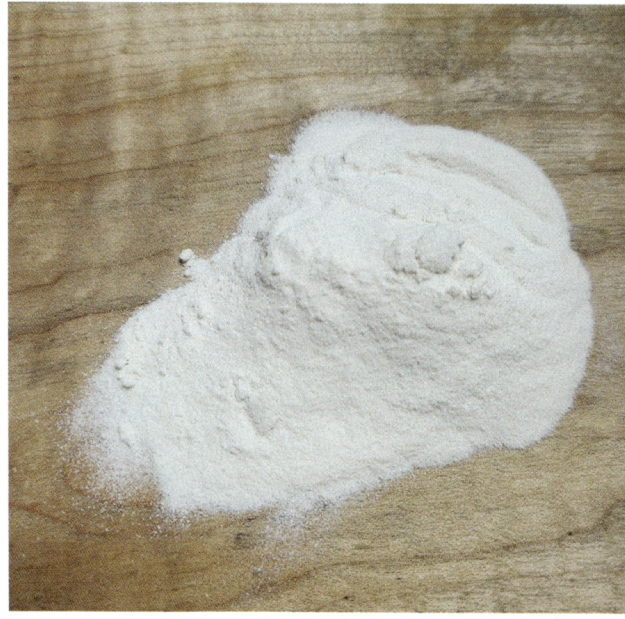

*Agar agar powder.*

## Understanding carrageenan

Like agar agar, carrageenan is derived from algae/red seaweed, albeit from a different species of seaweed. It is also a long chain carbohydrate (polysaccharide). Carrageenan is sometimes referred to as Irish Moss, as the variety of seaweed from which it comes is common on the coasts of Ireland and it has been used frequently in some parts of Scotland and Ireland in the making of a panna cotta-style dessert.

Carrageenan is a very popular additive in commercial food processes, especially in dairy food processes such as ice cream manufacturing (carrageenan reacts with dairy proteins and calcium and potassium ions in gel formation). It is generally used as a thickener, or gelling agent. Carrageenan has three primary forms, kappa, iota, and lambda, and each has different applications. For the purposes of quick firm vegan cheezemaking, kappa carrageenan is the preferred form and is the focus of this section. Kappa carrageenan forms strong, rigid gels and is sourced mainly from *Kappaphycus alvarezii* seaweed. It is generally sold in a powdered form.

**Adding Kappa carrageenan to recipes**

1. For use in quick firm vegan cheeze, kappa carrageenan can be added directly to the recipe mixture without heat activation. So, for recipes that are simple, without many ingredients, I recommend adding the carrageenan at the time of blending.
2. For recipes that have many ingredients, or ingredients such as nutritional yeast that require some breaking down time, I recommend heating up the ingredients first and adding the carrageenan during the cooling phase.

Your best results will come from experimenting with the kappa carrageenan and finding your preferences.

**Controversy and carrageenan**

I should note that there are some concerns about the prevalence of carrageenan in processed foods. There are some concerns that carrageenan may cause intestinal bloating and digestive difficulties for people. As for concerns about carrageenan as a potential carcinogen, this applies primarily to poligeenan, a degraded form of carrageenan. However, some concern exists about the prospect of carrageenan degrading once it makes contact with stomach acid in the human stomach. While this latter concern requires more evidence, I leave it to each user of this book to decide if carrageenan is something they wish to use.

## Understanding pectin

Another gelling agent that can be used in some semi-firm vegan cheeze recipes is pectin. Pectin is a structural heteropolysaccharide (that is, it is composed of more than one type of saccharide). Found in the cell walls of terrestrial plants, unlike agar agar and carrageenan, which are found in algae and seaweeds, pectin is most recognizably used in the making of jams, jellies, and in fruit related food processes. Commercially, the majority of pectin produced is made from apples and is combined with citric acid and dextrose as binders.

It has a shorter shelf life than agar agar and carrageenan, as its efficacy lessens over time with degradation of the pectin. It is best used in quick vegan cheeze recipes where you want more set than a spreadable cream cheeze has. For example, it can be used with an additional starch to make mozza-style cheeze.

Pectin added in too large an amount will not combine well with other ingredients and can result in a gummy texture or a granular texture.

I recommend experimenting with pectin and carrageenan in small batches or combining them with agar agar, as too much agar agar in a recipe can result in a rubbery texture. All three of these gelling agents are polysaccharides (carbohydrates), not proteins, so their use in quick vegan cheezemaking is very much the opposite idea of what occurs in cultured vegan cheese, which relies on the denaturing and coagulation of protein. All three will trap moisture in a matrix, and it will be important to add an acidic component to your vegan cheeze recipe to ensure some level of shelf life stability when using cheeze versus cheese recipes.

The recipes presented in this section provide a basis you can build on and expand through your own experiments.

---

3   Schulte, Erica M. et al. "Which foods may be addictive? The roles of processing, fat content, and glycemic load." PLOS ONE 10(2): e0117959. 18 February, 2015. doi:10.1371/journal.pone.0117959.

# Havarti/Gouda-style Quick Vegan Cheeze

Identifying this as a havarti- or gouda-style cheese is a very loose identification and really serves more as a broad reference. In general, though, havarti and gouda are mellow tasting cheeses with a soft, or grounded, acidity and a creamy but dense mouthfeel (I have had to ask many of my friends who still consume dairy or who have more recent memory of dairy cheese than me for help with this description). As such, I have chosen materials that provide more creaminess, muted sweetness, and mild acidity. Without the use of fermentation by microbes, flavor is built in quick vegan cheeze recipes through putting together ingredients that, when combined in favorable ratios, imply something familiar.

Like the other recipes in this quick cheeze section, the base recipes are intentionally plain, or non-flavored, so that you can focus on getting comfortable with blending and understanding the core ingredients on their own. Flavor-seasoning profiles are included at the end of the base method.

Note: Never add all the salt in a recipe at one time. You can always add more, but it is harder to balance if you have added too much. Likewise with moisture/water, always add in small amounts at a time during blending. You can always add more if you feel it is required.

## Tools and Equipment

High-speed blender (or food processor and less fancy blender)

Measuring spoons

Measuring cups

Spatula

Whisk or wooden or silicone spoon

Thick cast saucepan

Probe thermometer

Cheesecloth (not parchment or wax paper)

Mold (6–8-inch springform pan or loaf pan). Silicone molds can be used, but do not leave the cheeze in them for too long after it has set.

Bamboo mat or wooden board

## Ingredients

2 cups cashews (or 1 cup cashew/1 cup almond, or 2 cups almond, or 1 cup cashew/1 cup macadamia, or 1 cup cashew/1½ cups rolled oats)

2½ tsp salt

¼ cup apple cider vinegar

¼ cup nutritional yeast

1 cup coconut milk

1½ cups water (or coconut milk or another plant milk)

¼ cup softened coconut oil, or cacao butter

6 Tbsp tapioca starch

½ Tbsp agar agar powder (or 1 tsp kappa carrageenan)

## Method

Note: Using Agar Agar and Kappa Carrageenan.

This recipe can use either agar agar or kappa carrageenan as the gelling agent, but there are differences in how each of these agents behave, and the resulting cheese will differ based on which one you use.

Both agar agar and kappa carrageenan are derived from red seaweeds (rhodophyta) and are both thermoreversible (you can reheat them after they have set), but they express

## Making Quick Non-Cultured Cheeze

different characteristics as gelling agents. Agar agar tends to set very firm, and if you use too much of it, it will offer a rubbery, grainy texture that is not very pleasant. Agar agar activates at 185°F (85°C), so you must either disperse it in water, heat it, and then add it to your recipe or, as in this recipe, add it during the blending together of other ingredients. Agar Agar is sensitive to high acid, so if you are adding acid to your cheese such as apple cider vinegar or lemon juice, keep in mind the acid may weaken the agar agar and inhibit setting.

Kappa carrageenan tends to have better meltability than agar agar. It can tolerate pH from 4–10, so it is more stable when exposed to acids than agar agar is. Its gelling activity is promoted by the presence of potassium (which is found in high amounts in things like cashews and most plant materials), milk protein (which is why carrageenan is often found in dairy ice cream and yogurt), and calcium.

If you choose to use kappa carrageenan instead of agar agar in this recipe, you will need to disperse it in about ¼ cup of cool water, and then add it to the other ingredients during blending. Like agar agar, it is activated over heat, though its heat activation begins at 140°F (60°C).

1. Before beginning any recipe, ensure that you have all of the equipment and ingredients that you need. Wash and sanitize your preparation and storage area as well as the equipment you will use. Follow the steps for sanitizing in chapter 2.
2. Decide which substitutions you are going to make. If you decide to use oats in your version of this recipe, I suggest using hot water during the blending process because it will prevent the mixture from binding around the blades. Boil the hot water in advance and have it ready. Likewise, prepare your choice of coconut oil or cacao butter by softening it over heat in advance.
3. In a blender, add approximately half of the liquid ingredients except the softened oil. Add the nuts and dry ingredients, including the tapioca starch and agar agar. Begin blending on the lowest setting. If you have a blender with preset speeds for particular functions, start with the ice crush setting. Pulse a few times to allow the larger material to start breaking down into smaller pieces. This will aid emulsification of both the dry and wet ingredients.
4. Gradually increase the speed, or change the preset function to either smoothie or ice cream. As the speed increases, focus on observing the smoothness of the mixture. Add more fluid as you need.
5. Add the softened oil and reduce the speed of blending to allow the oil to bind with the mixture. Emulsification works best at low speed and when ingredients are at a similar temperature, so ignore your desire to get the blending over with, and pay attention to how the oil is combining. If it is too cold, it will clump in the warmer, already blended mixture.

6. Taste your mixture. If you want to adjust salt or acidity, now is the time to do it. Once you have adjusted the base seasoning, use a spatula to scrape the mixture from the pitcher, and place it in a thick cast saucepan. At this stage you may also fold in any dried herb or spice you wish to incorporate. If you wish to add solids (e.g., chopped dried fruit), wait until the mixture has finished heating up and is in the cooling process (at step 9).

7. Heat the mixture in the pot gradually. This allows all of the components to get heated evenly. Because you have starch and agar agar in this mixture, you will need to whisk or stir regularly to avoid clumping. As the mixture begins to heat, it will loosen and appear quite fluid at first. Be patient and keep whisking or stirring, and observing changes as it begins to thicken.

8. Gradually increase the heat to medium, and check the temperature of your mixture with a probe thermometer. If you do not have a thermometer, be sure to observe the mixture for the formation of bubbles. Remember, the agar agar needs to be heated to 185°F (85°C) and maintained at that heat for 5 minutes to become fully active. Because the agar agar is now within the mixture, the entire mixture needs to heat up evenly to ensure that the agar agar is properly activated. As it thickens, you should observe residue on the sides of the pot beginning to hold shape, which tells you that the mixture will set. The longer you heat it over low-medium to medium heat, the more moisture will evaporate from the mixture and the firmer the mixture will set.

9. Once the mixture is heated and you are confident it will set well, remove the pot from the heat. Use the spatula to scrape the mixture into a mold to hold the mixture in shape as it sets. If you use a silicone mold, you don't need to line it with cheesecloth. If you use a ring mold or springform pan, line it with cheesecloth (doubled up to ensure the weave is tight). If you use an open-ended ring mold, make sure you have the mold and cheesecloth set on a wooden board or other smooth firm surface that can be moved with the cheeze on top.

10. Allow the cheeze in the mold to rest at room temperature until it is noticeably beginning to set. If you refrigerate it too soon, the surface will cool too quickly, and heat retained within will cause cracking of the surface. Cooling at room temperature should be between 1 and 4 hours. Refrigerate the cheeze in the mold overnight, and check it the next day. If it is quite firm to touch, gently remove it from the mold and place on a wooden board or bamboo mat, top side down to allow the sides and bottom to begin to air dry, which helps remove excess moisture from the cooling process.

## Flavoring Options

When adding dry spices or herbs, dried fruit, or pepper flakes, it is better to fold them in after blending and the draining/moisture removal step.

# Making Quick Non-Cultured Cheeze

Dried fig and sundried tomato (softened in hot water and drained) can be added at the time of blending to integrate color and fruitiness.

Try your hand at one of the following suggestions or develop your own!

Spicy hot pepper: Add ¼ cup very finely sliced pickled hot peppers or dried hot pepper flakes. My preference is pickled: one, for flavor, and two, because they are less likely to impart foodborne pathogens. I also like to add 1 tsp powdered turmeric to change the color of the cheeze. If you use pickled hot peppers, add them after the mixture has cooked, folding them into the mixture before you place it in the molds to set. You can also use some of the pickle fluid in the base mixture during blending. If you add dried hot pepper flakes, add them to the mixture during the heating up and cooking process.

Smoked: One of the most popular flavor profiles, there are a number of ways to bring a smoky flavor into your cheeze.

a. Liquid smoke or smoked olive oil: Add ½ tsp of either directly to the mixture during blending. You can adjust according to your preference.
b. Smoked paprika: Add 1–2 tsp at the time of blending.
c. Cold smoking: If you have a smoking gun, you can smoke the mixture after you blend it, or after it has been removed from heat, or even after it has set.

You will need a container that you do not want to use for other purposes. Place your cheeze mixture or set cheeze inside the container, place the nozzle of the smoking gun hose inside the container, and cover the top of the container completely to ensure that the smoke does not escape. You can purchase containers for smoking, or you can use wax food wraps or plastic wrap to cover the surface. Smoking guns usually come with wood chips such as hickory, apple, mesquite, but you can also purchase wood chips for smoking from gourmet food shops. Cold smoking can take some practice to determine what strength of smoky flavor you want.

Apricot or cranberry: Add ½ cup chopped dried apricot or dried cranberry, ⅛ cup dried or preserved lemon zest, ½ cup white wine such as a Riesling or Viognier (which can replace some of the liquid component during blending). Add these elements when you add the cheeze mixture to the pot.

For additional flavor interest add an herbal component such as rosemary, thyme, sage, or marjoram.

## Storage

Store the cheeze on a bamboo mat or small wooden cheeseboard inside a closed container and in the refrigerator. The bamboo mat or cheeseboard will absorb extra moisture from the cheeze. Check the board or mat daily. This cheeze, stored properly and without cross-contamination from utensils and fingers, should keep well for up to 2 weeks.

> **Ways to use this cheeze**
> Sandwiches, burgers, pizza, flatbread, (raw or cooked)
> Torn into chunks in salads, but really, as you wish

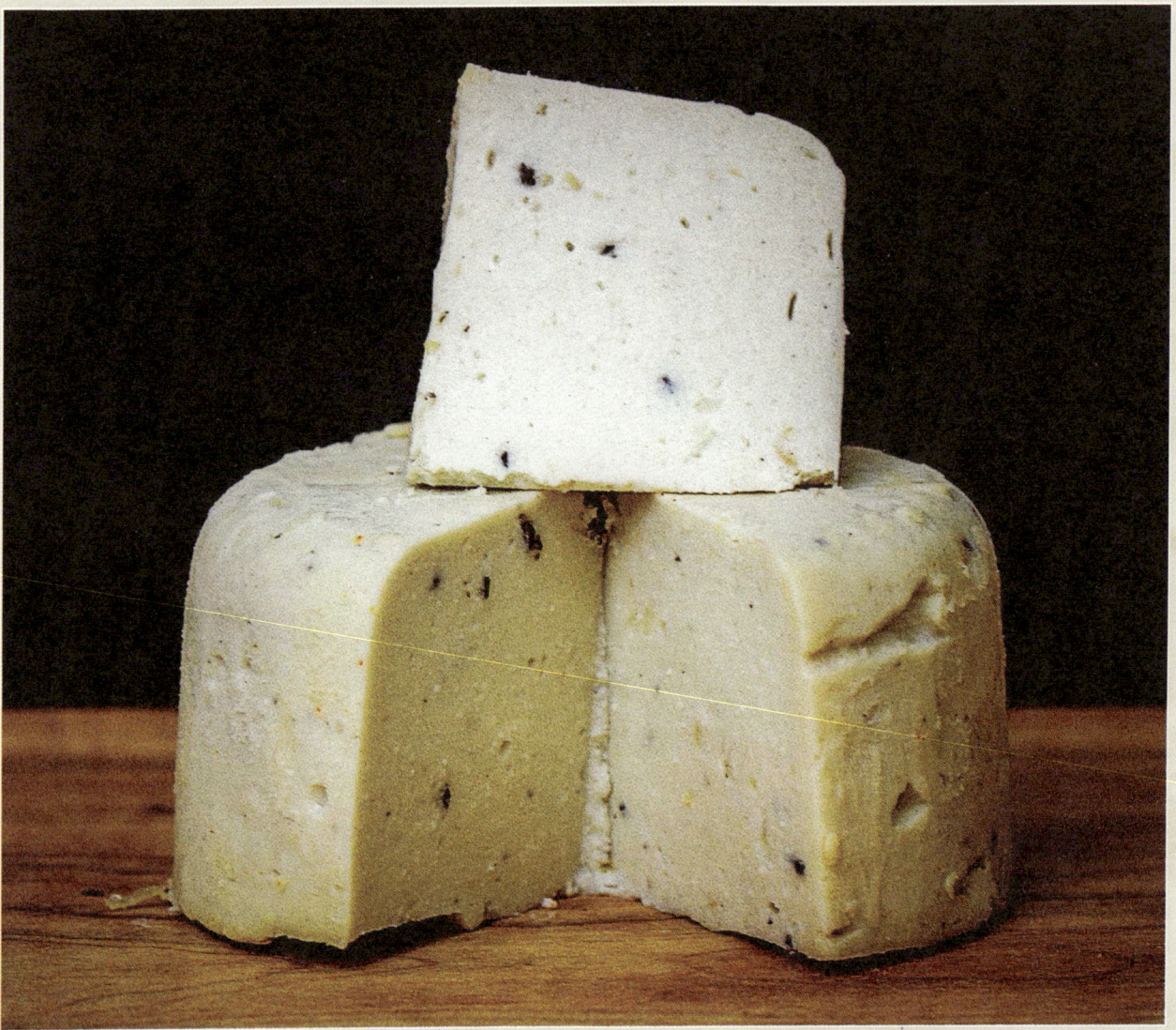

*The havarti/gouda-style quick cheeze can take on different flavor profiles. This one was infused with black truffle oil and shaved black truffle.* CREDIT: COLIN MEDHURST

Making Quick Non-Cultured Cheeze    51

# Semi-Firm Cheddar-Style Cheeze Base

This base is designed to allow you to create a semi-firm cheddar-style cheeze. This base includes more umami elements than the havarti/gouda-style base and you can amend it to add flavors. When adding flavor to cheeze that you wish to keep for more than 5 days, be sure to add only dried and dehydrated or otherwise preserved ingredients. Fresh herbs and garlic, for instance, can pose potential food safety risks by trapping pathogens inside a damp, fatty mixture.

## Tools and Equipment

High-speed blender
Measuring cups
Measuring spoons
Spatula
Wooden or silicone spoon or whisk
Thick cast saucepan
Springform pan, silicone mold, ring mold, or cheese mold
Probe thermometer
Cheesecloth
Bamboo mat or wooden board

## Ingredients

1 cup cashews
2 cups almonds (or substitute 1 cup macadamia nuts and 1 cup hazelnuts, toasted, with skins removed)
2½ tsp salt
⅓ cup apple cider vinegar (may also substitute a dry white wine or a white balsamic vinegar)
2 Tbsp miso*
¼ cup nutritional yeast
1 cup coconut milk
1⅔ cups water (filtered or rested tap water)
⅓ cup coconut oil, softened (or cacao butter or a blend of cacao and coconut oil)
3 Tbsp tapioca starch
1½ Tbsp agar agar (powdered, not flaked)

\* There are different types of miso such as red, white, brown, chickpea, and barley (which is quite dark in color and a little malty in flavor). Experiment with the different types of miso to see which you prefer.

## Method

1. Before beginning any recipe, ensure that you have all of the equipment and ingredients that you need. Wash and sanitize your preparation and storage area as well as the equipment you will use. Follow the guidelines for this in the section on sanitizing in chapter 2.
2. Decide which substitutions you are going to make. If you use oats in your version of this recipe, I suggest using hot water during the blending process because it will prevent the mixture from binding around the blades. Boil the hot water in advance and have it ready. Likewise, prepare your choice of coconut oil or cacao butter by softening them over heat in advance.

3. In a blender, add approximately half of the liquid ingredients except the softened oil. Add the nuts and dry ingredients, including the tapioca starch and agar agar. Begin blending on the lowest setting. If you have a blender with preset speeds for particular functions, start with the ice crush setting. Pulse a few times, to allow the larger material to start breaking down into smaller pieces. This will aid emulsification of both the dry and wet ingredients.

4. Gradually increase the speed, or change the preset function to either smoothie or ice cream. As the speed increases, focus on observing the smoothness of the mixture. Add more fluid as you need.

5. Add the softened oil and reduce the speed of blending to allow the oil to bind with the mixture. Emulsification works best at low speed and when ingredients are at a similar temperature, so ignore your desire to get the blending over with, and pay attention to how the oil is combining. If it is too cold, it will clump in the warmer, already blended mixture.

6. Taste your mixture. If you want to adjust salt or acidity, now is the time to do it. Once you have adjusted the base seasoning, use a spatula to scrape the mixture from the pitcher and place it in a thick cast saucepan. At this stage you may also fold in any dried herb or spice you wish to incorporate. If you wish to add solids (e.g., chopped dried fruit), wait until the mixture has finished heating up and is in the cooling process (at step 9).

7. Heat the mixture in the pot gradually. This allows all of the components to get heated evenly. Because you have starch and agar agar in this mixture, you will need to whisk or stir regularly to avoid clumping. As the mixture begins to heat, it will loosen and appear quite fluid at first. Be patient and keep whisking or stirring and observing changes as it begins to thicken.

8. Gradually increase the heat to medium, and check the temperature of your mixture with a probe thermometer. If you do not have a thermometer, be sure to observe the mixture for the formation of bubbles. Remember, the agar agar needs to be heated to 185°F (85°C) and maintained at that heat for 5 minutes to become fully active. Because the agar agar is now within the mixture, the entire mixture needs to heat up evenly to ensure that the agar agar is properly activated. As it thickens, you should observe residue on the sides of the pot beginning to hold shape, which tells you that the mixture will set. The longer you heat it over low-medium to medium heat, the more moisture will evaporate from the mixture and the firmer the mixture will set.

9. Once the mixture is heated and you are confident it will set well, remove the pot from the heat. Use the spatula to scrape the mixture into a mold to hold the mixture in shape as it sets.

If you use a silicone mold, you don't need to line it with cheesecloth. If you use a ring mold or springform pan, line it with cheesecloth (doubled up to ensure the weave is tight). If you use an open-ended ring mold, make sure you have the mold and cheesecloth set on a wooden board or other smooth firm surface that can be moved with the cheeze on top.

10. Allow the cheeze in the mold to rest at room temperature until it is noticeably beginning to set. If you refrigerate it too soon, the surface will cool too quickly, and heat retained within will cause cracking of the surface. Cooling at room temperature should be between 1 and 4 hours. Refrigerate the cheeze in the mold overnight, and check it the next day. If it is quite firm to touch, gently remove it from the mold and place on a wooden board or bamboo mat, top side down to allow the sides and bottom to air dry, which helps remove excess moisture from the cooling process.

## Flavoring Options

Smoky, cheddary cheeze: Add 1 tsp turmeric, 2 tsp smoked paprika, 2 tsp smoked salt (in place of the salt listed in main recipe), 1 tsp liquid smoke (optional depending on preference), 1 Tbsp extra nutritional yeast, 1 Tbsp extra apple cider vinegar. Add all of the elements at the blending stage. Taste after adding each ingredient to ensure that the mixture meets your flavor preference.

Roasted garlic peppercorn: Add ½ bulb of roasted garlic (make sure the garlic is fully roasted), peeled, and roughly chopped and 1 Tbsp coarse black peppercorns and 2 tsp pink peppercorns (or use your preferred mix of peppercorns). Substitute fermented black garlic if you want a deeper, more robust flavor. Black garlic is one of my favorite forms of garlic.

"Wenslydale": Add ⅓ cup chopped dried apricot, 1 Tbsp extra nutritional yeast, ¼ cup dry white wine. Reduce the amount of apple cider vinegar in the base recipe by half. Add the nutritional yeast and white wine during the blending process. Fold the chopped apricot into the mixture after it has been heated. Note that dried fruit has sugars, and sugars naturally want to ferment. Be sure to add the fruit at the lowest temperature possible. The fruit will also shorten the shelf life of the cheeze, but that is okay, you will probably eat it all before 2 weeks anyway!

Pseudo-blue: Blue cheeses are pungent, tangy, salty. Though this will not achieve the funkiness of a true blue as it is not cultured nor is it ripened with blue cheese mold, it is a fun cheeze just for appearances and the added nutritional benefit of blue-green algae. When you have made the base and are about to pour it into a form, add 1 Tbsp blue-green algae (I use E3Live) a little at a time, swirling it into the mix, but do not overstir or you will end up with the entire cheeze looking bluish rather than giving the impression of veins.

Sassy and spicy: Add 2 tsp chipotle or ancho powder or more if you use flakes, 1 tsp smoked paprika, and 1 tsp sriracha or other hot sauce during the blending process and if desired, slices of hot pickled pepper, which you add after blending spices into the cheeze mixture. This variation depends entirely on how spicy you like food. I like very spicy food, so I tend to veer toward the hotter end of the spectrum. Adding 2 tsp of dehydrated garlic powder grounds some of the spiciness. I also like to use brine from pickled hot peppers during blending to ensure spiciness and tanginess throughout this cheeze. If you do use pickled hot pepper brine, remove an equal amount of liquid in the base recipe so that you are not adding too much moisture.

## Storage

Keep the cheeze wrapped in cheesecloth for at least 3 days (change it once a day if particularly damp). Once the surface is dry to touch, not damp, wrap tightly in plastic wrap to keep air out. Now that the cheeze is fully cooled and most of the inherent moisture has evaporated, store the cheeze on a bamboo mat or small wooden cheeseboard placed inside a closed container. The bamboo mat or wooden board will absorb moisture, and this will help extend the shelf life of the cheeze. Turn the cheeze every day or every other day. You may also use waxed food wraps or plastic wrap (my least preferred option) for wrapping and storing the cheeze.

The cheeze is good for up to 2 weeks properly stored in the refrigerator.

# Mozzarella-Style Cheeze

Mozzarella is a mild flavored cheese, which, in traditional cheesemaking, is due to the short culturing time frame and thus, relatively low acidity. Mozzarella, like most short cultured, or fresh, cheeses, relies very much on the quality of the milk for its flavor. Balls of fresh mozzarella, rather than the shreds found in bags, tend to pool and settle when they melt, versus the dramatic stretchiness that is often associated with the shredded mozzarella.

Plant-based mozza alternatives usually focus on the so-called meltability or stretchiness of a mozzarella. Most of the commercially available plant-based mozza alternatives are attempting to replicate the shredded mozza often found in bags in grocery stores. This style of mozza (dairy or plant-based) does not reflect fresh mozzarella sold in soft balls either vacuum sealed or in brine.

The recipe below is intended to be made into balls of mozza or bocconcini (of whatever size you like).

## Tools and Equipment

Blender or mixing bowl
Heavy cast saucepan
Measuring cups
Measuring spoons
Metal whisk
Silicone or wooden spoon
Container for holding the setting fluid (Ensure this is large enough for the amount of cheeze you want to set, and keep in mind that as you add cheeze to the setting fluid, it will displace the fluid, causing the level to rise.)
Bamboo mat or wooden board

## Ingredients

2 cups coconut milk, high fat (or oat, almond, rice, or cashew milk)
1 cup coconut cream
½ cup tapioca starch (or modified tapioca starch or white rice flour)
1 Tbsp white balsamic vinegar (or apple cider vinegar)
2 tsp salt (adjust to your preference)
3 tsp–1 Tbsp agar agar powder

Optional: 1 Tbsp nutritional yeast or miso if you want a bit more umami
Setting brine: Place 5 cups water in a bowl, add ½ cup olive oil and 1 tsp salt and place in the freezer for 30 minutes or fridge for 1 hour. Keep in fridge until your cheese mixture is ready.

## Method

1. Combine coconut milk (or plant milk of choice), coconut cream, starch, agar agar, salt, and vinegar in a blender, and blend on low speed until well combined. You may also do this in a bowl with a whisk.
2. Place the mixture into the heavy cast pot on the stovetop. Turn the heat on low, and begin heating the mixture slowly. Whisk the mixture as it begins to heat to ensure that the starch and agar agar, which are dense, do not sink to the bottom of the pot.
3. Gradually increase the temperature to medium, and allow the mixture to come to a slow boil. As the mixture thickens, large bubbles should rise to the surface and pop.
4. Remember that agar agar needs to be heated to 185°F (85°C) and maintained at that temperature for at least 5 minutes to be fully activated. Do not rush this period.

Continue to whisk or stir, and pay attention to how the mixture feels while you are doing so. Is it thickening and offering more resistance? Is it still feeling very loose?

If it gets too thick too quickly, the agar agar may not activate fully, and this will result in a mozza that sets as gummy, rather than firm with a little bounce back. If it is feeling too thick too quickly, whisk in a little water or more plant milk.

If it is feeling too loose even after 15 minutes of heating, add a little more agar agar and or starch to absorb moisture. If you do so, pre-measure the dry material and mix with a small amount of moisture to make a slurry, and add the slurry into the hot mixture. This will ensure that it does not clump. Whisk vigorously after adding the slurry.

5. After the mixture has heated up for at least 15 minutes and has become thick enough to offer resistance while stirring:

   a. Use the spatula to scrape the mixture into a mold to hold the mixture in shape as it sets. If you use a silicone mold, you don't need to line it with cheesecloth. If you use a ring mold or springform pan, line it with cheesecloth (doubled up to ensure the weave is tight). If you use an open-ended ring mold, make sure you have the mold and cheesecloth set on a wooden board or other smooth firm surface that can be moved with the cheese on top. Allow the cheese to cool in the cheesecloth-lined molds in the refrigerator. Once the cheese has fully cooled, you will be able to handle it, and if you choose, you will be able to remove the cheese from the forms and hand mold it into balls. You can then store the balls in a seasoned or flavored brine in a sealed container.

   b. Allow the mixture to cool in the pot until very thick and easy to handle by hand. Use a scoop or measuring cup to measure out portions of the cheeze and drop each into the chilled water/oil/salt mixture that you had put in the fridge before starting the recipe. This will cause the cheeze to set relatively quickly in rounder shapes, which you can continue to gently mold into the classic mozzarella ball shape. Allow the balls to cool in the chilled water mixture for up to 20 minutes before removing.

   c. After the balls of cheeze have cooled (at least 20 minutes), remove them from the setting brine and lay them on a bamboo mat or cheesecloth and allow them to dry for up to 2 hours before you then store the balls of cheese in a seasoned brine, which can be a new batch of brine with your choice of herbs and spices added to it. You can refer to the section on brining in chapter 6 for guidance on how to make a light brine for storage.

## Ways to use this cheeze

In grilled cheese sandwiches, flatbreads, and other heat based recipes

Freeze until solid, and shred for use on pizza or nachos

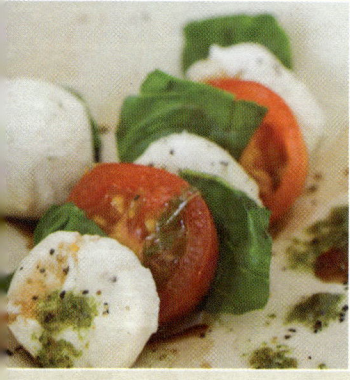

*Bocconcini caprese skewer. You can use the mozzarella recipe to form smaller balls.*
Credit: Colin Medhurst

## Storage

Stored in brine or olive oil, these will keep for up to 2 weeks. If you choose to store the cheeze in a container without brine, plan to use the cheeze within 7 days.

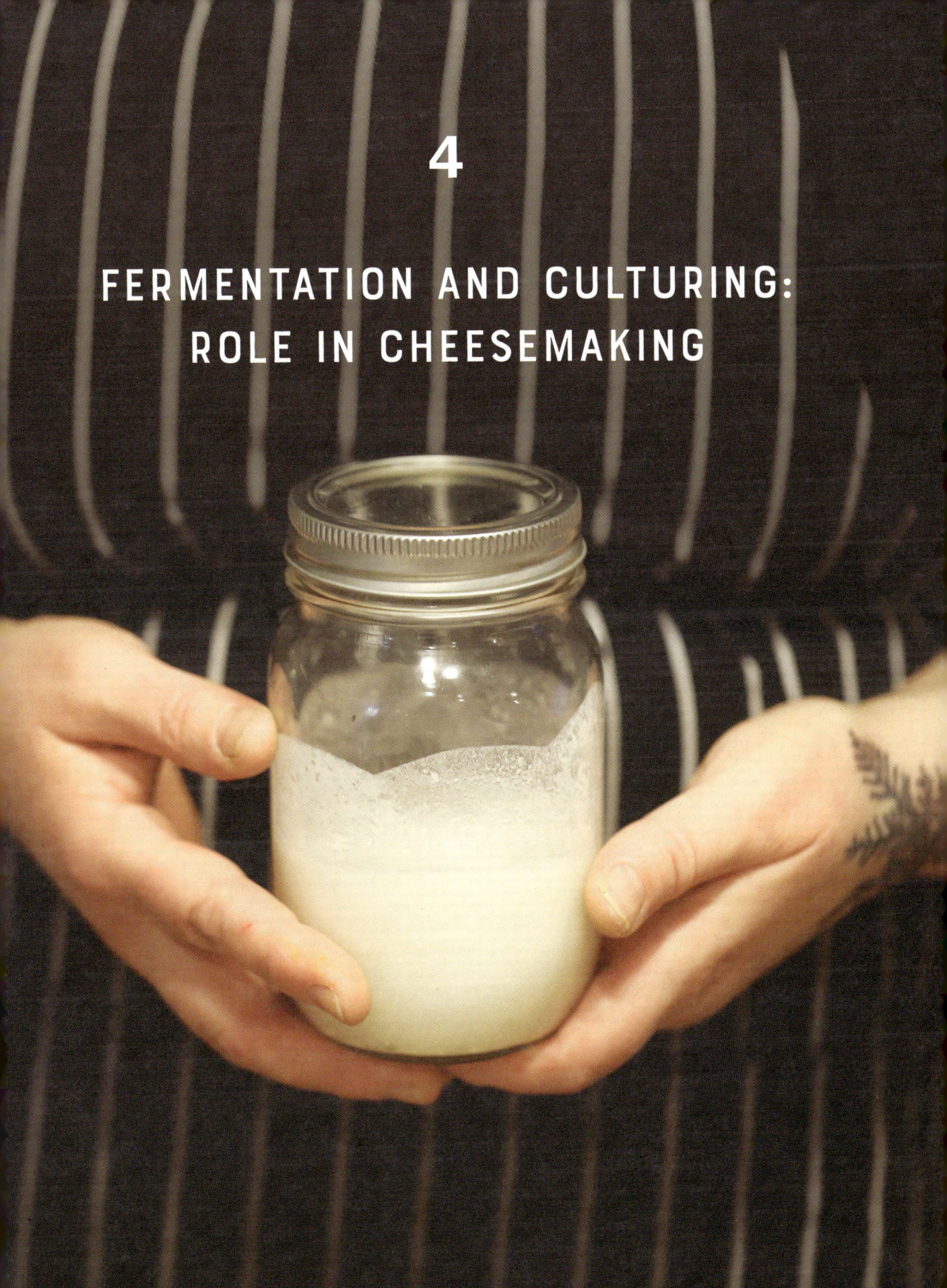

# 4

## FERMENTATION AND CULTURING: ROLE IN CHEESEMAKING

While I do discuss non-cultured cheeze in this book, my deepest appreciation and interest is in making cultured vegan cheese. I distinguish between the terms "cheeze" and "cheese" based on whether microbes are used in a process of fermentation. I spend my days exploring the ways microbes and fermentation can be utilized in the creation of unique, plant-based cheeses that are cheeses in their very own right. Once I began on my vegan cheesemaking path, I sought most of my information from traditional dairy cheesemaking methodologies, and even more so from the field of food science exploring the microbes responsible for so much variation of flavor and texture.

In traditional cheesemaking, different microbes (bacteria, yeast, and molds) are used at different stages of the cheesemaking process depending on what type of cheese the cheesemaker is making and what type of flavor, aroma, and texture they seek. The microbes used are often prepackaged in collections of cultures that work together to produce a particular set of outcomes.

Different types of lactic acid forming bacteria (LAB) are used in most styles of cheese to initiate acidification of the milk, which in turn results in the coagulation of the casein proteins (assisted by the use of rennet, a digestive enzyme typically obtained from calves or sometimes produced microbially). There are different types of bacteria that produce lactic acid, and some produce, in addition to lactic acid, other compounds that have identifiable aromas or produce other by-products that have an impact on how a cheese develops. Lactic acid forming bacteria are some of the most important microbes in use in commercial food production because many of them produce compounds that also protect against spoilage, molds, and yeasts.

Other microbes used in traditional cheesemaking include yeasts (used for many different reasons), molds like *P. roqueforti* and *P. candidum* (used in making blue and white mold ripened cheeses), and non-lactic acid forming bacteria such as *B. linens* (used as a wash on cheeses to create an orange rind and a funky smell, as in limburger).

At one time in the history of traditional cheesemaking, the microbes used were the result of accident, being naturally present on human skin, on the skin of the animals the milk came from, and in the environment in which the cheese was made. These days humans culture microbes for cheesemaking in labs. Microbes are prepared wet in a liquid solution and have a relatively short shelf life, or they are freeze-dried after being grown on nutrient plates. Freeze-drying results in microbes that are then vacuum sealed in foil packets and can be held (at correct temperatures) for much longer than the microbes in solution.

While microbes themselves are neither vegan nor non-vegan, the manner in which they are cultivated in the lab can determine whether they are suitable in making vegan cheese. Most of the microbes produced are fed on agar agar plates that also include animal product (offal from post slaughterhouse processes). Some are fed on plates that have tomato juice and yeast. Yet others are cultured on plates with dairy, and though only used as a nutrient source for the microbes, these packages of culture have to list dairy as a potential allergen.[4]

An issue of concern with the majority of pre-designed culture packages is that the feeding medium of the microbes is not listed on the package if there is no molecular presence remaining and if there is no presence of the top fourteen food allergens. When microbes metabolize they consume the feeding medium and convert that food into other by-products, which means that although many packaged cultures might be considered technically vegan (because there is no animal product inside), the production of the microbes will not meet ethical vegan requirements.

Indeed, Dupont, owner of Danisco, an established manufacturer of cheese cultures, has developed a culture line, identified as VEGE, set specifically for broad use in fermented vegan foods, but it is difficult to obtain, with few distributors carrying it in North America. It can be found in Europe, but shipping cultures can be tricky due to regulations. Later on, I discuss which commercial cultures are considered vegan friendly and their use, but I want to focus first on how to grow your own lactic acid forming cultures for use in vegan cheesemaking at home.

## Lactic Acid Fermentation

Lactic acid is the by-product of a carbohydrate metabolized by lactic acid forming bacteria, or LAB. Specific bacteria produce lactic acid after consuming carbohydrates. Some of these bacteria produce only lactic acid, which makes them homofermentative. Others produce lactic acid as well as other compounds such as $CO_2$, acetic acid, hydrogen peroxide, which makes them heterofermentative. Lactic acid fermentation is the process that uses LAB to make acid that then changes the material upon which it is acting and makes the environment generally hostile to pathogenic microbes.

Lactic acid fermentation is widely used in food processing. We enjoy the results of this process in cheese (dairy), sauerkraut, kimchi, beer, kombucha, sourdough bread, and sour pickles, for example. Lactic acid fermentation is commonly referred to as lacto-fermentation and has a very long history in human interaction with food. Although there are other forms of fermentation, I will not be discussing them in this book. So from here on when I refer to fermentation or culturing, I am referring to lactic acid fermentation.

Fermentation and culturing are related, and often the terms are used interchangeably by those experienced in these processes. However, there are some distinctions worth understanding.

Many of the foods we ferment in DIY home projects, or even in many commercial applications, rely on native or opportunistic bacteria, the bacteria that are already present on a foodstuff or in the environment. This is a form of "wild" fermentation. For a more comprehensive discussion of wild fermentation, Sandor Katz's *Wild Fermentation* and *The Art of Fermentation* are outstanding references. Certainly, there can be an element of wild fermentation in plant-based cheesemaking, and in fact one of the methods of growing a plant-based starter culture for your cultured cheese features a wild fermentation process: the making of rejuvelac.

Culturing relies on the use of bacteria and other microbes, often many of the same ones as in a wild fermentation process, but also sometimes employs technical species, that is, species of bacteria and other microbes that have been evolved in a lab space specifically for an industrial or commercial application. The formal distinction between fermentation and culturing is fluid and much more like a spectrum of activity, but the most significant distinction may be the degree of involvement required and the depth and specificity of knowledge of the microbes involved required for the cheesemaking process.

Certainly, wild fermentation involves the user as an active agent. Pascal Baudar, a wild food researcher and educator and author of *The New Wildcrafted Cuisine* and *The Wildcrafting Brewer*, provides an excellent example of this. However, often in wild processes there is a lack of knowledge regarding which specific bacteria or microbes are doing specific jobs, and the process relies on a degree of trust that all will work out well. Culturing is when we begin to refine or deepen this knowledge, adjusting variables like temperature and heat, identifying what species of microbes we are working with, learning what they do and what we do that allows them to perform optimally. The deep work of the folks at the Noma fermentation lab, led by David Zilber and René Redzepi, is an excellent example of this, and their book, *The Noma Guide to Fermentation*, is worth reading.

In both traditional cheesemaking and the processes I employ, acidification of the medium (milk in traditional cheesemaking, plant milk in mine) is achieved through applying a LAB culture. I outline two basic plant-based culture processes that you can do at home. These cultures are the by-products of fermentation processes on particular ingredients such as wheat berries in the production of rejuvelac and using water kefir grain to metabolize sugar and create a microbe rich solution.

## LAB Acidification

Acidification of the plant medium is crucial in culturing and fermentation. This action of the starter culture (microbes) on the medium is important for three reasons: one, it gives yogurt, kefir, and cheeses that familiar tangy taste; two, the lactic acid developed by the LAB creates a hostile environment for pathogens; three, the lactic acid also denatures, or breaks down, protein strands causing the medium to change from smooth and creamy to chunky and textured and to form a lactic acid curd. All three of these functions are essential to making a cultured vegan cheese.

Without the application of the starter culture, the medium will not be acidified and will be prone to contamination by the growth of unwelcome microbes. While the non-cultured cheezes discussed earlier in this book do employ acids like lemon juice, citric acid, and apple cider vinegar and that added acidity does add some protection as well as flavor enhancement, it is not the result of the metabolic process that LAB employ in the production of lactic acid. It is this process itself that is part of the transformative effect of lactic acid formation. The microbes digest material, and this act of digestion creates change. The lactic acid is formed from the very material that is to be converted to cheese rather than added in as an external ingredient.

In some cheeses, both dairy and plant-based, only a single culture is used in the process, while others may involve using other cultures at different stages such as washing a rind with a culture to create a surface-ripened cheese or adding a culture to the medium at a later stage to develop a different flavor or texture (these secondary cultures often feed off the by-products produced by the first cultures).

As this is an introductory book on the use of cultures, I do not delve too deeply into all of the ways in which cultures can be used, but I do discuss them as living organisms rather than as inactive ingredients. I also highlight the variables that have the greatest impact in growing your own starter cultures.

Since cultures are living organisms they must be grown and used with care; a reminder that sanitizing your equipment and tools is critical cannot be overemphasized. Make sure that all containers you will use in making rejuvelac or kefir are washed, sanitized, and air dried thoroughly.

## Rejuvelac

Rejuvelac is the microbe rich fluid produced by the sprouting and fermentation of grains such as wheat berries (soft), buckwheat groats, quinoa, rye, farro, spelt, millet, amaranth, and teff. Though mentioned earlier, it is worth saying again that making rejuvelac is an example of a wild fermentation process relying on opportunistic microbes present on the surface of the grains being used. The microbes present include a number of LAB as well as wild yeasts. The difference between rejuvelac and a lab grown culture is that we do not know what species of microbes are present without lab testing.

## Process for Making Rejuvelac

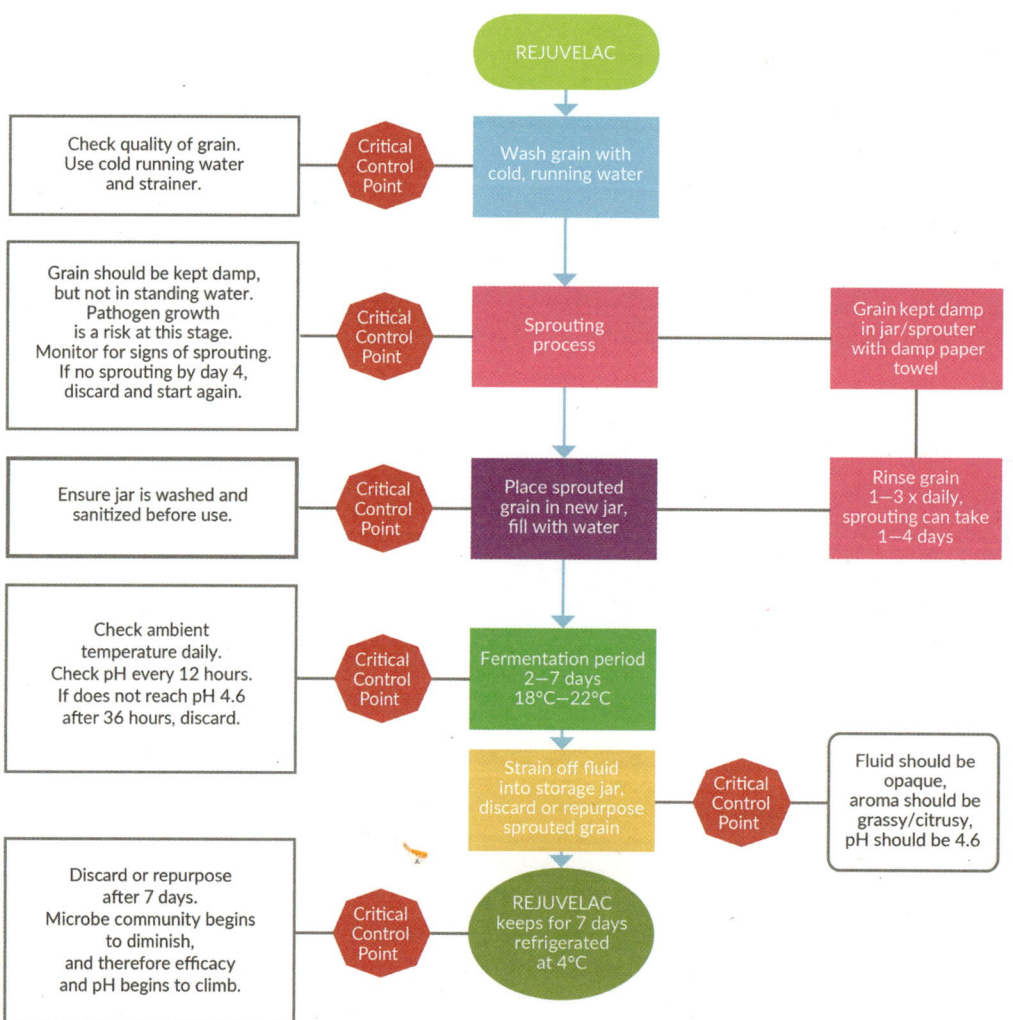

As a LAB and lactic acid rich fluid, rejuvelac is often consumed by health-conscious individuals as a way of maintaining a healthy digestive system. Many of the microbes found in rejuvelac are present in or related to strains of microbes in the human gut microbiome.

As a tool in cheesemaking, rejuvelac serves as a LAB starter culture that can be used to acidulate (make acidic) a nut/seed/legume-based milk or paste. This is significant in terms of distinguishing cheeze from cheese, as the use of a lactic acid or starter culture (not just the addition of lactic acid powder) is an essential component of the process-oriented definition of cheese. The bacteria consume and metabolize nutrients found inside the grains after the grains have begun the sprouting process, thereby producing lactic acid.

Each type of grain produces a culture that has different types of bacteria, which produce different results in terms of culturing strength, aroma, flavor, and texture depending on the manner in which the bacteria perform their metabolic functions. The bacteria (and yeasts) reside on the surface of the grains.

Wheat berries make a particularly potent rejuvelac that is highly effective for culturing plant mediums, but I have found it useful to explore using other types of rejuvelac in specific combinations. For instance, when culturing almond paste, I have found it preferable to use a farro or quinoa rejuvelac, as the stronger wheat berry one in combination with the sulfur compounds of almonds can yield a particularly strong odor and a tendency to overculture, creating an almost unpleasant flavor.

## *Making rejuvelac*

In order to make rejuvelac several steps need to be followed closely. The following steps for wheat berry rejuvelac can also be used with the other grain or groat choices.

### Step 1: Purchasing grains or groats

Ensure that the wheat berries or other grains are from reliable sources and are organic, if possible. Unless you purchase grains from local growers or from resellers who are focused on supply chain transparency, you will likely be obtaining grain from bulk bins or from regular grocery stores. Generally, grain is harvested from multiple locations and stored in large silos, and the length of time that the grain spends in storage before being sold is not listed. Coaxing older grain to sprout can be a futile effort. Additionally, while irradiation may not be of particular concern (it inhibits unwelcome pathogens and sprouting during storage), it may impact the degree to which sprouting will occur. All of this can affect the quality of the grain you purchase, so look for grains that are plump, do not appear shrivelled or too thin, and look at how they are packaged or stored. Since the primary objective with this grain is to sprout them for the purpose of making rejuvelac, I suggest purchasing organic grain or purchasing grain from smaller scale shops focused on supply chain transparency of their inventory. In Vancouver, British Columbia, where I live, I am fortunate to be able to source my grains and groats from Flourist, a local shop whose owners purchase grains only from Canadian farmers they know themselves.

### Step 2: Sprouting

Sprouting ability is important because the microbes that live on the surface of the grains or groats feed on the carbohydrate rich interior of a grain, groat, or seed. The LAB digest the carbohydrates and then reproduce, producing more

LAB and lactic acid needed for use as a starter culture. Grain, groats, or seeds must be soaked and rinsed before sprouting can happen. Moisture helps leach away inhibiting enzymes such as phytic acid that protect the grain from digestion in an animal or human gut and allow them to pass through. From the perspective of plant evolution this allows the grain, groat, or seed to land in a nutrient rich fertilizer and begin growing into a new plant, thus fulfilling its evolutionary purpose.

Once the grain has been rinsed and soaked properly, the sprouting process begins. The sprouting process can take several days, and it is important during this time to ensure a high degree of food safety. Much of the grain that is available for purchase—barring nearly direct from single source growers—has traveled large distances, been stored in various places, and has come in contact with numerous people and other living creatures. This means that there is the, albeit relatively low, possibility of a pathogenic microbe also being present alongside the ones we seek to grow.

The sprouting phase of making rejuvelac presents the highest degree of risk and, therefore, is where we should focus closely on following good procedure. Microbes thrive in a moisture rich environment, so both the ones we want and the ones we do not want may grow simultaneously. The sprouting process presented here is updated and is more cautious and more specific than the method outlined in the first version of this book.

Sprouting can be done safely, of course, and doing so makes for better outcomes all around. If you are an experienced sprouter and have a safe method, please follow it. The method below relies on a mason jar and a sprouting mesh or cheesecloth, but you can purchase small, tiered sprouting devices that make sprouting and water control very easy.

### Tools and Equipment

2 × 500 mL or 1 L glass jar, washed and sanitized
Fine mesh sieve
Mesh sprouting jar top, or cheese cloth
Measuring cups
Measuring spoons

### Ingredients

1 Tbsp–¼ cup wheat berries or your grain of choice

### Method

1. Wash and sanitize all the equipment.
2. Rinse the grain under cold running water. Allow the grain to drain off excess water. Rinsing helps to eliminate any chaff or debris that may be present.

3. Place the rinsed and drained grain in a clean, sanitized jar. Add 1 cup of filtered water or tap water that has rested for 45 minutes. Cover the jar and allow the grain to soak for a minimum of 1 hour at room temperature or overnight in the refrigerator.

    It is critical to ensure a safe process is followed. If you wish to soak the grain longer than 1 hour, ensure that it is done in the refrigerator. During this time, fermentation has not yet begun. Only the leaching of phytic acid and other inhibiting enzymes is taking place. If the grain is left soaking in standing water at room temperature (especially temperatures warmer than 72°F/22°C), it is possible that pathogens that are present may start to replicate. Soaking the grain in a covered jar in the refrigerator overnight will ensure that the inhibiting enzymes are removed and that growth of pathogens such as listeria or salmonella is prevented.

4. After the short soak is over, drain the grain, discard the soaking fluid, and rinse the grain again. The damp grains are now ready for sprouting.

5. Place the grain in another clean, sanitized jar and spray the grain with filtered water or tap water that has rested for 45 minutes. DO NOT leave the grain soaking in standing water. Cover the top of the jar with cheesecloth or a mesh sprouting lid. Leave the jar at room temperature, ideally between 62°F and 72°F (17°C and 22°C), and ensure that it is placed out of range of potential contaminants.

6. Each day for the next 2 to 4 days rinse the grains 2 to 3 times a day, and drain the excess water off each time, leaving the grain damp. Keep the grain in the jar.

7. Watch for signs the grains are beginning to sprout (you'll notice the little tails of the sprouts beginning to emerge from the seed coat). When approximately 50% of the grain has sprouted, you are ready to begin fermenting the rejuvelac.

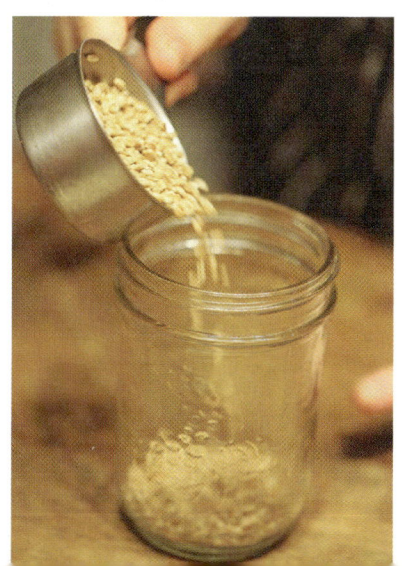 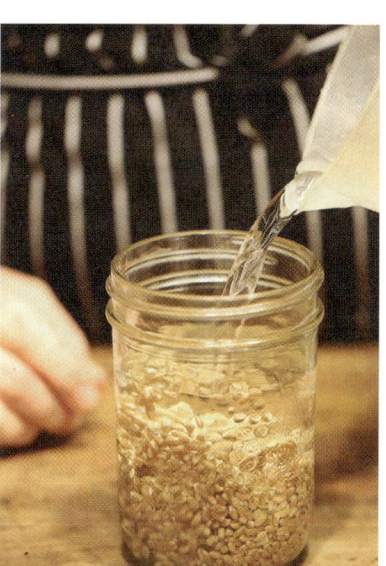 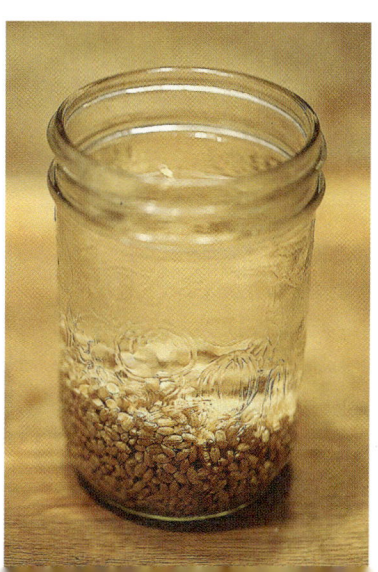

Left: *Wheat berries added to jar.* CREDIT: CATHERINE DOWNES

Center: *Pouring water into the jar for a short soak of the grain.* CREDIT: CATHERINE DOWNES

Right: *Water-covered wheat berries.* CREDIT: CATHERINE DOWNES

## Step 3: Fermentation

**Tools and Equipment**

1 × 500 mL or 1 L jar
Impermeable lid for jar
Measuring cups

**Ingredients**

Drained, sprouted grain

**Method**

1. Wash and sanitize a jar.
2. Place the sprouted grain in the jar. Add water (filtered or rested tap water) to the sprouted grain at a ratio of approximately 4:1 water to grain.
3. Ensure that you have about ⅓ of the jar as headspace above the surface of the water to allow for gas exchange during the fermentation process.
4. Cover the jar with an impermeable lid such as a plastic mason jar storage lid. Make sure that the lid is not metallic as moisture released during fermentation can react with the metal.
5. Place the jar in an area of your kitchen (or wherever you do your ferments), that has an even room temperature. An optimal temperature is between 62°F and 72°F (17°C and 22°C). Avoid leaving the jar in an area that will experience large temperature fluctuations.
6. Allow the sprouted grain to ferment at room temperature for 2 to 7 days. This process may take longer during cooler weather periods or be quite fast during warmer periods.
    a. Monitor the progress daily. You will be looking for the fluid to become slightly cloudy and for little bubbles to begin forming. The formation of bubbles indicates the bacteria that form $CO_2$ are present and active. The opaqueness of the water indicates that microbes are populating the water.
    b. It is very important during this fermenting period that you taste and smell the fluid that is fermenting. The rejuvelac is this liquid. It should smell somewhat citrusy to mildly vinegary; the aroma will depend on what grain you use. Quinoa rejuvelac, for instance, smells a little bit lemony and grassy, while buckwheat rejuvelac has an earthy aroma. Some rejuvelac, especially that made from wheat berries, can present quite a strong odor.
    c. If you notice mold growing on the surface (this will appear as spots that gradually become larger before uniting), discard and start again.
    d. If you notice a thin whitish to light pinkish or orange film that is evenly spread across the surface and not just distinct circular spots, scrape it off

the surface. This is a wild yeast called kahm and generally poses no risk, but it is best to remove it for the overall quality of the rejuvelac.

7. When the rejuvelac is ready, you will need to drain the fluid into a new, clean, sanitized jar. Cover the jar with an impermeable lid, and store it in the refrigerator. The liquid is your starter culture. This liquid is full of LAB and lactic acid and is what you will use to make cultured vegan cheese.

**Storage**

Rejuvelac keeps in the refrigerator for a maximum of 2 weeks at 39.2°F (4°C). Discard after 2 weeks and make a fresh batch.

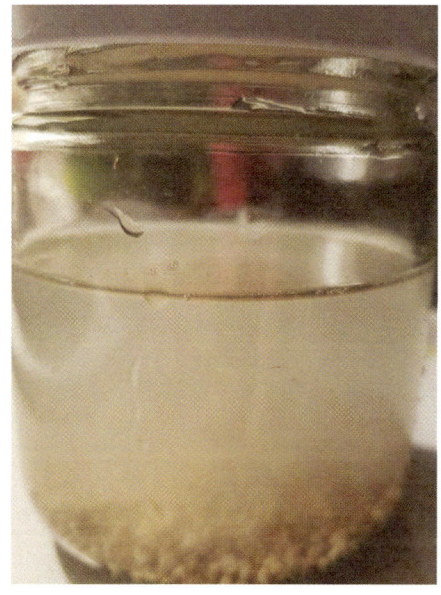

*Quinoa rejuvelac at 3 days of fermentation.*

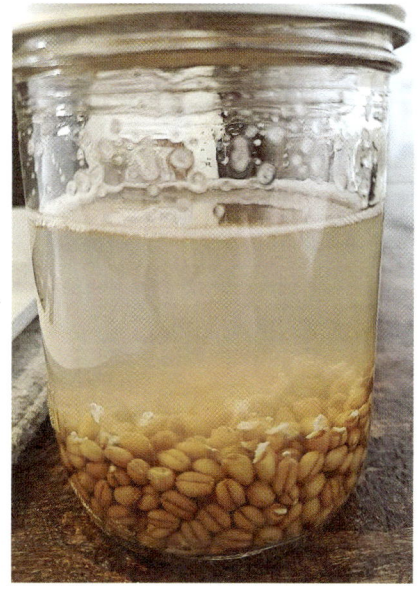

*Wheat berry (kernel/grain) rejuvelac at 3 days of fermentation.*

### Ways to use this rejuvelac and sprouted grain

**Rejuvelac:**

In smoothies

In juice

On oatmeal

In making pancakes

In making dehydrated raw breads and crackers

**Sprouted grain:**

In salads

Baked in crackers

Repurposed in some other food applications

Composted

## Kefir: Water Kefir Versus Dairy Kefir

Kefir itself is a beverage similar to a drinkable yogurt and typically has been a dairy-based beverage. Thought to have origins in the Caucasus region, Eastern Europe, and Russia and possibly to be related to a Turkish fermented milk product known as kopur, kefir has been consumed widely in these regions since at least the 1880s. Made from goat, cow, or sheep milk and a mesophilic culture of symbiotic bacteria and yeast, the process of making it results in a product rich in gut friendly microbial flora (probiotics).

The culture used to make kefir is now primarily cultivated in labs and freeze-dried (you can order wet cultures, but I do not favor these). The globules formed by the bacteria and yeast are referred to as grain. They are obviously not a true grain, but rather the interaction of the bacteria and yeast results in the production of a biomatrix of proteins, lipids, and polysaccharides that unites the microbes. The species of bacteria in kefir grains are, typically, *Lactobacillus, Lactococcus, Streptococcus,* and *Leuconostoc*. The yeast strains present are commonly *Saccharomyces, Candida,* and *Kloeckera*. Each species of organism performs different functions in metabolizing lactose in milk, but all include the formation of lactic acid, which in turn leads to protein breakdown, and this produces other by-products. The overall result is a tangy, slightly thickened yogurt-like fermented milk product.

### *Experimentation*

I began testing kefir cultures in 2013 while investigating different options for making cultured vegan cheese. As I am allergic to dairy and have chosen to live a vegan plant-based lifestyle, I wanted to make a plant-based version of kefir, and I began experimenting with kefir on different plant mediums.

My first experiment was in converting some dairy trained kefir grain given to me by a friend. Kefir grains are somewhat gelatinous looking, almost clear (once they are rehydrated). I set up to test several kefir options: cashew, almond, coconut, coconut water, and water.

With the assistance of Katie, a stage in the Graze kitchen, we set out to see if we could, one, successfully train the dairy-fed kefir grains onto a plant-based medium, and two, make a kefir/yogurt/probiotic beverage that would work successfully as a starter for further cheese tests.

Dividing the grain among five 1-liter jars, we added 2 cups of a test medium to each of the five jars (one jar with coconut milk, one jar with cashew milk, etc.). We also added 1 tablespoon of maple syrup to help feed the kefir grains. We then put lids on the jars and kept the jars in a container set on top of the convection oven where it was warm but not hot (maintaining 100°F/38°C), and left them to culture for 24 hours.

After 24 hours, the coconut milks had cultured, with the kefir grains having multiplied quickly. We were able to strain off the coconut milk and save the grain for making another jar of coconut milk kefir in which we used less maple syrup. We repeated the coconut milk process two more times until the kefir grain was trained onto just coconut milk, with no added sweetener.

With each subsequent batch we saved the grain and evaluated the results of the cultured coconut milk for texture, taste, and that bright, somewhat effervescent quality of kefir beverages. Because the goal was to produce kefir grain fed only plant-based mediums, we discarded the first two rounds of the kefir. After batches three and four we reserved grain by straining the coconut milk through very fine mesh sieves and retrieving some of the grain.

We added the reserved grain to a small amount of coconut milk with a small amount of maple syrup in order to store the kefir culture for a longer period of time in the refrigerator.

As for the other kefir efforts, the cashew and almond milks we made ourselves in order to avoid the extra stabilizers and to be able to control the amount and kind of sweetener that we wanted to use. The cashew milk was a success, but it did take a little longer (36 hours) to culture to the same degree of tanginess or sharpness as the coconut milk. It produced a thicker substance than the coconut milk, more like a very soft yogurt. The individual kefir grains, however, were much smaller and slower to replicate, and we were not able to culture subsequent batches of cashew kefir as quickly as with the coconut milk.

For the purposes of being able to maintain a supply of cashew kefir, we decided to culture cashew milk using coconut milk kefir as a starter. This worked well, and is still the method I use when making large batches of cheeses.

The almond milk was more challenging. Of the milks, it took the longest and had the least pleasant taste. This could be a result of the culture struggling with the sulfur compounds in almonds. We found that adding 2 tablespoons of maple syrup to 1 liter of almond milk gave the kefir grain more to feed on and resulted in a better tasting product.

Lastly, with respect to the coconut water and water kefir tests, these took longer than all of the milks. The weaning process started with higher amounts of maple syrup (our sweetener of choice, though some people use raw cane sugar) and we reduced the amount with each subsequent batch until we found the minimum we could use and still get the results we were seeking.

## *Water kefir as bulk starter*

I have moved away from my experiments weaning dairy kefir to plant mediums and now use water kefir to culture coconut kefir and other plant milk kefirs.

Water kefir has proven to be a consistent and excellent acidifying culture and is generally easy to obtain. Some places, such as Cultures for Health (www.culturesforhealth.com), sell coconut milk kefir culture, but I still prefer to make my own coconut milk or other plant milk kefir using water kefir grain as a starter.

Water kefir is known as tibicos, California bees, and Japanese water crystals, among several other names, and like milk kefir it seems to have entered popular use in the 1880s. Like milk kefir grain, water kefir grain is a symbiotic community of bacteria and yeast, and the types of bacteria and yeast found in water kefir grain are the same although the species differ somewhat. Water kefir is NOT a result of simply adding a probiotic capsule to sugar water and allowing that to ferment, and in many ways that is not a useful way to create a starter, something I will discuss a little later on. It is the specific relationship between the bacteria and the yeasts that form the globules that become the kefir grain.

The origin of water kefir is not 100 percent confirmed, but interestingly, hard granules, called tibicos, were found on the pads of the Opuntia cactus (found in Mexico), and have been observed being used to make fermented beverages.

Water kefir, as its name suggests, grows in a medium of water and sugar. The primary bacteria, like milk kefir, are lactic acid forming bacteria, and they metabolize the sugar in the water solution, and this acidifies it, making a lightly carbonated, tangy beverage that also contains large amounts of gut friendly microbes.

Since 2015, I have been consistently using water kefir to ferment coconut kefir, cashew kefir, and other plant milk bases to amplify different members of the microbial community and therefore the different by-products (flavor, texture, and aroma) for making different types of cultured vegan cheese. Though I have used water kefir grain to directly ferment coconut milk, I have found that using the grain directly in the other nut-based plant milks is less successful than using water kefir in a solution.

For the vegan cheesemaker, the nice thing about using water kefir instead of weaning milk kefir onto new mediums is that it is plant-based from the beginning, and once you have a healthy batch of water kefir, you can use it (even without the larger pieces of kefir grain) to culture vegan cheese batches. The water kefir solution serves as a sort of bulk starter that can keep virtually indefinitely provided you care for it properly.

Feeding water kefir grain is important and different sugars will have different impacts on the symbiotic community of bacteria and yeast because certain members of the community may change how they behave according to the type of sugar.

## Sugar Feeds for Water Kefir

| Sugar type | Effect on water kefir |
|---|---|
| White sugar | Grains remain quite tight and are slow to activate/ferment.<br>    Though slow, this feeding medium does allow for a neutral flavor base. |
| Evaporated cane sugar crystals | Not optimal, approximately the same kind of response as to white sugar. |
| Raw cane sugar (brownish in color, indicates presence of minerals, less refined) | Water kefir microbes generally do very well with a high quality raw cane sugar. Level Ground brand sells a raw cane sugar that has good mineral content. The grains are responsive, become quite plump and activate well. |
| Coconut sugar | Water kefir becomes VERY active, but there can sometimes be too much mineral content, and while the grain will plump up quickly, some detritus (will look a bit sandy) will develop.<br>    This can be strained out, but another alternative is to combine coconut sugar with some raw cane sugar or white sugar to reduce the mineral load. |
| Maple syrup | This works well when combined with another sugar.<br>    Maple syrup has a high level of minerals and can overwhelm the grain.<br>    Water kefir fed on maple syrup does produce a nice flavor, but the maple note remains. |
| Date sugar | Again, like coconut and maple syrup, it is used best when in combination with another sugar with less mineral content. Similar flavor and behavior to coconut sugar. |
| **Avoid using**<br>Honey (anti-microbial properties)<br>Stevia (does not offer an appropriate sugar food source for the microbes)<br>Synthetic sugars<br>Xylitol<br>Blended dates or other fruit (too much fiber and mineral content) | |

Next I detail how to rehydrate freeze-dried water kefir grain, ferment water kefir, store water kefir, and use water kefir to make coconut kefir.

## Making water kefir

Before starting any food preparation process, wash and sanitize your work surfaces and all related tools and equipment.

### Tools and Equipment

2 × 500 mL jar or 1 L jar (depending on how large a batch you wish to make)
Impermeable lid for jar
Measuring cups
Measuring spoons
Kettle (or means of boiling/heating water)
Probe thermometer
Spoon

### Ingredients

1 package (or less) water kefir grain (preferably freeze-dried)
1 Tbsp sugar (Choose type of sugar from recommendations in table Sugar Feeds for Water Kefir.)
½ cup water (filtered or rested tap water)

### Method: Rehydration

Freeze-dried grain must be rehydrated, but this initial step also works well when you want to help new grain (obtained from friends etc.) adjust to your home.

1. Wash and sanitize work surfaces and equipment.
2. Decide which sugar you want to feed the water kefir.
3. Pre-measure tap water if you are using that, and allow it to rest for 45 minutes.
4. Measure out the sugar and place it in a clean, sanitized jar.
5. Heat the water but do not boil it. You want it just warm enough to dissolve the sugar. Pour the warm water over the sugar, and stir until dissolved.
6. Check the temperature of the sugar water mixture to ensure that it is less than 105°F (40°C).
7. Add the water kefir grain to the solution. Ensure there is headspace between the top of the jar and the surface of the water for gas exchange. Cover the jar with an impermeable lid, and allow the grain to rehydrate for 24 hours at room temperature.

### Method: Fermentation

1. Observe the grains after the rehydration period. They should be plumped up, and less golden in color than when they were dry. They should be opaque

and whitish in color. Strain the grains from the rehydration solution, and discard that solution.
2. Place the strained grain in a fresh, clean and sanitized jar, 500 mL to 1 L in size (depending on the volume of water kefir you intend to make).
3. Make a new feeding medium. Pour it over the rehydrated grain.
a. 500 mL jar: 1¼ cups warm water with 1 Tbsp sugar dissolved in it.
b. 1 L jar: 2½ cups warm water with 1½ Tbsp sugar dissolved in it.
4. Cover the jar with an impermeable lid to inhibit other microbes in the environment from joining the solution.
5. Leave the jar at room temperature (optimal temperature for fermentation is between 62°F and 72°F (17°C and 22°C). Allow the mixture to ferment from 24 hours to 5 days. I sometimes ferment mine longer depending on how fast it is metabolizing the sugar and how it tastes. Check the solution every 12 hours, or at least once a day. Taste and smell in order to observe changes in acidity, which you will notice as it becomes tangy. During this time you should also notice the water kefir grains replicating and increasing in number.
6. After the water kefir has become more tangy than sweet, refrigerate it. This is now the starter culture for making cultured vegan cheese.
7. Water kefir grains can be kept indefinitely. Once they are refrigerated, check them every 2 weeks to once a month. Observe their physical condition to ensure they are still plump and are not disintegrating. Taste the solution, and if it is very tangy, bordering on sour, remove them from the refrigerator. Make a new batch of feeding solution, and transfer them to that new solution in a new jar. When the solution is too tangy, it means the microbes have digested most of the food available, and this situation could end up with members of the community consuming each other. Simply follow the instructions for making water kefir to make a new solution for the grains.

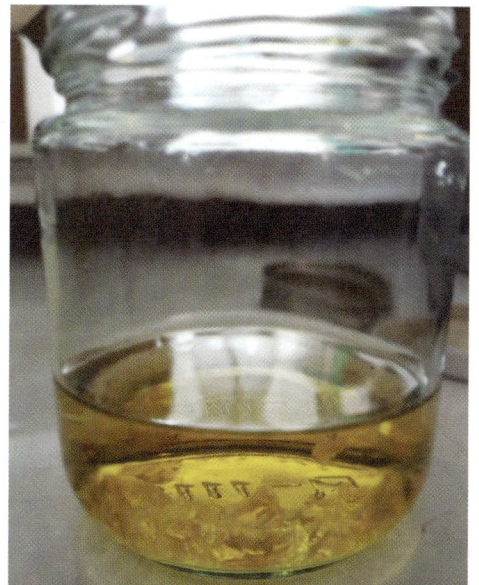
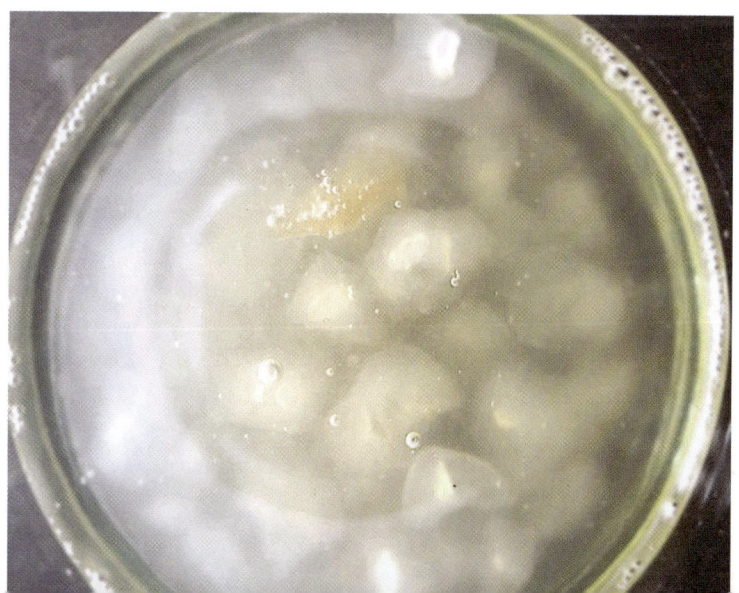

Left: *Rehydrating water kefir grain.*

Right: *Water kefir grains fermenting in sugar water solution.*

### Making coconut kefir using water kefir

One of my favorite things to make just for its own sake is coconut milk kefir. I love the bright, tangy flavor and light effervescence. I make small batches weekly at home for myself and use it in smoothies, salad dressings, cultured vegan cheesecake, add it to oatmeal, use it to leaven biscuits and to make fermented crepe and pancake batter. I find it indispensable.

It also makes a great starter culture for cultured vegan cheese. When making coconut kefir the bacteria and yeast from the water kefir produce compounds that are different from those produced when digesting only sugar. In cheesemaking this translates into a depth of flavor and a buttery mouthfeel and flavor.

When selecting the coconut milk you will work with, seek high fat coconut milks. All coconut milk is a combination of coconut milk and water. Check the ingredient label for percentage of coconut milk fat and for the extraction percentage. I find a great deal of success using Aroy-D coconut milk in Tetra Pak form, but you will need to read the labels of the coconut milk brands available in your area.

If you have personal concerns about using coconut milk with stabilizers in it, avoid brands that have guar gum or maltodextrin cellulose. Both of these are used to prevent separation by binding water molecules with the coconut milk. Not all brands use these, so, again, check the label.

Avoid using low-fat coconut milks or 100% coconut cream. It has too much fat. The bacteria will not be able to metabolize all of the fat, and this will lead to a sour, rancid product. Too little fat will lead to very low yields, though you will still be able to use that as a starter culture or as a culture boost to beverages like smoothies. I look for coconut milk that has 17% or higher coconut milk fat and an extraction percentage of 60–85%. This tells me that I will be getting enough fat to work with.

Having this third home-grown starter culture gives you more options for experimentation. You can also make coconut milk kefir yogurt with the method below.

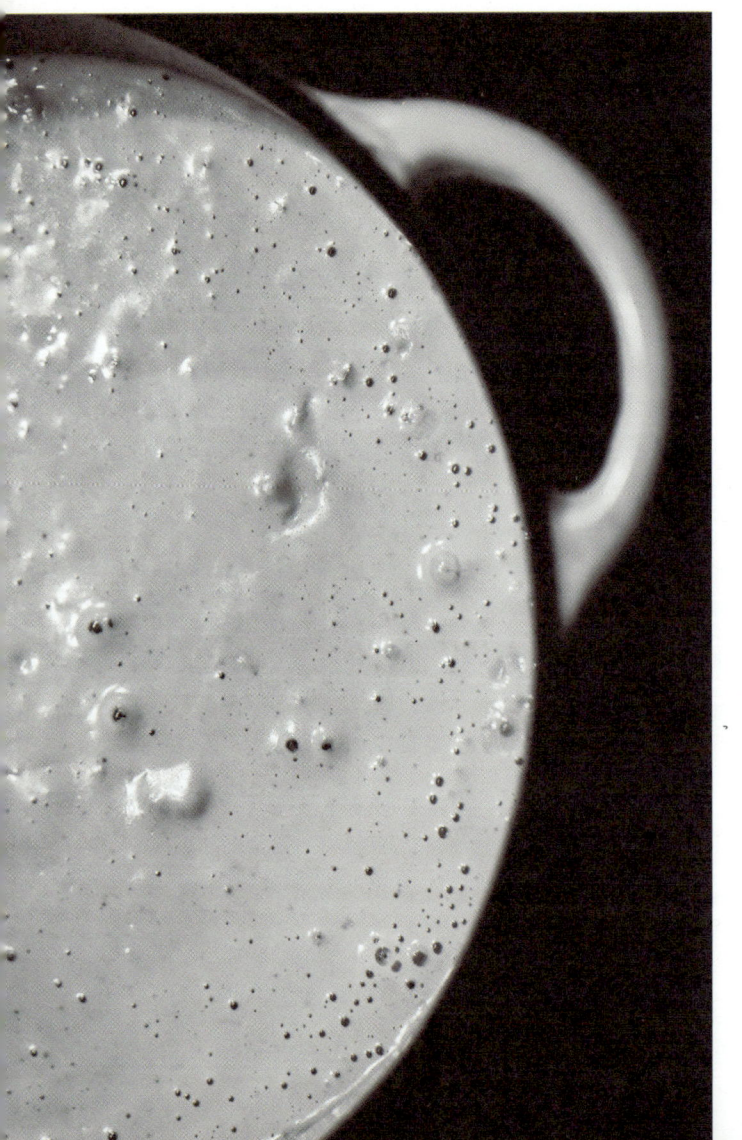

*Culturing coconut milk with kefir grain.*
CREDIT: CATHERINE DOWNES

Fermentation and Culturing: Role in Cheesemaking 75

## Tools and Equipment

Thick cast sauce pot, medium
1 L jar, washed, sanitized
Impermeable lid (for the jar)
Measuring cups
Measuring spoons
Probe thermometer
Fine mesh strainer (optional)

## Ingredients

500 mL high fat coconut milk
1 Tbsp water kefir (from the water kefir you have made, with or without some of the grain)
Optional: 1 tsp sugar (or any of the options that you would use to feed water kefir)

## Method

1. Wash and sanitize all surfaces and tools you will be working with.
2. Heat 500 mL of the coconut milk to 185°F (85°C). Do not boil the coconut milk.
3. Remove from heat, and using active cooling processes (e.g., place on an ice bath, or stir), cool the coconut milk to 105°F (40°C). Active cooling is important because it either cools the coconut milk down quickly (ice) or allows the hot coconut milk beneath the surface to come to the top and the excess heat to evaporate (stirring). Allowing the coconut milk to cool by just standing on the counter means that the surface cools while the middle stays hot, and this puts the surface milk at risk of becoming host to unwelcome microbes.
4. OPTIONAL. At just over 120°F (about 50°C), add 1 tsp of sugar (use the same kind of sugar you fed the water kefir with). Stir until the sugar is dissolved. This is not necessary, but it can help the water kefir microbes replicate quickly when you add them. The coconut milk is a richer medium than the sugar/water mixture the microbes feed on, so the added sugar helps them take to the new medium.
5. At 105°F (40°C) place the coconut milk in the 1 L jar and add the water kefir (with or without the grain). Cover the jar with the lid, and place the mixture in an area of your kitchen that is even in ambient temperature (no large temperature changes). The kefir microbes are mesophilic, meaning

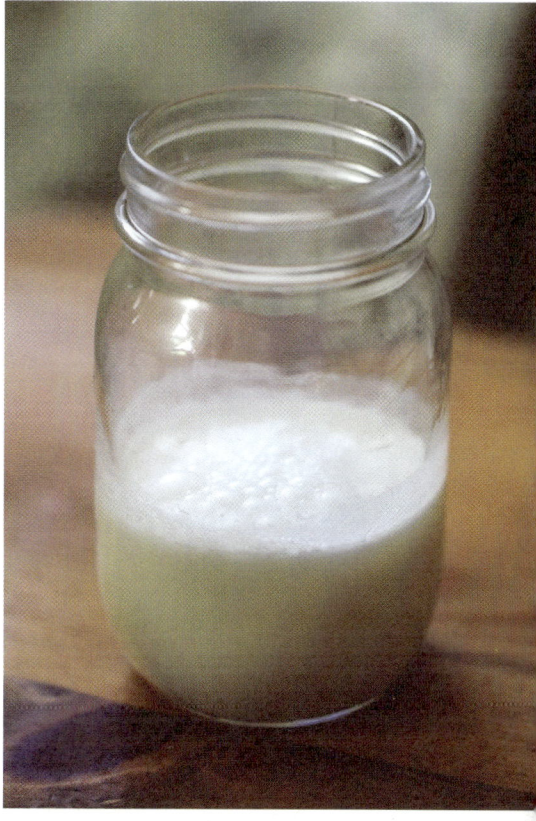

*Coconut kefir starter in a jar.*
CREDIT: CATHERINE DOWNES

they do their metabolizing work at room temperatures, so you want to avoid keeping them near too much heat. However, in cooler months or if you do not do a lot of culturing in your environment, you can place the jar in the oven with the oven light on (not the heat) and use this as an incubator for the fermentation period.

6. Allow the mixture to ferment for 24 to 48 hours. Check the mixture every 12 hours, or at least once a day. Visually, you are looking for signs of change, and that will include some small bubbles. Taste and smell the mixture. It should start to smell a little tangy, or bright, and the flavor should be mildly to moderately acidic.

7. The longer you culture, the more you will notice changes to the surface of the coconut milk kefir and the thicker it will get. Depending on the inherent water content of the coconut milk you use, you will notice varying degrees of separation as the thicker fat component rises and the water settles. This is normal, and in fact indicates that the microbes are doing their job.

8. If you want a thicker texture, allow the mixture to culture the full 48 hours. If you want the coconut milk kefir only for use as a starter culture, stop the culturing anywhere between 24 and 36 hours and refrigerate.

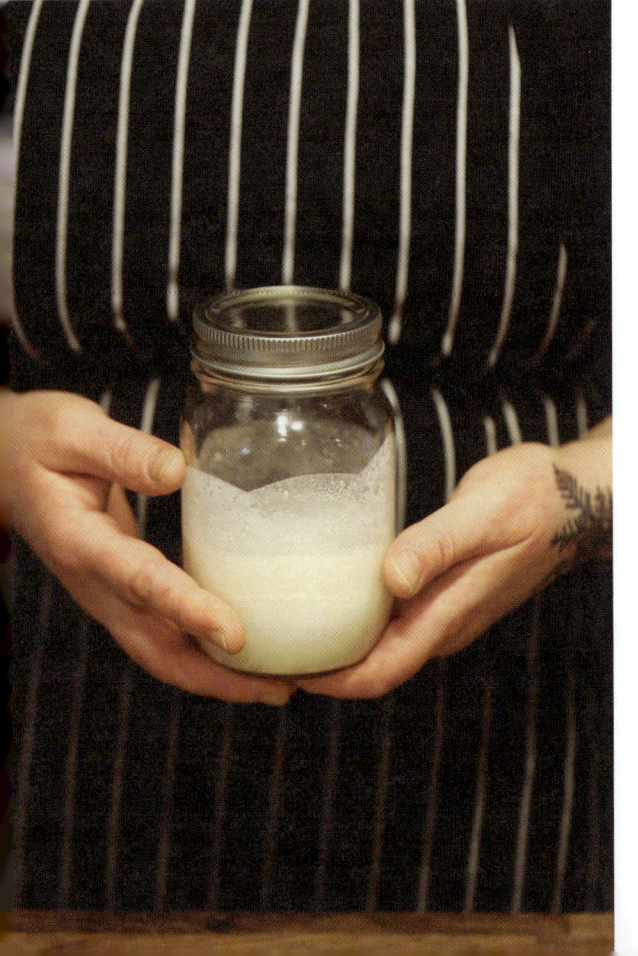

*Coconut Kefir in a jar, ready for storage in the refrigerator.*
Credit: Catherine Downes

9. Transfer the coconut milk kefir to a new, clean, sanitized container for storage. Less headspace is needed than in the culturing jar. It must be kept in the refrigerator after the culturing process is finished. You will notice it thicken up after cooling.

10. If the surface of the coconut milk kefir is starting to buckle but there is no unwanted growth, it is usually a sign that it has been heavily cultured and that the microbes have produced enough acid to break down any proteins. Check the surface for any color changes. If there is a light pinkish, beige, tan, or orangish color evenly spread on the surface, this is wild yeast. Simply scrape off and discard. If you find bright pink spots (not an even spread) or other colored spots, they are molds and you should discard out of an abundance of caution and start again.

**Storage**

Coconut milk kefir can keep properly stored in the refrigerator for up to 30 days (with no cross-contamination from double-dipping etc.).

## *Back slopping*

"Back slopping" is a term used to describe the act of using a small amount of a fermented item to help start the next batch of the same item. It is often employed in DIY yogurt making and can be used in the case of coconut milk kefir to make several subsequent batches of coconut milk kefir. The back slopping process starts with making a new batch of coconut milk kefir similar in size to the original one, but instead of adding the water kefir, add 1 Tbsp of coconut milk kefir.

Back slopping can be repeated a limited number of times. I suggest up to ten times, after which, I recommend you return to making a batch of coconut milk kefir using the water kefir. Each time you back slop, you change the community of microbes a little, as the ones who do best in the new environment thrive, while others that would have thrived in the water kefir sugar/water solution become less active. This alters what by-products they produce and can affect their efficacy in terms of acidification.

I do use back slopping at home when I just want to get a new batch of coconut kefir going, and I have found that the coconut milk kefir produced from this approach is optimal around the third or fourth batches but starts to move away from my personal flavor and texture preferences in batches five to ten.

The amount of time it takes to ferment a batch of coconut milk kefir using water kefir or some starter from the previous batch of coconut milk kefir is comparable, so it does not save time.

## Other Starter Cultures

In this section I discuss other starter cultures that can be used for making cultured vegan cheese. In the first edition of this book, I included probiotics, sauerkraut brine, miso, and tempeh cultures. In this edition, I provide clarification and updated information about starter cultures, beginning with retracting some of my previous recommendations. Experimentation, research, and newer materials coming to market mean that cultured vegan cheesemaking will be evolving.

## *Probiotic capsules*

In my first edition of this book, I did suggest that probiotic capsules could be used, and although they will provide some level of acidification when used, I have moved away from recommending them for many reasons.

"Probiotic," as a term means very little scientifically, but is defined by the World Health Organization as "live microorganisms that when administered in adequate amounts confer a benefit on the host."[5] This definition, though, is not accepted by some such as the European Food Safety Authority because the health claim embedded in the definition is not measurable, a problem that persists across arenas concerned with regulating products labeled probiotic.

"Probiotic" is a term that has migrated from the wellness industry to describe products featuring bacteria and yeasts purported to support the human gut microbiome and offer human health improvements. The term itself does not actually mean anything in terms of microbiological understanding of bacteria and yeasts. While the impact of the human gut microbiome on overall health is becoming better understood, the usefulness or effectiveness of probiotic products still requires substantial research.

Probiotic products are produced by a poorly regulated industry, and probiotic products can vary significantly in performance and activity. When making cultured vegan cheese, we should use cultures that we know work well for food culturing. Probiotic powders and capsules contain many types of bacteria and yeasts, but not all are suitable for the act of lactic acid fermentation. Growing your own lactic acid starter cultures either from rejuvelac or from water kefir will yield more consistent results and better tasting ones.

### *Miso*

A fermented paste made from soybeans, brown rice, barley, and sometimes legumes (there is a great chickpea miso made in Canada by Feeding Change), miso is fermented using the fungi *Aspergillus oryzae* and is a staple food item in Japanese cuisine. In the first edition, I did suggest that it could be used to make a cultured vegan cheese. However, I now recommend that its use in making cultured vegan cheese be more about it amplifying a sense of umami rather than fulfilling an acidification process, which is what culturing does. In other words, I suggest using miso as an additional ingredient, not as an active culturing agent.

### *Sauerkraut brine*

Sauerkraut has long been understood to be a digestive aid and has seen a resurgence of popularity with the increasing awareness of its nutritional benefits and of how easy it is to make. Sauerkraut brine (the fluid in which sauerkraut is stored) is full of lactic acid forming bacteria and naturally occurring yeasts. It is very tangy and will certainly culture a nut or seed base. Pascal Baudar, a wild foods chef from California, often uses it as a starter culture for the wild foods nut cheeses that he teaches about in his workshops. However, and this is something to be mindful of, it will impart a cabbage-like flavor to your cheese. If you use sauerkraut brine as a cheese culture, use it the same way you would use rejuvelac.

## Tempeh culture

When this book was first published in 2017, I had only begun testing the use of tempeh culture in a cultured vegan cheese context. Tempeh making is an entirely different fermentation process from lactic acid fermentation. It relies on *Aspergillus oryzae* mold, and thus requires very different fermentation conditions.

The potential use of tempeh processes in cultured vegan cheesemaking is more likely to be as a secondary culturing process (after an initial acidification process). I am still testing the use of tempeh culture, but sharing insights from these experiments would be presumptive at this point.

## Mesophilic direct-set culture

In traditional cheesemaking, mesophilic starters are used for acidification (just as rejuvelac, water kefir, and coconut kefir cultures would be). These culture sets combine a number of different lactic acid forming bacteria, all of which perform slightly different functions (fast acidification, slower acidification, production of diacetyl, a buttery flavor compound, etc.).

The culture sets are sold in prepackaged arrangements and their purpose and performance are well understood in traditional cheesemaking. They are most often sold in a direct-set format, meaning that you cannot back slop with them or make bulk cultures with them (water kefir would be an example of a bulk culture, in that you can make a batch of it and keep using it to culture). They are usually sold freeze-dried on a feeding medium, often a carbohydrate, that allows them to activate and replicate quickly when used in culturing.

Although a number of vegan cheesemakers, me included, have tested these traditional cultures in plant-based mediums, it has been with the knowledge that these cultures are not always assuredly vegan. (I do not use any cultures that are NOT 100% vegan friendly in the Blue Heron cheeses that I make, but I have tested the cultures to better understand what they do and how they behave.) Sometimes the agar agar culturing plates they are grown on involve animal components such as sheep brain or cow parts. The website www.realvegancheese.org provides good information about feeding mediums for cultures, and although it still takes a little detective work to figure out which brands of mesophilic direct-set starters are considered vegan friendly, it is possible to find some.

Many direct-set cultures do not contain actual dairy in the freeze-dried form but have been fed dairy during the culturing/growth phase and usually list dairy as an allergen caution on the information sheet that accompanies them.

There are two thermophilic lactic acid starters from Danisco Choozit that are accidentally vegan, (they do not use any dairy as part of their feeding medium), but they are not suitable for mesophilic (room temperature) culturing processes.

Thermophilic cultures require warmer temperatures to activate than do mesophilic cultures, so you cannot use one of these thermophilic cultures in the same way you use water kefir or rejuvelac. You need to heat the mixture you wish to culture first and then add the thermophilic culture.

The good news is that due to the continually expanding demand for better quality vegan cheeses and for cultured vegan cheeses in general, some producers of traditional cheesemaking cultures are starting to see the potential in this market. Danisco, a producer of traditional cheese cultures, now makes a line of cultures identified as VEGE (and then the identifying culture number follows), that are designed for creating different flavors and textures or outcomes in making cultured vegan foods. This particular culture line is a little difficult to access because very few cheesemaking supply shops sell it (a few in Europe do) to the DIY consumer. These cultures are just now becoming available for commercial sector producers, but are, again, a little challenging to source.

Interestingly, The Cheesemaker (www.thecheesemaker.com), a US-based cheesemaking supply shop maintains a section titled Vegan on its website and includes starter cultures that are accidentally vegan, including two thermophilic (not mesophilic) cultures that can be used. It is important to note that using thermophilic cultures requires a process slightly different from culturing at room temperature.

In the recipes following, I highlight a number of the different starter cultures. Have fun!

---

4   See www.realvegancheese.org for information on what particular cultures are fed in the lab process.

5   Food and Agricultural Organization of the United Nations and World Health Organization. "Health and nutritional properties of probiotics in food including powder milk with live lactic acid bacteria." World Health Organization [online], (2001).

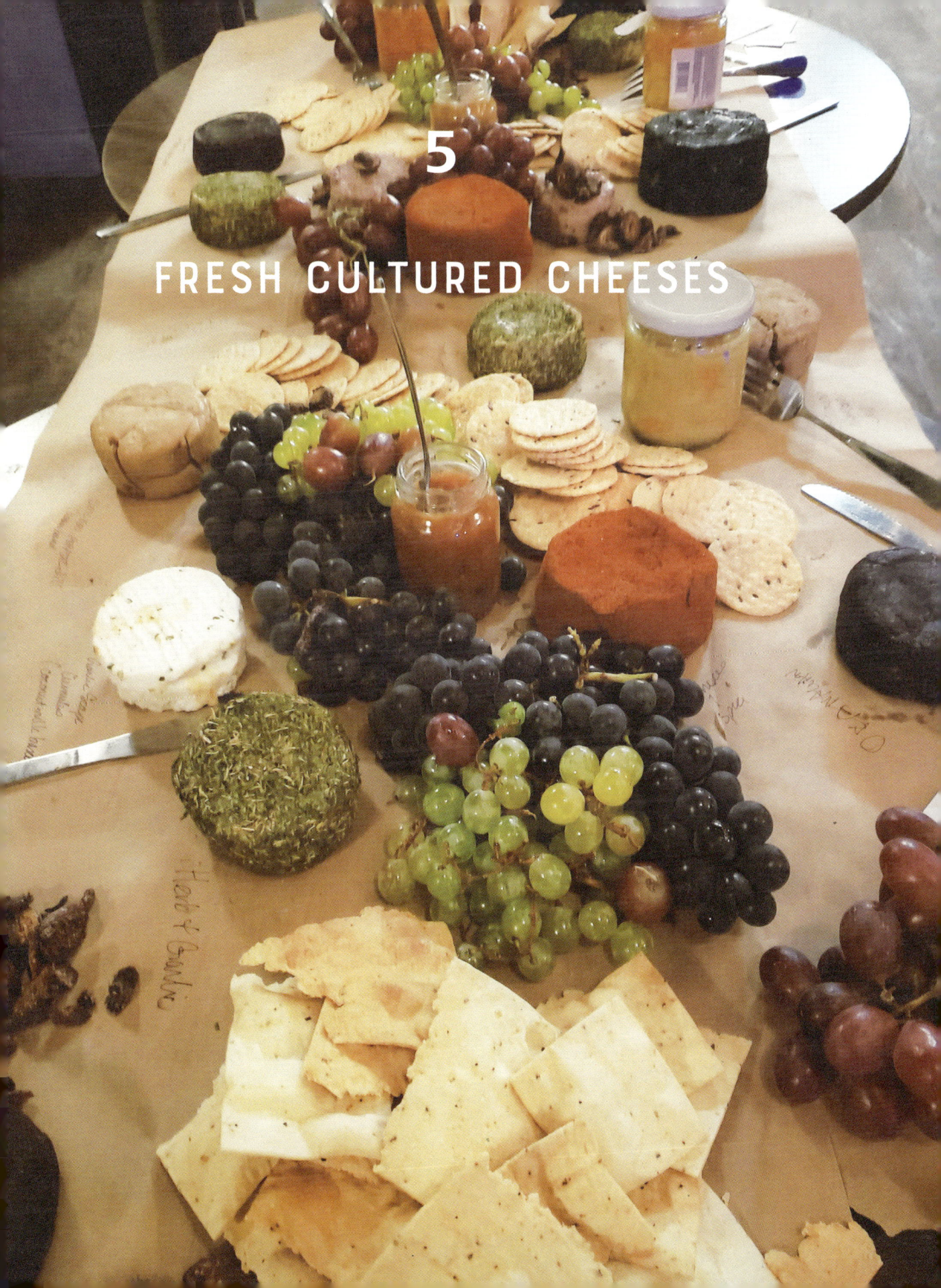

# 5

## FRESH CULTURED CHEESES

This chapter presents several recipes for cultured cheeses that are easy to make and take very little time. They will still take more time than the non-cultured cheezes, but it is worth the waiting time for the cultures to do their work! These recipes are intended to get you comfortable with the culturing process, with testing the different starter cultures, and with recognizing the taste and textural changes that culturing delivers.

The recipes use different materials, and you can experiment with them in the culturing process to see how they respond and find out what this means. Not all nuts, seeds, and legumes will make successful cheeses, and some will certainly produce better results than others. Cultured vegan cheesemaking, like all food work, is an empirical process, and for your experiments, I suggest keeping a notebook handy for recording dates, times, and observations.

These cheeses mirror their dairy-based versions to the extent that they are shorter-term cultured cheeses, soft, and typically made with just a mesophilic lactic acid starter. Texturally, these will be somewhat familiar to those who are nostalgic for soft, fresh, dairy cheese, but not perfectly so. However, and much more importantly, they begin to truly demonstrate that plant-based cheese can indeed be a "thing," despite the hard and fast definition of the Codex Alimentarius.

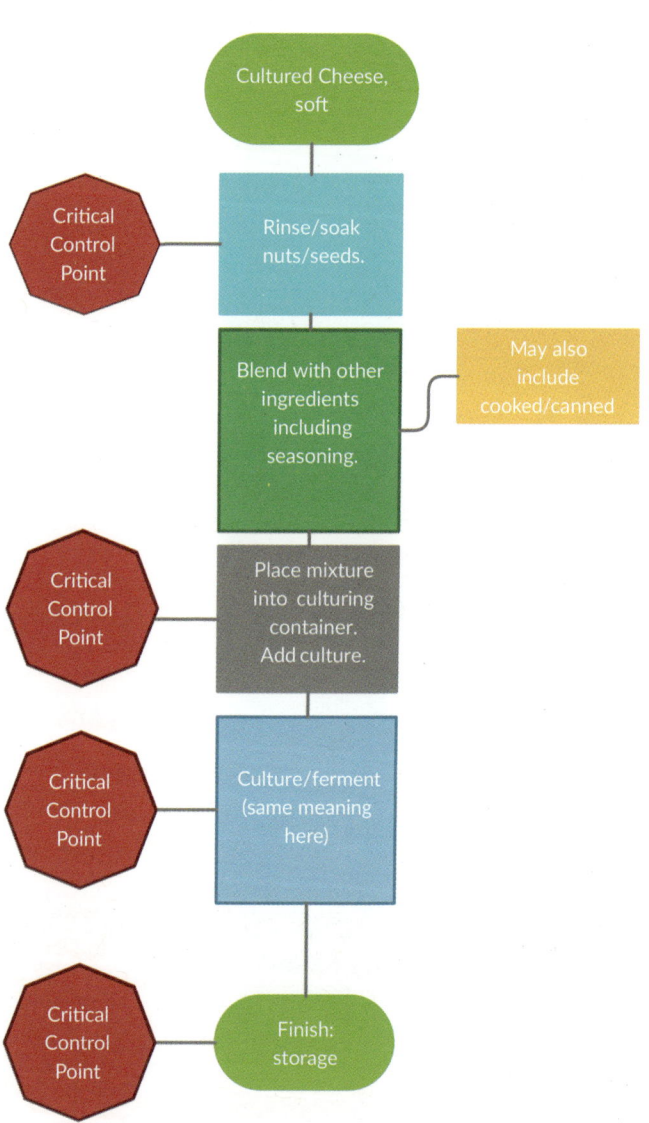

# Cultured Almond Ricotta, non-cooked

This remains one of my favorite quick-cultured cheeses to make, and I use it as an assigned recipe in the four-week cultured vegan cheesemaking class that I teach. It differs from a traditional dairy ricotta in that it is not cooked, and I use LAB cultures for acidification rather than lemon juice or vinegar.

I use it in so many applications, including raw vegan savory dishes like raw cannellini, and in many warm dishes such as lasagne, ravioli filling, spinach and artichoke dip, and in a baked almond ricotta tarte tatin that I like to make several times a month.

I have modified the method of this recipe significantly. Almonds contain sulfur and can, when cultured for too long, produce an eggy aroma. Also, almonds tend to culture very quickly, and with too long a culturing period, or too much culture, protein breakdown happens too quickly and bitter notes arise. I have simplified the process overall.

Other nuts can be substituted for the almonds: macadamia nuts, pine nuts, and even pistachios. You may also use Brazil nuts, but I highly recommend using those in combination with other nuts because Brazil nuts are high in selenium and it is easy to overconsume when they are blended. Selenium, while beneficial for thyroid function, can lead to toxicity when overconsumed, and although selenium toxicity is considered to be a rare occurrence and one mostly caused by the use of supplements, it is still wise to moderate the use of Brazil nuts in vegan cheesemaking.

You may also use rolled oats to make a ricotta-like cultured cheese, though I do recommend combining oats with another seed or a nut so that the stickiness of the oats is reduced.

## Tools and Equipment

High-speed blender (or combination of food processor and lower quality/less fancy blender)
Measuring cups
Measuring spoons
Colander or fine mesh sieve
Spatula
Food grade plastic bowl or container
Reusable food wrap or other ability to seal the container during fermentation
Cheesecloth or butter muslin

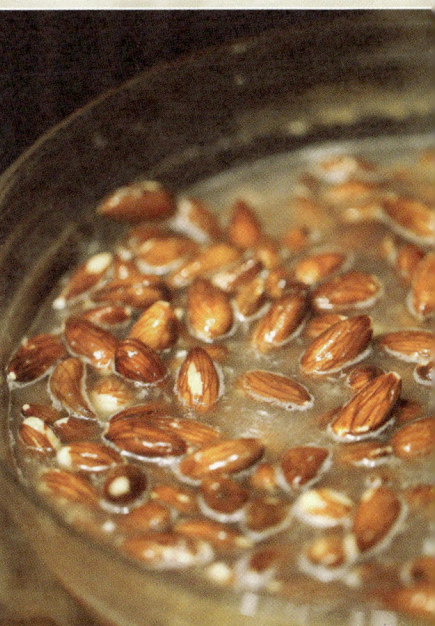

*Soaking almonds.*
CREDIT: CATHERINE DOWNES

## Ingredients

2 cups almonds (See Soaking Guidelines in chapter 3.)
1½ cups water (or equal amount oat milk or coconut milk for a richer, creamier ricotta)
1 tsp salt (non-iodized), adjust salt to suit your preference
starter culture: ½ tsp water kefir or coconut kefir, or ¼–½ tsp raw apple cider vinegar (Flavor and texture outcomes will vary according to the choice of starter culture.)

## Method

1. Wash and sanitize all work surfaces and tools to be used.
2. Soak the almonds 1 hour to overnight in filtered water or rested tap water. If soaking overnight, do so in a covered container and in the refrigerator. If soaking at room temperature, do so in a covered container.

3. Peel the almonds. Use a little hot water to help during the peeling process. I usually add a little boiling water, and the skins pop off easily. Save skins for the compost.
4. In a high-speed blender, add some of the water (or choice of plant milk) and then the almonds.
5. Start at low speed, pulsing several times to gradually break down the almonds. This will ease the work of your blender and will produce better emulsification results.
6. Gradually increase speed. A preset function such as smoothie or ice cream can be helpful because the speed profile is intended to do emulsifying. Blend until smooth.

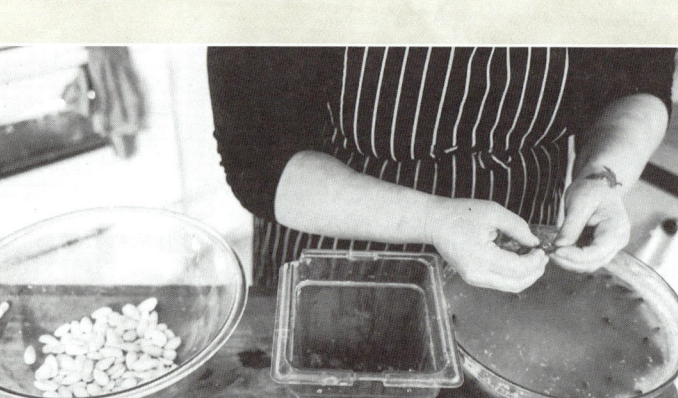

Left: *Peeling almonds.*
CREDIT: CATHERINE DOWNES

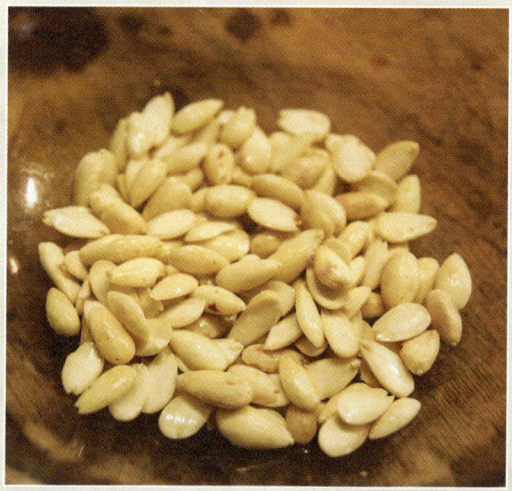

Right: *Peeled almonds.*
CREDIT: CATHERINE DOWNES

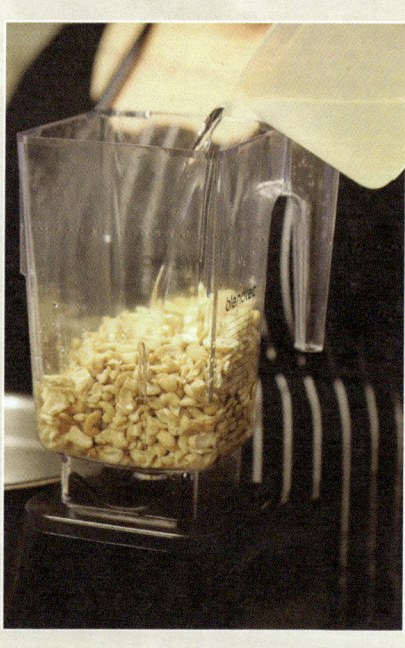

Left: *Adding water to the blender.*
CREDIT: CATHERINE DOWNES

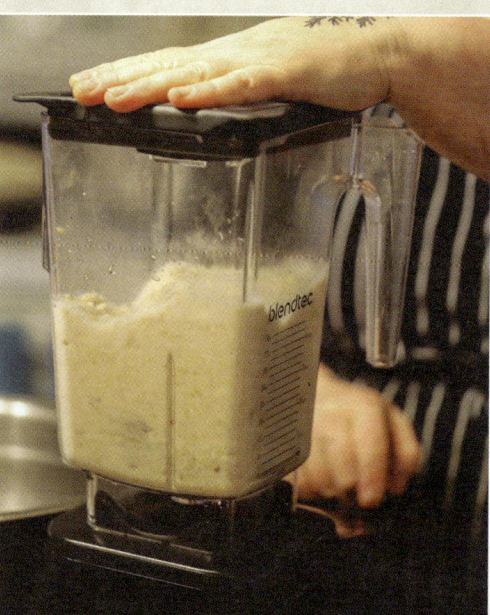

Right: *Blending almonds.* CREDIT: CATHERINE DOWNES

7. Scrape the mixture into a food grade container, and add the starter culture. Gently fold in. Place the lid on the container, ensuring that there is a space of ⅓ of the jar above the surface of the mixture for gas exchange.
8. Allow the mixture to culture 4 to 6 hours at room temperature (but if the room temperature is over 77°F (25°C) during summer months, reduce this to 2 to 4 hours) or in the refrigerator overnight if using water kefir coconut kefir or apple cider as culture.
9. After the mixture has finished culturing, place a sieve or colander over a bowl. Line the sieve or colander with cheesecloth or butter muslin. Using a spatula, scrape the cultured mixture into the cheesecloth. Sprinkle the salt over the top and gently fold into the mixture. Allow to drain for 1 to 3 hours at room temperature or in the refrigerator. Taste to adjust the salt flavor. The ricotta should be slightly tangy, have a creamy, non-grainy texture and a mellow flavor overall.

Insider tip: Save the strained fluid. It acts similarly to buttermilk and can be used in baking recipes!

## Storage

After draining the ricotta, store it in a covered container and in the refrigerator or use it in a recipe. Stored appropriately, it will keep for up to 5 days before it becomes too tangy, or sour. This is a fresh cheese and as such is meant to be consumed shortly after making.

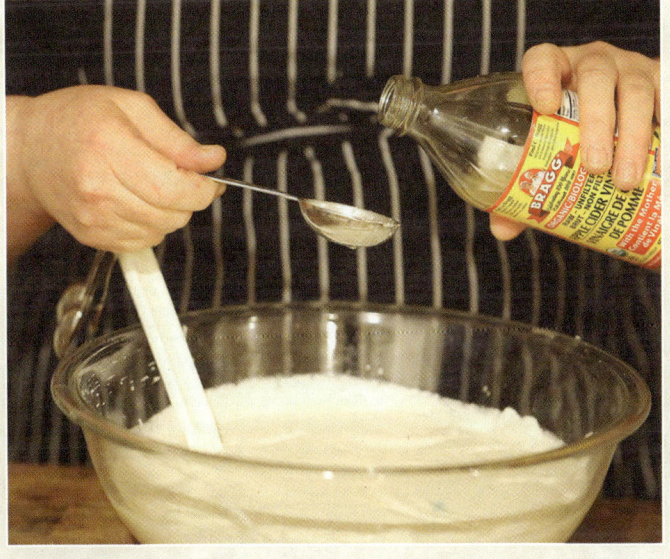

Above: *Adding apple cider vinegar as a starter culture to blended almond mixture.* CREDIT CATHERINE DOWNES

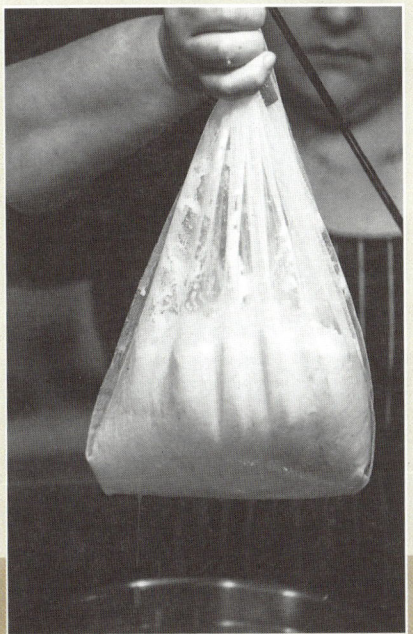

Left: *Draining cultured almond mixture.*
CREDIT: CATHERINE DOWNES

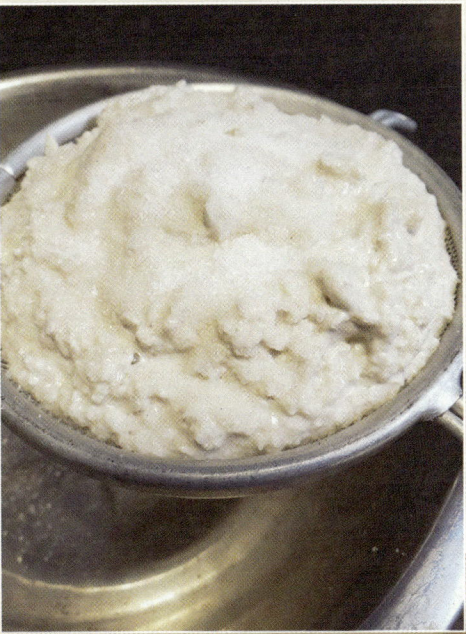

Right: *Texture after culturing and draining.*
CREDIT: CATHERINE DOWNES

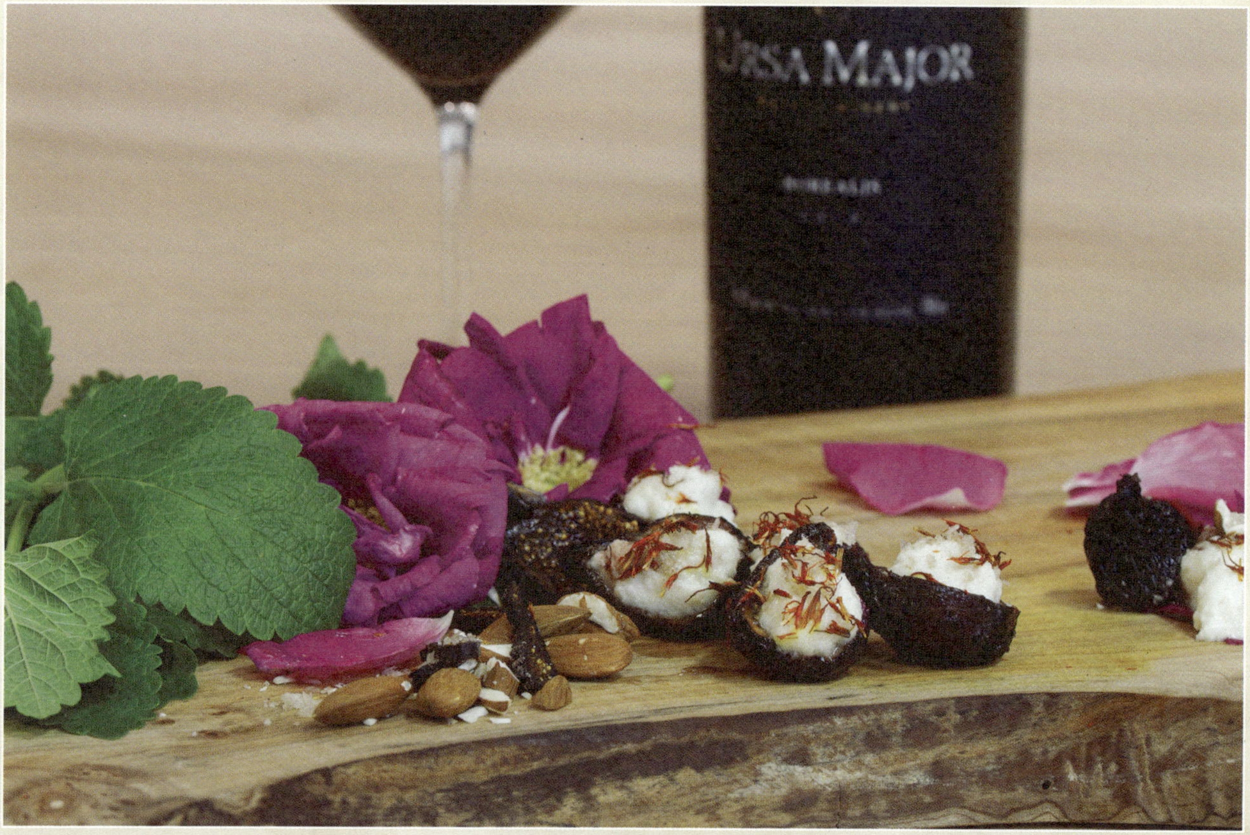

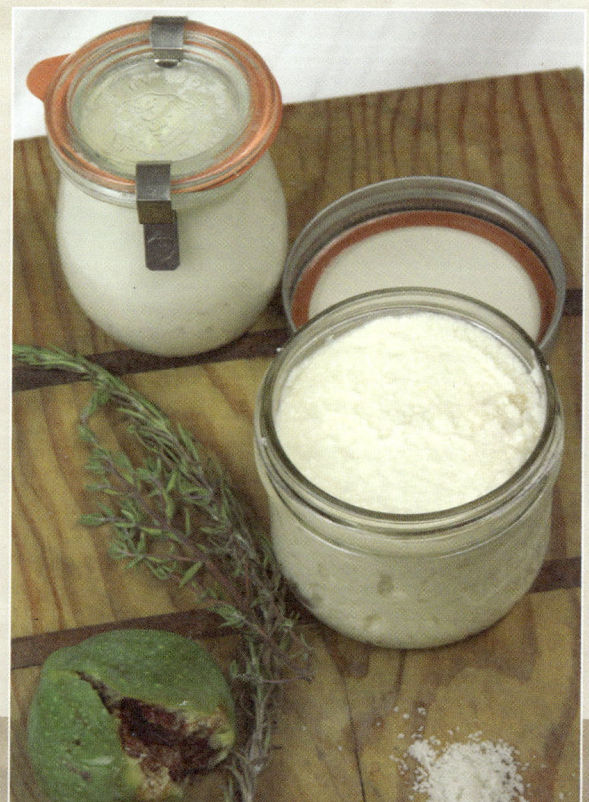

Above: *Almond Ricotta stuffed figs.*
CREDIT: COLIN MEDHURST

Right: *Jars of almond ricotta to be stored in refrigerator.* CREDIT: COLIN MEDHURST

# Farm-Style Cheese

This is a simple method for making a fresh, cultured soft cheese that can be flavored or used on its own. Its simplicity belies the possible applications. Mirroring the approach taken in traditional dairy cheesemaking, this cheese begins by heating up the matrix before adding the culture and relies on the acidity produced by the bacteria to create a curd. There is no additional use of enzymes to assist with further denaturing the proteins. This could be considered a lactic acid curd. The curd will not look like the curd formed by dairy milk in a similar process.

In dairy cheesemaking there are many versions of fresh, farm-style cheese that contain living cultures, all made slightly differently depending on regional traditions and preferences: quark, queso fresco, fromage frais, cottage cheese.

Macadamia nuts can be substituted for the cashews or combined with them, and white beans can also be combined with cashews. Use macadamia nuts as a straight substitution for cashews or use them in equal parts with cashews.

Use white beans such as lima or cannellini half and half with cashews or macadamia nuts. Note that white beans must be cooked before using, not just soaked.

### Tools and Equipment

High-speed blender (or food processor and less fancy blender)
Spatula
Thick cast saucepan
Probe thermometer
Container with lid for culturing
Cheesecloth or butter muslin
Measuring cups
Measuring spoons
Colander or fine mesh sieve
Bowl

### Ingredients

3 cups cashew nuts (or suggested substitution/combination above)
½ tsp salt (you may add more if you like)
1¼ cups water (filtered or rested tap water) plus more for blending as needed
½ cup high fat coconut milk or coconut cream
starter culture: 1 tsp rejuvelac, water kefir, or coconut kefir

### Method

1. Wash and sanitize all work surfaces and tools to be used.
2. Add the water and nuts (or nuts and cooked beans) to a high-speed blender. Starting on low speed, pulse several times to break down the solid materials.
3. Gradually work up to higher speed, stop periodically and scrape the mixture down the sides of the pitcher. If it is too thick and binding around the blender blades, add small amounts of water and blend at low to medium speed until the mixture is very smooth.
4. Scrape the mixture into the thick cast pot. I usually add about ¼ cup of water to the pot first to create a barrier between the bottom of the pot and the mixture during the initial heating process. Heat the mixture over low-medium heat, and stir occasionally. Use a probe thermometer to check the temperature,

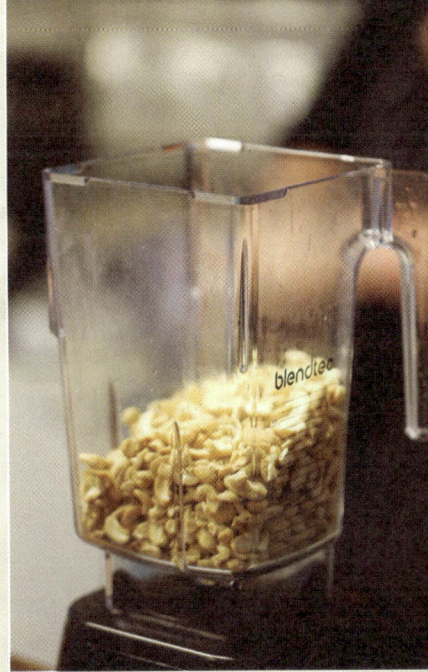

*Cashews in blender.*
CREDIT: CATHERINE DOWNES

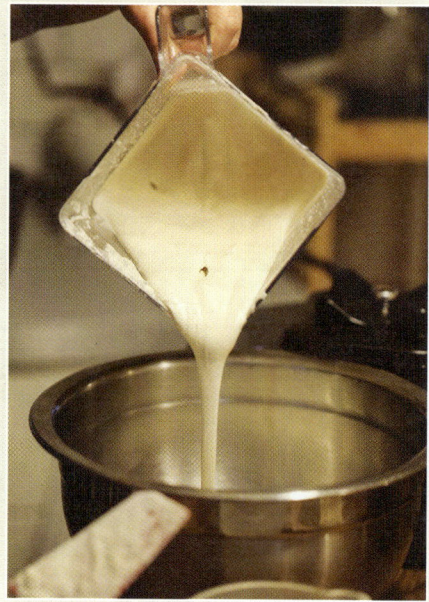

*Pouring blended cashew mix into a bowl prior to adding culture. The texture is thick but pourable.*
CREDIT: CATHERINE DOWNES

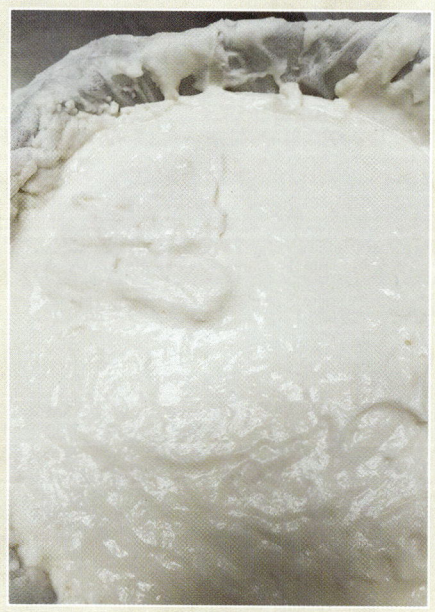

*Cultured mixture (after culturing period is finished).*

and once the mixture reaches 200°F (93°C), adjust heat levels to keep it at temperature or just below it. Do not allow the mixture to boil.

5. After 2 hours, remove the mixture from the heat and allow to cool to 105°F (40.5°C). When the mixture reaches this temperature, gently fold in the starter culture and place the mixture into a clean, sanitized container for the fermentation/culturing period. Cover the container with a fitted lid or otherwise impermeable covering. Leave the container in an even temperature area of the kitchen, making sure that it will not experience severe temperature changes. You are working with mesophilic cultures, which means the optimal range is between 62°F and 72°F (17°C and 22°C). Up to 77°F (25°C) can be okay for short periods of time, around 4 to 6 hours. Allow the mixture to culture from 24 to 48 hours.

   Note: When ambient temperature becomes a challenge during summer months, I break up the culturing period allowing the mixture to culture for a 12-hour period, refrigerate, and then remove from the refrigerator and allow it to culture for another 24 hours. This helps prevent the microbes from metabolizing the carbohydrate content too quickly, leading to overculturing. Generally, in a warmer ambient temperature the culturing time is shorter than in a cooler ambient temperature.

6. Check the mixture every 12 hours. You should observe small bubbles or expansion of the mixture. It should smell pleasant, from sweet-tangy to cheesy. You should taste it to ensure that acidity is forming. It should taste tangy. The mixture should start to appear clumpy like cottage cheese.

7. The longer the mixture cultures the greater the amount of moisture is released from the mixture, and it will become firmer.

8. After the culturing period has finished, you have a lactic acid cultured curd. Lactic acid powder alone will not give you this transformation. The physical change in the mixture from blended smoothness to cottage cheese-like is a result of microbes metabolizing the carbohydrates and lactic acid produced by the bacteria breaking down protein.

9. Place a colander or fine mesh sieve into a bowl and line with cheesecloth or butter muslin. Scrape the mixture into the cheesecloth and sprinkle salt over the surface. Gently fold the salt into this lactic acid cultured curd. Allow the mixture to rest in the cheesecloth in the sieve for up to 4 hours at room temperature, or overnight in the refrigerator. The longer it rests in this stage, the more moisture it will lose, and the firmer it will become.

10. After draining, or what I call moisture removal, (because the moisture loss from the curd will be more from evaporation and absorption of moisture by the cheesecloth than from loose draining) you can then shape the curd by rolling it into a log shape in cheesecloth or placing it inside a shaping mold for 1 to 2 days. If you choose to do this, place the cheese in the mold or in the log shape on top of a bamboo mat or small wooden board, put into a container, and keep in the refrigerator. This will give you a soft, but nicely shaped fresh cheese that will look good for presentations.

You may also choose to forego the above step and simply keep the cheese stored in a sealed container in the refrigerator.

## Storage

This cheese can keep, stored properly, for up to 30 days.

**Ways to use this cheese**

Tacos

Flatbreads

As a spread

As a base for cultured vegan cheesecake

With fresh fruit and maple syrup

However you wish

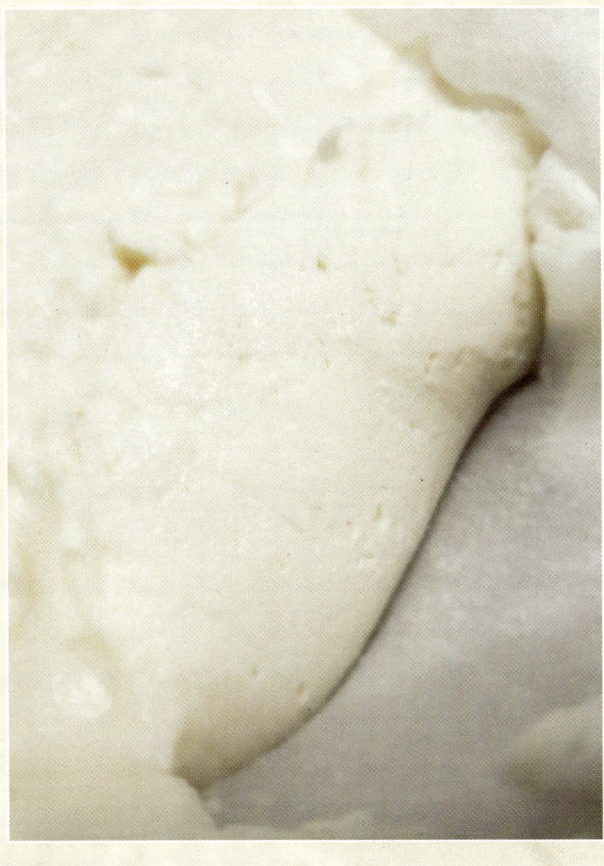

*Drained lactic acid curd/fresh cheese.*

# Chèvre-Style Cheese

This is another soft cultured cheese that can be aged up or consumed right after the culturing period. The primary difference between this method and the previous one is that this one does not require you to heat the mixture before adding the starter culture. They both use mesophilic cultures. Making each of these recipes allows you to compare and contrast the impact heat has on the ingredients and subsequently on the overall outcome of the cheeses.

I use the term "chèvre-style" here only to reference the general similarity of texture in the cheese after a short aging period. It does not taste like chèvre, obviously, as it is not made with goat milk.

## Tools and Equipment

High-speed blender (or food processor and less fancy blender)
Food-grade plastic bowl or container for culturing
Spatula
Measuring cups
Measuring spoons
Colander or fine mesh sieve
Bowl
Reusable food wrap to cover culturing container
Cheesecloth or butter muslin

## Ingredients

2 cups macadamia nuts, soaked*
1 cup cashews, soaked* (or substitute 1 cup of cooked white beans in place of the cashews. The flavor of the cheese will be a little more earthy/umami than sweet/tangy.)
½ tsp salt
1½ cups water (filtered or rested tap water) plus more for blending as needed
starter culture: 2 tsp coconut kefir or ⅛ tsp direct-set mesophilic culture

*The cashews and the macadamia nuts should be soaked separately. See Soaking Guidelines in chapter 3.

## Method

1. Add the water and nuts to a high-speed blender. I usually start with the macadamias first and pulse a few times before adding the cashews, as the macadamias are harder than the cashews.
2. Start on low speed and gradually work up to higher speed, stopping to periodically scrape down the mixture from the sides of the blender. If it's too thick and binding around the blender blades, add small amounts of water and blend at low to medium speed until the mixture is very smooth.
3. Scrape the mixture into a clean and sanitized container. Add the starter culture and gently fold into the mixture.
4. Cover the mixture in the container and allow it to culture at room temperature 24 to 48 hours. Check every 12 hours.
5. If you chose coconut kefir as your starter culture, you should observe bubble activity (evidence the culture is happy and healthy) and find it tastes mildly to moderately tangy. If you chose the direct-set mesophilic starter, bubbles are less likely, but you

will definitely notice changes in aroma. In either case, make sure to taste and smell the mixture each time you check it.

6. After the culturing period is finished, place a sieve inside a bowl, and line the sieve with cheesecloth or butter muslin. Place the cultured mixture into the cheesecloth.

7. Sprinkle salt lightly over the surface of the curd, and gently fold in. Allow the mixture to drain/lose moisture for up to 4 hours at room temperature. If you wish to evaporate more moisture, place the bowl/sieve/cheese in the refrigerator and allow it to continue to lose moisture for up to 24 hours (or longer if necessary).

8. After draining, you can elect to keep the cheese as is and store it in a clean, sanitized, covered container in the refrigerator. This can keep for up to 30 days. Flavor will continue to develop over time, and the cheese will continue to firm up.

9. Alternatively, you can also elect to form the cheese. I like to roll the cheese into logs and garnish with fresh herbs on the surface. To shape, place the curd onto cheesecloth on top of a bamboo mat. Fold the cheesecloth over the cheese, and gently encourage it into a log shape and roll it. Place the cheesecloth-wrapped cheese on the bamboo mat (or a small wooden board), place inside a larger container, and store in the refrigerator. Turn the cheese over each day during this aging time, and check the container daily for moisture, removing excess moisture as necessary. Remove from cheesecloth after 5 to 7 days or when the cheese feels firm enough to touch that you can handle it without it squishing in your hand.

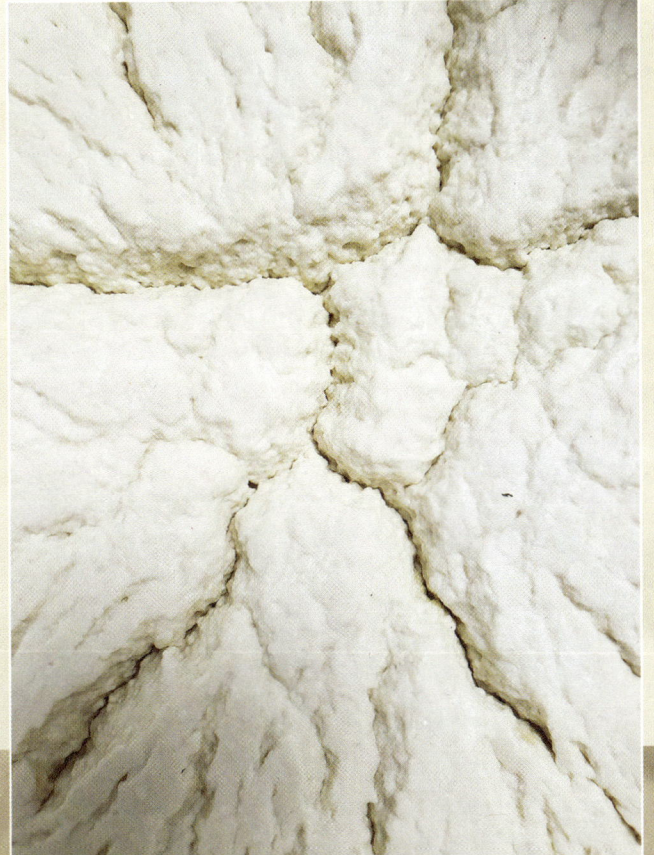
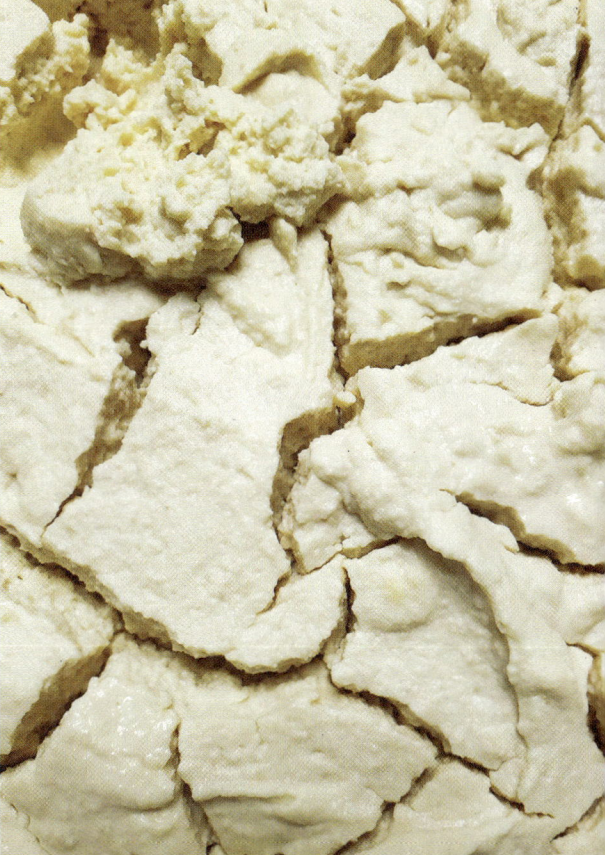

Bottom left: *Lactic acid cultured cashew curd (42-hour ferment at 66°F/19°C).*

Bottom right: *Lactic acid cultured oat and cashew mixture (46-hour ferment at 66°F/19°C).*

The flavor should be lightly salty and moderately to slightly more tangy. It should have a creamy mouthfeel and hold together when picked up with your fingers. It should also hold shape under heat and sustain a bit of torching when heating it up in the oven. It will melt more readily than traditional goat cheese but should still retain some form. This is a good base cheese to use for exploring flavor profiles and aging times.

## Flavoring Options

This is an easy cheese to modify, and you can be creative with your choices; however, there are some limitations to consider in making your choice of modifications.

Fresh ingredients: You may add ingredients like fresh garlic or fresh herbs like basil, but if you do, the cheese will need to be consumed within 5 days. Fresh ingredients trapped in a wet, fatty mixture, can increase the risk of pathogen growth. So, fresh ingredients mean you consume this as a young, fresh cheese. Fresh herbs can be applied to the surface of the cheese, as they will air dry.

Dried ingredients: Adding dried herbs, spices, dried fruit, sundried tomatoes, or dried mushroom or pepper flakes is recommended for cheese that will age longer than 5 days. The inherent moisture of these ingredients has been removed, making them less risky. Do note that adding dried fruit will stimulate the living cultures in the cheese, and can produce some enzymatic and wine notes.

Preserved/brined ingredients: You can also add ingredients such as preserved lemon, rind and some flesh are okay, or ingredients such as pickled hot peppers and olives. They have been fermented or preserved in a salt brine, which protects them from pathogen growth. Keep in mind that should you add ingredients from this spectrum, you may want to add a little less salt at the salting stage.

Truffle and black pepper: Before draining the cultured curd add 1–2 tsp crushed black peppercorns (or rainbow mix peppercorns), 1 tsp white or black truffle paste, or 1 Tbsp shaved then crumbled fresh truffle. Fold these into the curd gently, ensuring even spread throughout. Then proceed with the draining/moisture evaporation process for the next 12 to 24 hours in the refrigerator. After the moisture evaporation process you can consume the cheese or follow step 9 above to age the cheese for up to 30 days.

Fig and cassis: I love dried fig or cherry compote made with cassis, a black current liqueur, a cheeseboard condiment I make frequently for when I am catering special events. This modification is based on that.

1. Add ⅛ cup very finely diced dried fig at the time of blending and culture it along with the rest of the mixture. This will add a mildly wine-type flavor.
2. After the culturing phase is completed add another ⅛ cup of chopped fig mixed with 1 Tbsp cassis, and 2 tsp maple syrup. Proceed with the draining/moisture evaporation steps.

Preserved Lemon and Sage: At Blue Heron we make a seasonal cheese, our Winter Cheese, which features preserved lemon (that we make in advance), and sage. While I will not provide the full recipe for that particular cheese, I will share a modification featuring these two ingredients that pair so well together.

After the culturing phase and at the same time that you add the salt, add 2 tsp chopped preserved lemon zest (or 1 tsp dried lemon zest), and 1tsp sage powder. Fold the ingredients into the curd, and proceed with the draining/moisture absorption steps. If you decide to roll the cheese into a log shape, you can place fresh sage leaves on top and allow them to dry in place.

## Storage

This cheese can age up to 30 days in the refrigerator, but it can be eaten any time before that.

## Forming and Aging for Short-Term Aging

This particular cheese can be served young (after 48 hours of culturing) or can be aged for a short amount of time, up to 30 days, in the home refrigerator.

I provide more in-depth information on specific cheese aging processes further on, but to start, here is an outline of the steps for shaping and initial aging of chèvre-style cheese (with or without modifications).

1. Once the initial culturing, salting, and draining has occurred, form the cheese into logs (do this after you add other elements if using one of the above amendments).
2. Set up a bamboo mat or small wooden cheese board, and lay out some doubled up cheesecloth or butter muslin.
3. Place the drained, salted curd (with or without additions), in the center or just off center of the cheesecloth. With your clean, washed hands, gently shape the curd into a log. I fold a portion of the cheesecloth overtop, gently roll the mixture into place, pat the ends, and continue to do this until I have an even shape. I then roll the cheese in the cheesecloth and fold the ends over until the cheese is fully swaddled.
4. Place the bamboo mat/board with the cheese on top inside a container large enough to allow for airflow. Place this in the refrigerator, making sure there is nothing that will touch the cheese. Do not cover fully; leave the cover on top of the container a little ajar to allow for airflow.
5. Allow this air drying to occur for up to 5 days. Then remove the cheese from the cheesecloth. During the aging time, check the container each day and wipe away any moisture from the container or from the bamboo mat/wooden board. Flip/turn the cheese to allow for even removal of moisture.

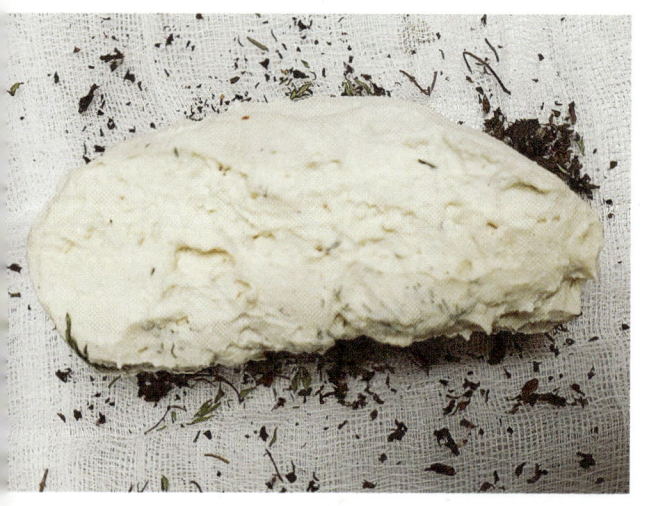

Top: *Placing the loose lactic acid curd into the cheesecloth with herbs.*

Bottom left: *Beginning log rolling.*

Bottom right: *A slightly different approach to rolling the cheese in cheesecloth.*
Credit: Andre Shepperd

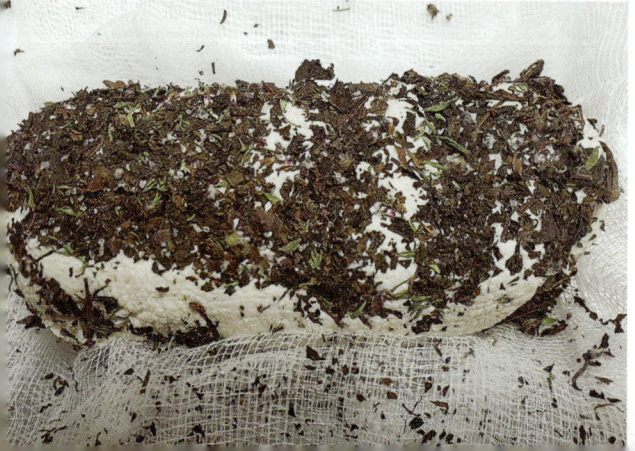

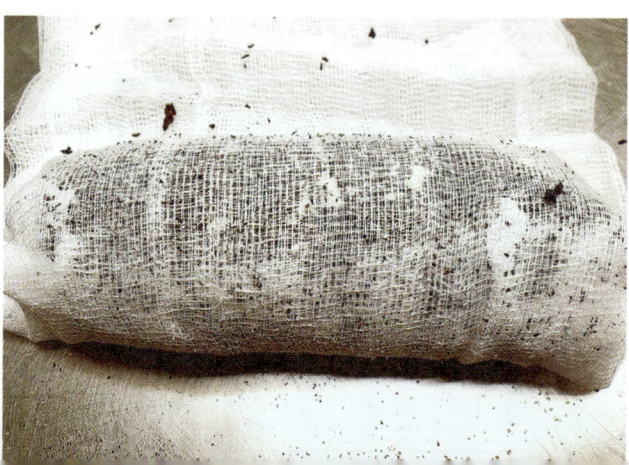

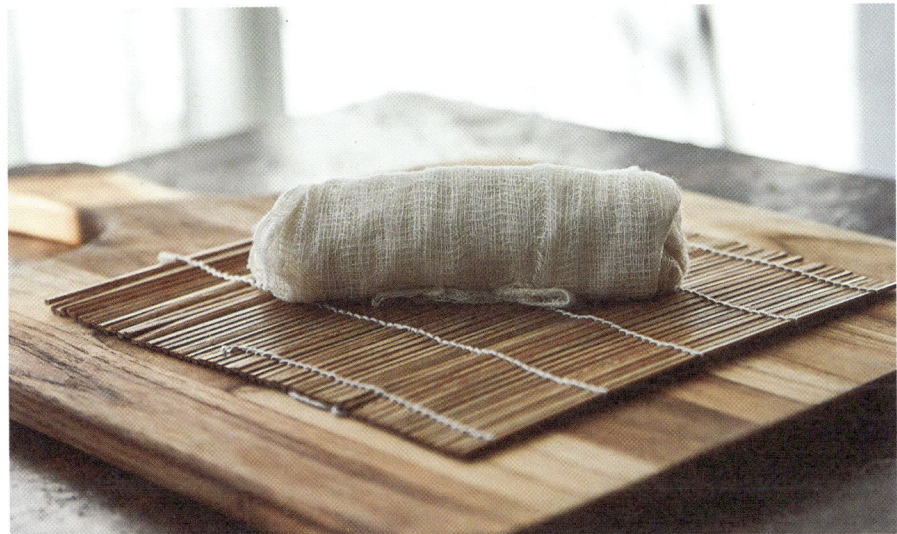

*Cheese wrapped in cheesecloth sitting on a bamboo mat prior to being placed in a ripening box and then in the refrigerator.*
Credit: Andre Shepperd

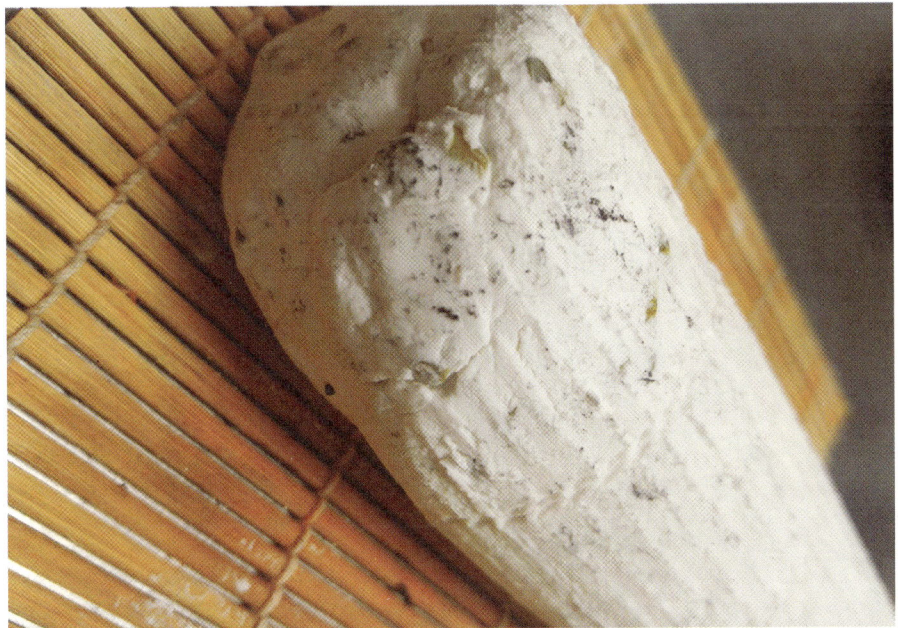

*Cheese removed from cheesecloth and resting on bamboo mat.*

6. Once the cheese is out of the cheesecloth, you can continue to age it on the bamboo mat or wooden board (inside the larger container or ripening box), in the refrigerator, allowing you to keep it longer than the fresh cheeses or cheeze, up to 30 days in ideal conditions. Continue to check the cheese daily, and sprinkle a small amount of salt on the surface every 2 to 3 days. This will continue to pull moisture out of the cheese and protect the surface.

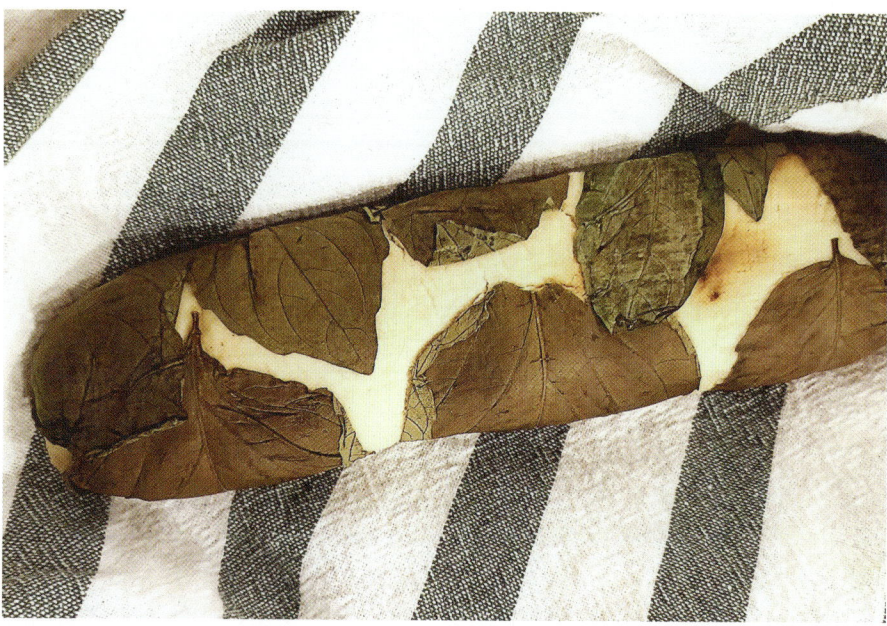

*Basil leaf wrapped chèvre-style cheese, from a student in my course The Art of Plant-based Cheesemaking, 2019.*

## Coconut Kefir-based Cheeses

It should be apparent by now that my approach in this book is to focus on method and understanding how materials behave and is not about any personal inspiration stories I might have. I will leave the combination of storytelling and recipes to those in the food blogging realm or maybe for my students.

Developing vegan cheese styles and nomenclature that can be understood globally, a language of our own that parallels and intersects with the traditional dairy cheesemaking terminology, is an ongoing project that I pursue with other vegan cheesemakers. An important part of developing practice specific language is doing the experimental work. There is nothing like working with live cultures and different mediums without the infrastructure of a funded research lab to teach you that you know very little about many things.

With more mediums to test than dairy cheesemaking has, there is a wide realm of prospective outcomes to explore. Animal milks, while differing somewhat, are on the whole more consistent and similar in their molecular content and behavior in culturing than the difference, for instance, between cashew and any of sunflower seed, white bean, lupini, or coconut milk. Each of these has different kinds of protein, different kinds of polysaccharides (carbohydrate), and different types of fat, never mind amounts. How cultures behave in mediums made from these will differ, and the outcomes will vary more significantly from one another than would, for example, fresh cheeses made from cow milk and sheep milk.

# Coconut Kefir Cheese: three ways

In this section I provide some simple coconut milk based cheeses. These can be made as written, or you can include nuts or legumes in the culturing stage to create different profiles of cheese. I recommend making these as written first so that you can see how coconut milk changes with culturing and understand how it ages.

Use high quality coconut milk, high fat, with a good extraction rate. This information can be found on the nutritional panel of the can or Tetra Pak. In terms of coconut milk fat percentage, I recommend 18% or higher and in terms of extraction rate, 60% or higher. See the section on making coconut kefir for more detail about sourcing coconut milk and making coconut kefir, which will serve as your starter culture for these methods.

This one approach can be used to create three different styles of cultured vegan cheese: labneh, soft cream cheese, and semi-firm cheese. Each of these requires a different method for aging after the culturing period, and these are excellent examples of how a common curd can produce different styles of cheese based on how you age it.

If you have read the first edition of this book, you will notice that this section is significantly different. I have eliminated the non-heated coconut milk approach for two reasons: one, the potential for food safety issues (though I have had none occur, I prefer to err on the side of caution) and two, the heated milk method produces much better taste and textural results.

**Tools and Equipment**

Thick cast sauce pot
Food-grade plastic container for culturing
Measuring cups
Measuring spoons
Probe thermometer
Wooden or silicone spoon
Spatula
Cheesecloth or butter muslin
Fine mesh sieve
Bamboo mat, cheese aging mat, or small wooden cheese board (for making semi-firm cheese after the main process is finished)
Container for storing cheese during ripening/aging in refrigerator

## Ingredients

2 L coconut milk, full fat
2 cups coconut cream
starter culture: ¼ cup coconut kefir
2 tsp maple syrup
½–1 tsp salt

## Method

1. Wash and sanitize all work surfaces and all equipment that you plan to use.
2. Empty the coconut milk and coconut cream into a thick cast sauce pot.
3. Heat the coconut milk to 185°F (85°C) over low-medium heat. You want to heat moderately slowly to avoid reaching the boiling temperature. Use the probe thermometer to check the temperature during the heating process.
4. Once the coconut milk and cream mixture has reached the prescribed temperature, remove it from heat. Begin an active cooling process: set the pot on an ice bath, or use frequent stirring to cool the mixture to 120°F (49°C). Add the maple syrup and

stir in. The maple syrup will serve as extra food for the culturing microbes when you add them.

5. Continue active cooling until the mixture reaches 105°F (40.5°C). Add the 1/4 cup coconut kefir (this is the starter culture), and stir in.

6. Pour the mixture into a food grade container that has a lid. Make sure that you have ⅓ of the container as headspace space above the top of the mixture to allow for gas exchange.

7. Cover the container and leave it to culture for 24 to 48 hours in an area of your kitchen that maintains an even temperature. In cooler weather, you may place the covered container in the oven with just the oven light on. Just be sure to leave a note telling others in your household that you have a sensitive culturing project in the oven. The optimal temperature range for culturing this cheese is 62°F–72°F (17°C–22°C). It can sustain temperature exposure up to 77°F (25°C), but it will start to acidify too quickly if it cultures at too warm a temperature for too long.

8. Check the mixture every 12 hours during the culturing period. Observe the mixture for changes in appearance, smell, and taste. If it is not developing acidity quickly enough, which you will notice when you taste the mixture, you can add a bit more maple syrup to encourage the culture to feed, or wrap the container in a thick towel to increase the temperature. This is more of an issue in cooler months.

9. After the culturing period is finished, place the mixture in the refrigerator and allow it to rest overnight. Sometimes you will observe separation of the cultured solids from the whey, or liquid. This is normal, and the amount of separation depends upon the quality of the coconut milk and cream that you use.

Left: *Coconut kefir culturing in jar.*

Right: *Coconut kefir draining in cheesecloth-lined sieve.*

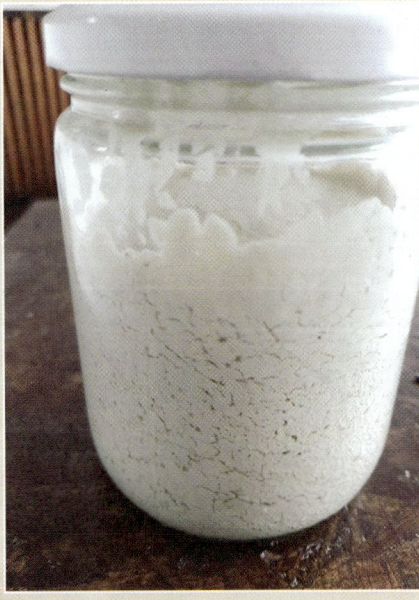
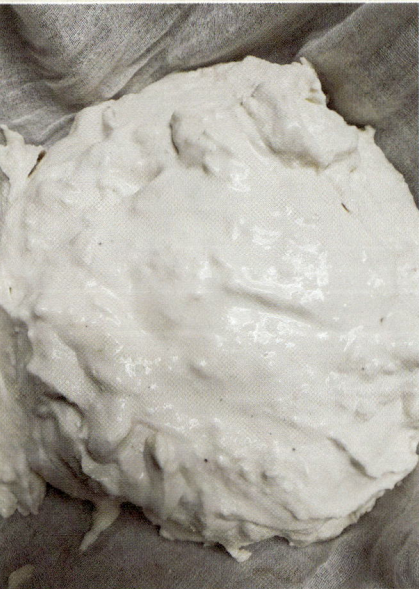

10. After the refrigeration period, decide which direction you want to take your coconut kefir curd:
    a. labneh, a pressed yogurt, soured milk fresh cheese, common in Middle Eastern and Jewish cuisines;
    b. soft cream cheese style, ages longer than the labneh, a good base for cultured vegan cheesecakes;
    c. semi-firm cheese, slices well but does not hold well under heat and is best used for uncooked dishes or eating on its own.

## Labneh

Labneh, as mentioned, is used widely in Middle Eastern and Jewish cuisines. It is a salted, strained yogurt that is used as an addition to many meals. While this coconut milk kefir curd is not a true labneh (yogurt is made with thermophilic cultures; kefir is made with mesophilic cultures), this will give you a similar result and usefulness.

## Method

1. After step 9 above, set up a bowl and place a fine mesh sieve inside it. Line the sieve with cheesecloth or butter muslin.
2. Place the coconut kefir in the cloth, and sprinkle salt over it. Use the spatula to fold the salt in. Wait 30 minutes and taste to see if you need more salt.
3. Allow this mixture to drain/lose moisture for up to 4 hours at room temperature, and overnight in the refrigerator, if not already quite thick.
4. After the salting and draining, the labneh/pressed sour cream is ready to use.

## Storage

Store in a clean, sanitized, covered container in the refrigerator for up to 30 days.

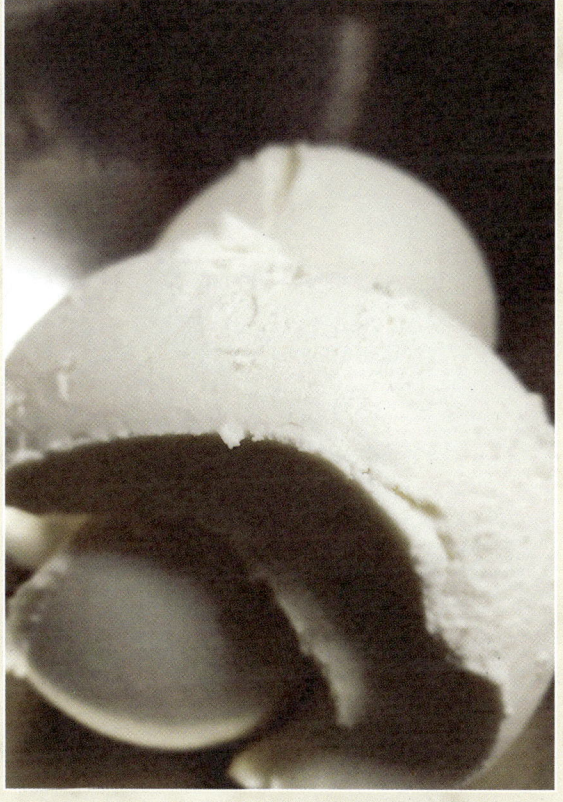

*Labneh-style coconut kefir after being drained for 30 hours.*

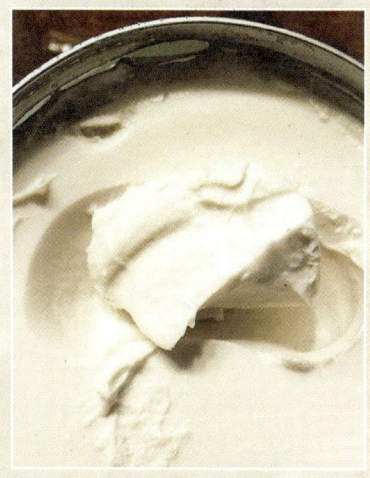

*Coconut kefir cultured 48 hours and rested in the refrigerator overnight.*

## Soft cream cheese

Aging the coconut kefir curd a little longer than for labneh produces a cream cheese style cheese. The primary difference between this and the labneh is the amount of time you allow the curd to lose moisture. The longer you focus on helping the curd evaporate moisture, the thicker the cream cheese will be. You can add herbs, spices, or dried fruit to it before aging it. It makes a very nice, bright, tangy, herb and garlic cream cheese, perfect on toasted bagels or sourdough bread. This also makes a delicious tzatziki!

### Method

1. After step 9 (refrigeration of the coconut kefir after culturing), set up a bowl and place a fine mesh sieve inside it. Line the sieve with cheesecloth or butter muslin.
2. Place the coconut kefir inside the cloth, and sprinkle salt over it. If you are adding dried herbs or spices, now is the time to do so. Use the spatula to fold the salt (and herbs or spices) into the mixture. Wait 30 minutes and taste to see if you need more salt.
3. Allow the mixture to drain/loose moisture for 2 to 4 days in the refrigerator. Leave the mixture in the cloth-lined sieve and bowl setup, and place a light covering overtop.
4. Each day check the consistency of the cream cheese. When it is as thick as you want, you can store it or use it. If you wish to add ingredients like dried fruit or preserved lemon, now is the time to do it. Fold in any additions.
5. Store the coconut kefir cream cheese in a sealed container.

### Storage

This cheese should be stored in the refrigerator. If fresh herbs or garlic have been added, this cheese should be consumed within 7 days.

## Semi-firm cream cheese

By now, you should be identifying a theme in the progression from coconut kefir curd to different thicknesses or firmness of the cheese you wish to make. The key concept in this progression is the amount of time needed for moisture removal. Moisture removal can be straining, draining, evaporation, absorption, or pressing, and oftentimes two or more methods are used simultaneously.

The coconut kefir curd ages up quite well and is a relatively safe cheese to age in the home environment without fancy equipment or a refrigerator specifically used for aging cheese. This cheese has a high acidity, and this helps protect it from pathogens.

### Method

1. After step 9 (refrigeration of the coconut kefir after culturing), set up a bowl, and place a fine mesh sieve inside it. Line the sieve with cheesecloth or butter muslin.

Fresh Cultured Cheeses    101

2. Place the coconut kefir in the cloth, and sprinkle salt over it. If you are adding dried herbs or spices, now is the time to do so. Use the spatula to fold the salt (and herbs or spices) into the mixture. Wait 30 minutes and taste to see if you need more salt.
3. Allow the mixture to drain/loose moisture overnight in the refrigerator. Leave the mixture in the cloth-lined sieve and bowl setup, and place a light covering overtop. Check the mixture the next day. If you wish to add dried fruit at this time, do so, and fold in. Sprinkle an additional ½ tsp salt into the mixture.
4. You may need another layer of cheesecloth at this point to assist with moisture removal. Take the cheese in cheesecloth and remove it from the sieve. Place another layer (or two) of cheesecloth in the sieve, and then return the cheese in cheesecloth, and leave in the sieve in the refrigerator for another 12 hours or overnight.
5. After the main drainage/moisture removal period is over, you are ready to shape the cheese. On a bamboo mat or small wooden board, lay out clean cheesecloth or butter muslin, place the salted, drained cheese onto the cloth, and shape it into an even round or a log. You may also use a stainless steel hoop or cheese mold to shape the cheese. Line the hoop or mold with cheesecloth or butter muslin

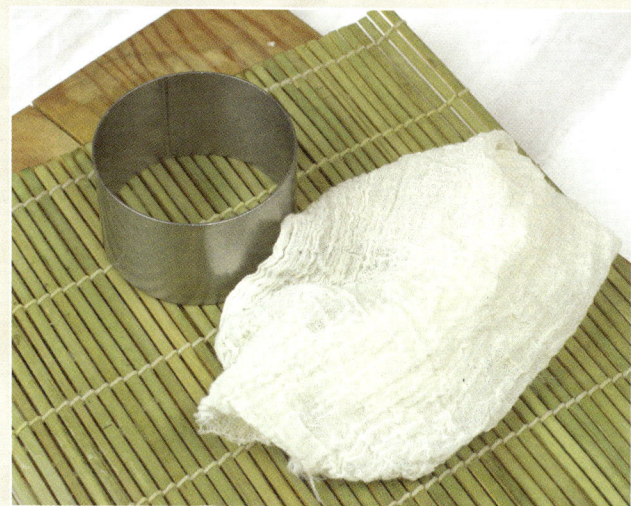

*Stainless steel ring mold, bamboo mat, cheesecloth.*
CREDIT: COLIN MEDHURST

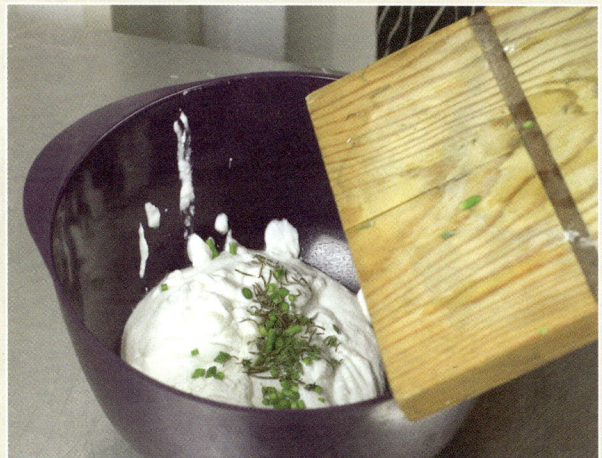

*Adding herbs and chopped garlic scapes to cheese.*
CREDIT: COLIN MEDHURST

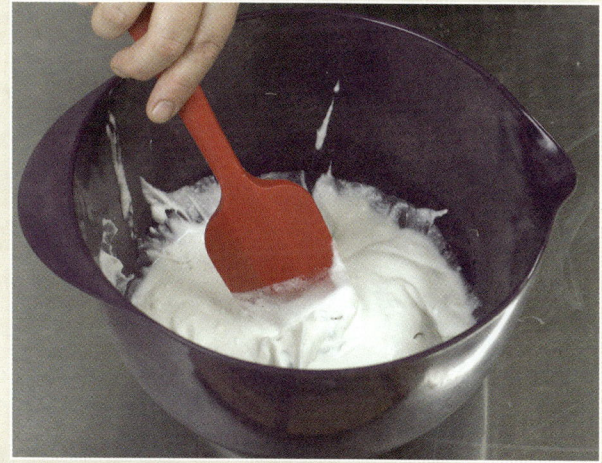

*Folding in herbs and chopped garlic scapes.*
CREDIT: COLIN MEDHURST

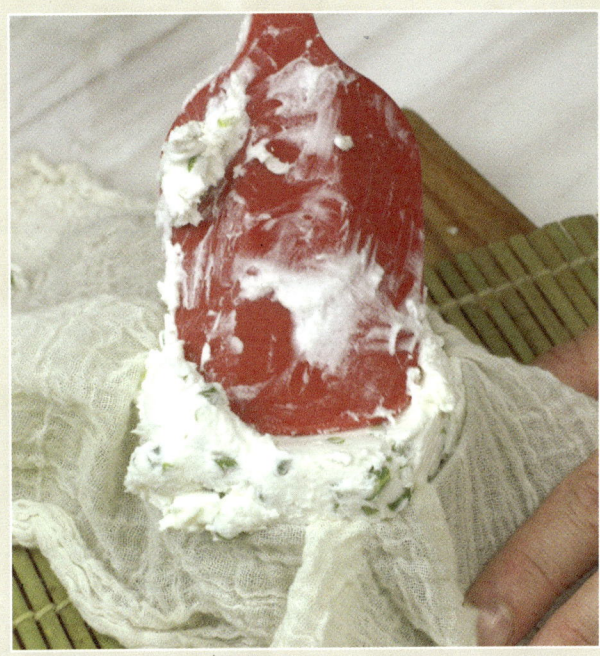

*Pressing coconut kefir cheese with garlic scapes and herbs into a cheesecloth lined cheese mold.* CREDIT: COLIN MEDHURST

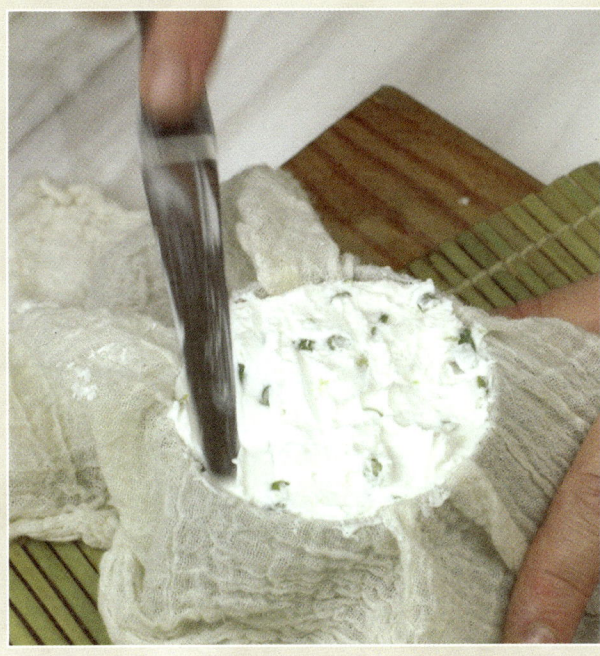

*Smoothing top of coconut kefir cheese.* CREDIT: COLIN MEDHURST

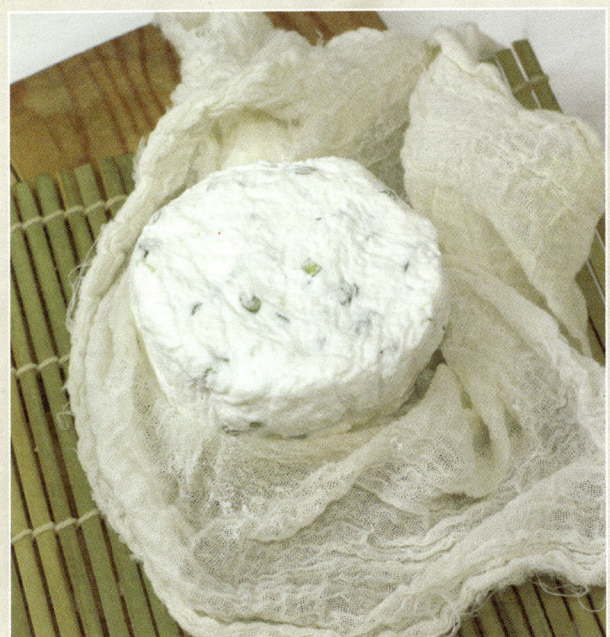

*Removing the cream cheese from the ring mold and cheesecloth.* CREDIT: COLIN MEDHURST

and add the cheese. Ensure the cheese surface does not have cracks or fissures. You will likely have enough to make 1 or 2 cheeses.

6. Place the wrapped cheese or the cheese mold or hoop on the bamboo mat or the board, and put this inside a container large enough to allow for airflow. Place this entire setup in the refrigerator.

7. Check the cheese daily, and flip and turn it. Wipe away excess moisture from inside the container, and when the bamboo mat becomes too wet, change it out.

8. Do this daily for 2 to 5 days. By day 3 or 4 you should be able to remove the cheese from the cheesecloth and allow it to continue to air dry (in the container, in the refrigerator) for another 7 to 14 days. Every few days, check there is no unwelcome growth on the surface. Pat down the surface with a little salt or brine (see section on brining in chapter 6 for instructions for making brine). Light salting or a brine wash protects the cheese from unwanted surface growth.

9. This cheese should be semi-firm to firm and be sliceable. This also makes a great base for cultured non-baked vegan cheesecakes.

## Storage

Store this cheese in the refrigerator and on a piece of cheese aging mat, butter muslin, or on a small wooden board or bamboo mat and place inside a covered container. The cheese will keep for up to 30 days (after aging is finished).

## Flavoring Options (for soft cream cheese and semi-firm cheese)

The soft cream cheese and the semi-firm cheese are well suited to the addition of herbs, spices, dried fruit, and ingredients like dried olives and pickled peppers. Modifications should be made based on how you intend to use the cheese and on how long you want to age it for.

Fresh ingredients can be used, but only if you plan to consume the end result within 5 to 7 days.

Dried, preserved, or fermented ingredients should be used for anything that you wish to age beyond 5 days. Recommended flavor additions are: black peppercorn, cumin seed, dried garlic, dried onion, your favorite mixture of dried herbs, dried marigold, dried fruit such as apricot, cherry, blueberries, figs, and candied ginger.

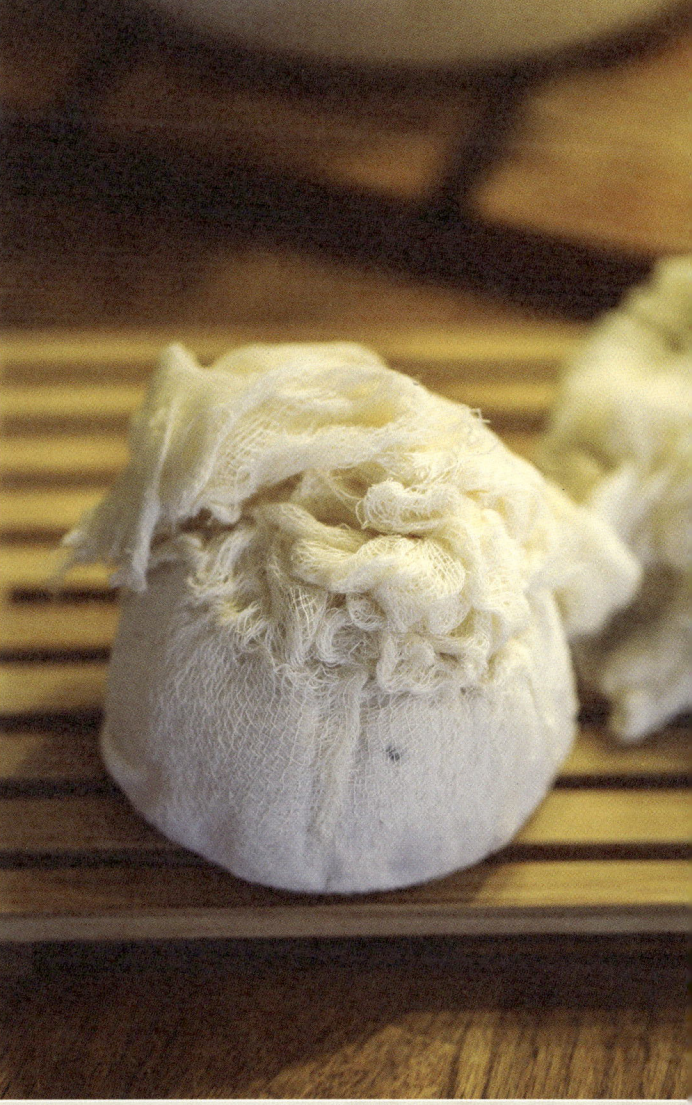

*Rounds of coconut kefir cheese in cheesecloth on aging mat.* Credit: Catherine Downes

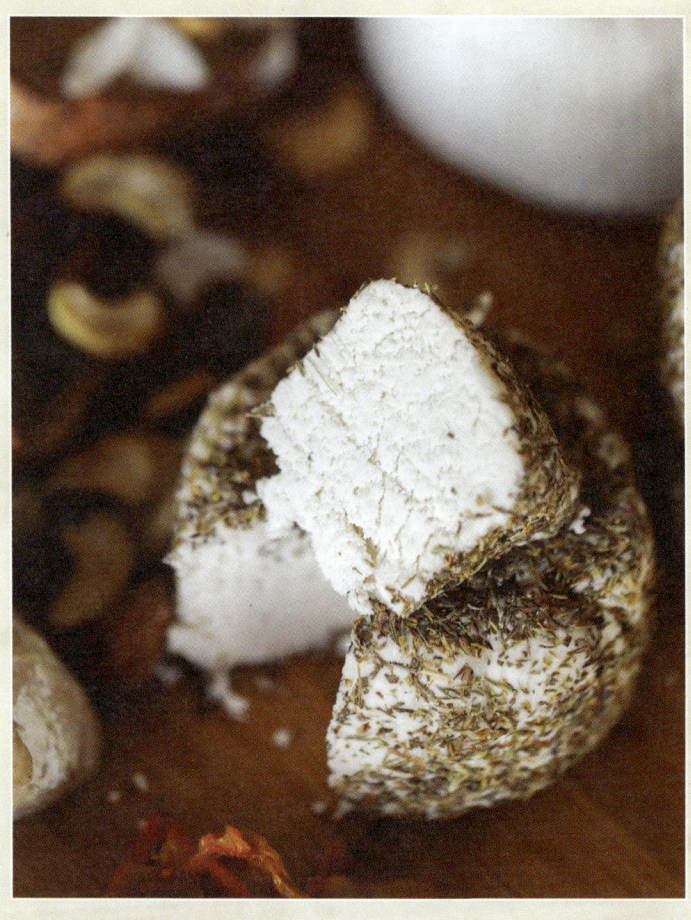

This semi-firm cheddar-style cheese can take on different flavor profiles. The cheese on the right has an herb rind, and the cheese below is infused with spices and finished with a smoked paprika rind. CREDIT: CATHERINE DOWNES, COLIN MEDHURST

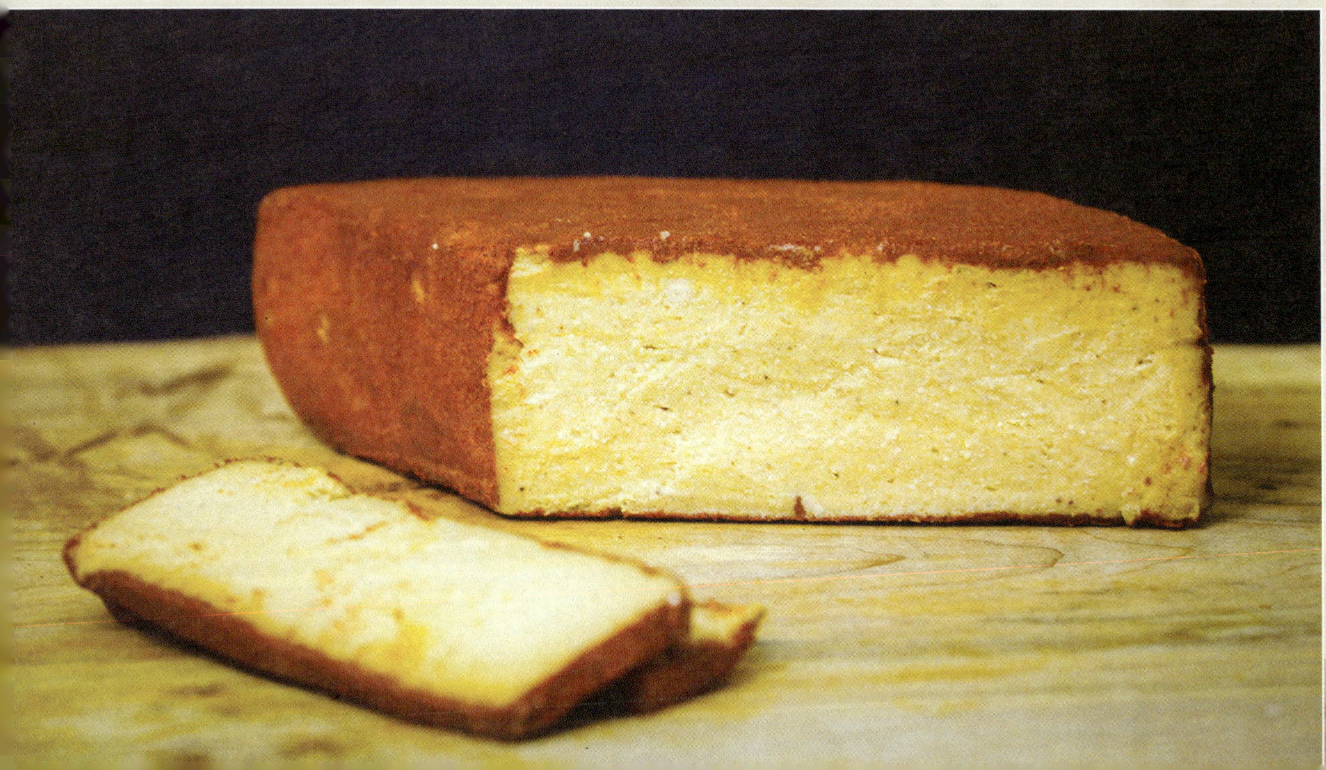

# Lemon-Garlic-Herb Coconut Kefir Cheese with Macadamia

This cheese is a perfect light fresh cheese that does develop a bit more complexity if you choose to age it. If you avoid the lemon, garlic, and herb, the base makes an excellent cultured vegan cheesecake. As it is, with the lemon, garlic, and herbs, it makes a lovely vegan frittata or quiche.

**Tools and Equipment**

High-speed blender
Bamboo mat or wooden board
Cheesecloth or butter muslin
Cheese paper
Cheese mold or stainless steel ring
Fine mesh sieve
Thick cast pot
Ripening box
Food grade container

## Ingredients

2 cups macadamia nuts, soaked
2 cups coconut kefir curd
2 tsp salt
1 Tbsp lemon zest (wash the lemon first) or dried lemon zest
2 tsp garlic powder
2 Tbsp herbs of your choice (I like to use rosemary, dill, tarragon.), fresh, minced (or 3 Tbsp dried herbs)
1 cup water (filtered or rested tap water) for blending

## Method 1

1. Soak the macadamia nuts overnight.
2. In a high-speed blender add ½ of the water and all the macadamia nuts.
3. Start on low speed, progressing gradually to high speed. Blend the nuts until very smooth. Add the lemon juice, salt, garlic, and more water if needed.
4. When blended completely, add the coconut kefir curd and pulse until the mixture is emulsified. Scrape from the pitcher into a food grade container, cover and allow to culture at room temperature, between 62°F and 72°F (17°C and 22°C) for 24 to 30 hours. During the culturing phase, be sure to taste, smell, and observe how the mixture is changing. If it is becoming too acidic too quickly, refrigerate overnight and check it the next day. Because the coconut kefir curd is already cultured, it is not likely the mixture will need to culture for a full 30 hours.
5. After the culturing period is complete, scrape the mixture into a cheesecloth-lined sieve. Make sure there is at least a double layer of cheesecloth. Add the salt and herbs and fold into the cheese. Allow this to drain, or lose moisture, for up to 4 hours at room temperature. If you wish to have the mixture lose more moisture, continue the process in the refrigerator. Make sure that the top of the cheese is lightly covered by cheesecloth or other light covering.

6. After the cheese has finished this initial moisture loss, place a stainless steel ring or cheese mold on top of a bamboo mat or wooden board. Line the ring or mold with cheesecloth and place the curd in the form, pressing down gently to remove air pockets or cracks. Place the cheese in its form and on the bamboo mat or wooden board within a ripening box (a container large enough to hold this setup and allow air flow) and then place the ripening box in the refrigerator to begin aging.
7. Check the cheese every day. Likely after day 2 you will be able to remove the mold or ring and allow the cheese in cheesecloth to sit directly on the bamboo mat or wooden board. Flip or turn the cheese over every day, check the bottom of the container for fluid and wipe clean. After another 2 to 3 days you should be able to remove the cheesecloth, and if you wish, you can cover the surface of the cheese in more dried herbs. You can choose to eat this cheese at this stage or to age it for a week or two longer.
8. The longer this cheese air dries, the longer it keeps. This cheese ages quite well, and whether you choose to eat it soft or firmer and more crumbly is up to you. After you have aged it to the hardness you like, wrap it in cheesecloth or cheese paper (a paper designed specifically for storing cheeses, which you can find at gourmet shops, cheese shops, or online) and keep it refrigerated.

### Storage

Kept wrapped in cheese paper and refrigerated, this cheese will keep for up to 30 days.

### Method 2

An alternative method is to blend the macadamia paste first without the other ingredients except the salt, mix it with the coconut kefir curd, and allow that mixture to culture together in a pot, over low heat for 90 minutes. After this heat aided culturing, place the mixture into a food grade container and culture at room temperature (62°F–72°F/17°C–22°C) for 12 hours

After this culturing process is finished, pick up from step 5 above and follow the same process. When using this method note that you will likely see more moisture separation from the solids and a somewhat more jiggly texture. Initially, this curd will feel a bit more delicate, but it knits up well during aging.

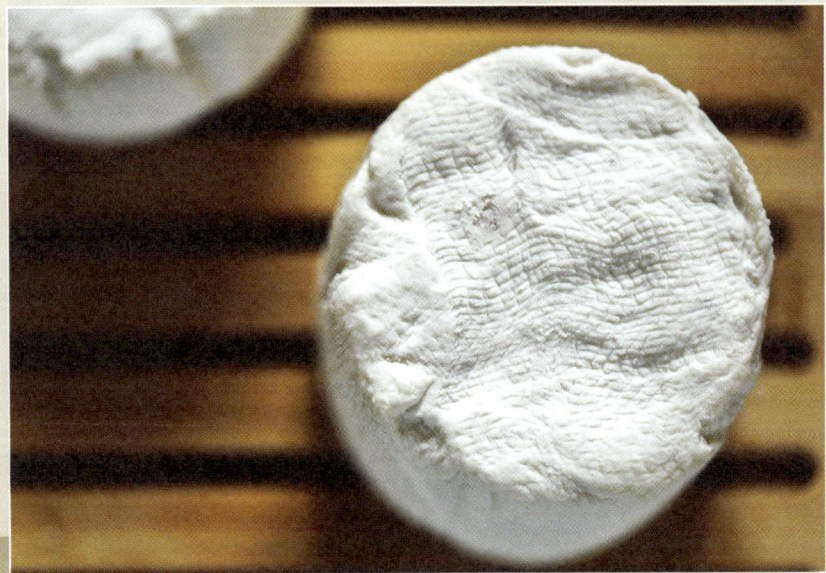

*Kefir/macadamia cheese unwrapped and on aging board, before adding herbs.*
CREDIT: CATHERINE DOWNES

## Lactic Acid (cultured) Almond Curd

I use almond curd in several of my Blue Heron cheeses and find that cultured almond offers some of the funkiness and pungency that occurs in dairy-based cheesemaking. Of the nut-based curds I use, it is the most finicky, but as long as you check frequently for taste and texture, it can yield very good results.

Almonds contain a significant amount of sulfur (the amount will depend on the quality of the soil that they are grown in), and the breakdown of protein during culturing creates a by-product of hydrogen sulphide that produces an "eggy" smell.

This tendency can scare folks off from using almonds in longer aging cheeses, and for the most part I do not recommend doing long-aged almond based cheeses at home unless you can do so in an environment in which you can control temperature and humidity during aging.

However, because almonds also have a high percentage of protein, using an almond curd in combination with other ingredients such as cashew, coconut milk, or white bean can produce some pleasantly pungent and sharp tasting cheeses.

I have amended the almond curd process from the first edition so that it will be more usable as a base for combining with other ingredients, as in the almond-white bean cheddar recipe in the cheddar-style cheese section. It also differs from the cultured almond ricotta recipe earlier in the book in that the almond base is heated first.

**Tools and Equipment**

High-speed blender
Thick cast pot
Probe thermometer
Food grade container for soaking almonds
Food grade container for culturing
Measuring cups
Measuring spoons
Wooden or silicone spoon
Spatula
Cheesecloth or butter muslin
Fine mesh sieve
Bamboo mat/wooden board
Bowl

## Ingredients

3 cups almonds, soaked and peeled

1½ tsp salt

1 Tbsp maple syrup

starter culture: ¼ cup coconut kefir culture or thermophilic TA061 (Danisco Choozit)

3–4 cups of water (filtered or rested tap water) for blending (may substitute 1 cup of oat milk or coconut milk for a portion of the blending water)

## Method

1. Wash and sanitize all work surfaces and all of the tools you plan to use.
2. Soak the almonds as per the Soaking Guidelines in chapter 3.
3. Add ½ of the water for blending (or 1 cup water and 1 cup oat milk or coconut milk), to the high-speed blender, and then add the peeled and soaked almonds.
4. Begin by pulsing the mixture in the blender several times before moving to continuous blending. This will ensure that the almonds break down into small enough pieces to prevent binding around the blades. Gradually increase the speed of blending, but check frequently to observe the texture of your mixture. Add water/fluid in small amounts.
5. Keep increasing the blending speed, and occasionally use the spatula to scrape the mixture on the sides down. You want the mixture to be thick, a little loose, and creamy with no grainy texture.
6. When you are finished blending, place the mixture into the thick cast pot. Heat the mixture on low-medium heat until it reaches 185°F (85°C). Use the probe thermometer to check the temperature. Monitor the mixture while it is heating, and stir frequently to prevent it from scorching or burning.
7. Remove the mixture from heat, and begin one of the active cooling processes (placing the pot on an ice bath or stirring frequently). When the mixture reaches 120° F (48.9°C) add the maple syrup and stir in. (If you use the thermophilic culture, add this now.)
8. Continue cooling and at 105°F (40.5°C) add the starter culture.
9. Place the mixture into a clean, sanitized container for culturing. Ensure the top ⅓ of the jar is empty to provide headspace above the surface of the mixture to allow for airflow and gas exchange. Cover the container, and allow the mixture to culture at room temperature (optimally between 62°F and 72°F/17°C and 22°C) for 12 to 36 hours.
10. Check the mixture every 12 hours. Look for the presence of bubbles (this will be more likely if you use the coconut kefir starter culture). Taste the

mixture and assess it for acidity. If it is beginning to become more sour than tangy, stop the culturing process and place it in the refrigerator. If I use coconut kefir starter, I allow the almond curd to finish culturing in the refrigerator after the first 12 hours because the yeasts in the starter will continue culturing at the lower temperature of the refrigerator and acidification will slow. The yeasts will also offer a mellow, implied sweetness.

11. After the mixture has finished culturing, set up a bowl, and place a fine mesh sieve in it. Line the sieve with cheesecloth or butter muslin, and put the cultured almond mixture into it. Sprinkle it with salt, and fold in. Allow it to drain overnight (and for up to 2 days) in the refrigerator with the top covered lightly.

The almond curd is now ready to work with.

**Storage**

Store the curd in a sealed container and save it to make cheese. It will keep for up to 2 weeks in the refrigerator.

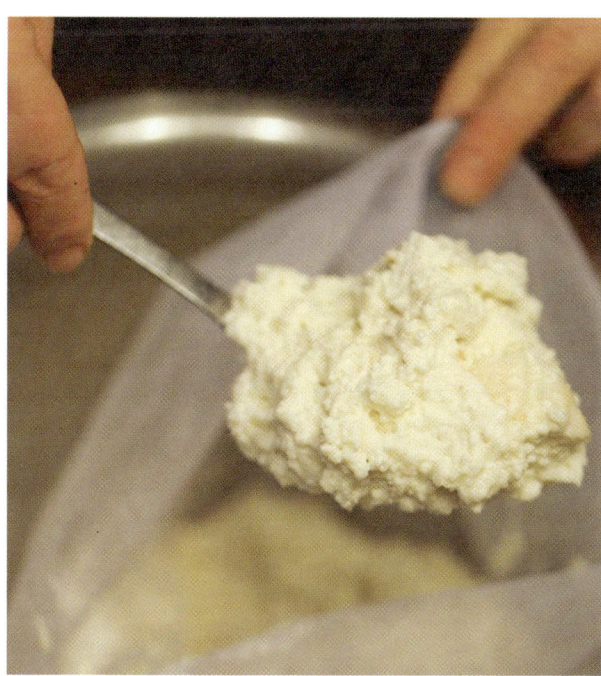

*Texture of cultured almond curd.* CREDIT: CATHERINE DOWNES

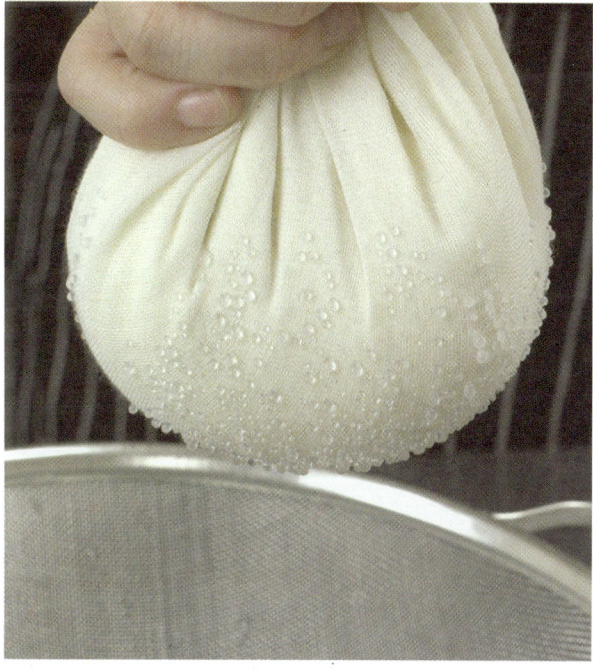

*Gently squeezing curd to demonstrate how much moisture curd retains. Avoid using this method to rush the process of moisture loss.* CREDIT: COLIN MEDHURST

# Soft, Short-aged Cultured Almond Cheese

## Tools and Equipment

Cheesecloth or butter muslin

Bamboo mat or small wooden cheese board

Spatula

Cheese mold or stainless steel ring

Container for ripening

There are a number of ways to use the lactic acid almond curd, and the recipes for feta-style cheese and cheddar-style cheese demonstrate two of these methods. Here is a simple method for making a short-aged cultured almond cheese that can be used like a drained and set ricotta or as a chèvre-style cheese.

Follow steps 1 to 11 for Lactic Acid (cultured) Almond Curd. After step 11 taste the curd to see if it needs more salt. Season accordingly. If you wish, you can add dried herbs, spices, fruit, olives, sundried tomatoes, or any similar ingredients to the cheese at this time. My favorite combinations in this cheese are black olives and sundried tomatoes, and porcini powder and preserved lemon.

## Method

1. Lay some clean cheesecloth or butter muslin on top of a bamboo mat or small wooden board. Scoop the almond curd into the cheesecloth.
2. Shape the cheese, using your hands to guide the curd into shape. You can roll it into a log, or you can use a cheese mold or stainless steel hoop that is lined with cheesecloth to absorb moisture from the cheese.
3. Place the shaped cheese on top of the bamboo mat and place inside a container (ripening box) and place in the refrigerator. Leave a top on the container askew to allow for airflow.
4. Check the cheese daily for 2 to 4 days, taste to ensure flavor is not evolving in an unpleasant (too sour or bitter) way. I recommend using the cheese after this time period is up, but you could age/cure it for a few more days, if you wish.

## Storage

When the cheese has reached the flavor and texture that you prefer, place it on a bamboo mat or wooden board and keep it in a large enough container that good airflow will keep the cheese surface from becoming damp. If the container is too small, humidity in the container will soften the cheese. Be sure to leave the lid off the container for an hour a day to allow humidity to escape.

### Ways to use this cheese

In a vegan frittata when combined in a chickpea batter

In a sweet baked almond tart

## Feta-style cheeses

I am including three cultured/fermented feta-style recipes. While none of them follow a traditional dairy feta process, the results are cultured vegan cheeses and one fermented tofu recipe that fulfill the desire for a dense, crumbly, salty cheese.

## Coconut Kefir Curd Feta-Style Cheese (Macedonian-style feta)

I have made this feta-style cheese multiple times. It does take several weeks to make, but the results are worth it. A good friend of mine, who still loves dairy cheese and is familiar with a wide range of them, told me that this recipe reminds her of a Macedonian style rather than a Greek feta. The primary difference between the two styles is that Macedonian feta is creamier and less crumbly. This coconut kefir curd feta-style cheese achieves density as it loses moisture and is very creamy. This feta will be best used in uncooked recipes, or crumbled on top of cooked food.

### Tools and Equipment

Container large enough to hold the cheeses and allow good airflow
Bowl
Fine mesh sieve
Cheesecloth or butter muslin
Bamboo mat or small wooden cheese board
Measuring cups
Measuring spoons
Knife
Jars with lids or container with lid for storage

### Ingredients

4 cups coconut kefir curd (follow coconut kefir curd process)
2 tsp salt (you will use more during the aging process)
10% saline brine: 1 L water and 100 g salt
Herbs, dried (I also like to use some preserved lemon fluid)

### Method

1. Wash and sanitize all work surfaces, tools, and containers that you will use during this process.
2. Fold the 2 tsp salt into the coconut kefir curd; do not whip it or stir vigorously.
3. Place the fine mesh sieve inside the bowl, line this with doubled up cheesecloth or butter muslin. Place the salted coconut kefir curd in the cloth.
4. Allow the coconut kefir curd to lose moisture in the refrigerator (cover the top of the curd lightly) for 24 hours. Check the progress of moisture loss every 12 hours. Sprinkle a small amount of salt over the top of the surface to encourage moisture loss.
5. After 24 hours, place fresh, clean cheesecloth or butter muslin on a bamboo mat or wooden board. You can make 1 larger cheese or 2 smaller cheeses (divide the cheesecloth/muslin accordingly). Place the coconut kefir curd into the new cheesecloth. Roll it into a log ensuring it is wrapped entirely in cheesecloth. Alternatively, if you have a square shaped cheese mold (with perforations), you can place the curd in cheesecloth inside the mold.
6. Place the shaped cheese on its bamboo mat or small wooden board inside the larger container that will then go into the refrigerator.
7. The cheesecloth will help in moisture loss via absorption. After 2 days, unwrap the cheese, sprinkle some very fine salt over the surface, and rewrap in fresh cheesecloth. You will also want to change the board or mat as it will have absorbed moisture.

8. Place the rewrapped cheeses back into the refrigerator, and repeat this process every 2 days for up to 10 days. After about 5 days, if the surface of the cheese is dry, use a piece of clean cheesecloth to wash the surface with salt brine, or salt and rewrap the cheese. Check the cheese daily, and turn it over.
9. Once the cheese is firm to touch and you can't leave fingerprints on the surface, remove it from the refrigerator and cut into 1-inch cubes/chunks. The cheese may be softer than you want or expect it to be, and you can continue to air dry the cubes until they are quite firm. They can then be stored in a sealed container and kept for up to 2 weeks.

## Storage

If the cheese is dry and firm enough, you can consider storing it in olive oil with herbs in a sealed container in the refrigerator for up to 30 days, but be sure to check for quality of flavor, and make sure the cubes are not disintegrating. You may also store the cubes of feta in a salt brine with added herbs. I often use a salt brine with added preserved lemon fluid replacing ¼ of the brine amount.

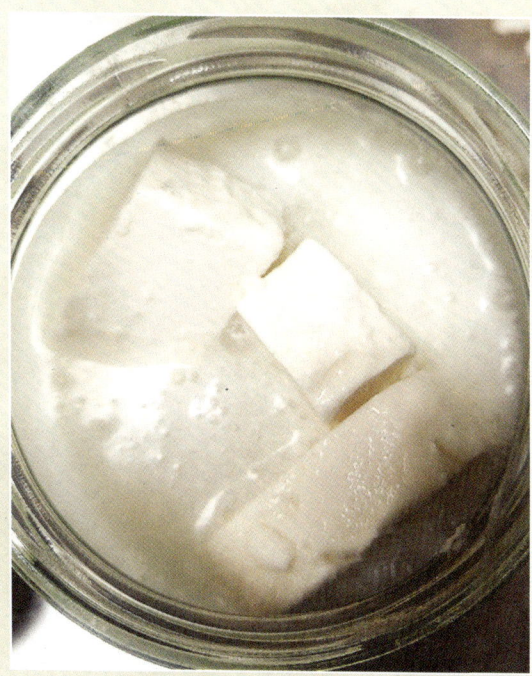

Cubes of coconut kefir feta in brine. This feta is creamier than a Greek feta. It is closer to a Macedonian-style feta and is best used on fresh dishes.

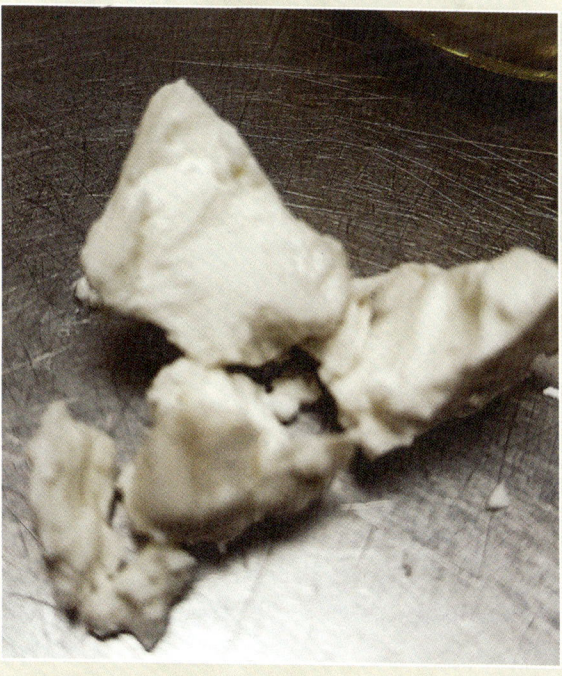

Coconut kefir feta removed from brine. This cheese is dense and creamy.

# Almond Curd Feta

This cheese employs the cultured almond curd (uses heat prior to adding culture) and not the cultured almond ricotta.

## Tools and Equipment

Container for storing the ripening cheese in the fridge
Bowl
Fine mesh sieve
Cheesecloth/butter muslin
Spatula
Measuring cups
Measuring spoons
Bamboo mat/small wooden board

## Ingredients

3 cups almond curd (You may substitute 1 cup of coconut kefir curd for 1 cup of the almond curd to make a feta. The fat of the coconut milk helps the cheese form a nice density.)

¼ cup miso (This is your choice of type of miso, but just note that each type of miso has a different flavor, so you may want to amend the amount of miso you use if you choose something like a barley miso.)

2 tsp salt

brine for washing/storage: 1 L water and 100 g salt

## Method

1. Wash and sanitize all work surfaces and equipment you plan to use.
2. In a bowl, place a fine mesh sieve and line it with cheesecloth or butter muslin. Fold in the almond curd, salt, and miso, until miso is fully integrated. Lightly cover the top of the mixture and allow it to drain/evaporate moisture in the refrigerator for 24 to 30 hours. Check the mixture every 12 hours. Gently turn the mixture over at each 12-hour check. This encourages even moisture loss. Sprinkle a pinch of salt (¼ tsp rubbed between fingers), over the surface at every second check.
3. Place fresh cheesecloth or butter muslin on bamboo mat or small wooden cheeseboard, and place the almond curd onto the cheesecloth. It is up to you whether you make 1 or 2 cheeses. For more than 1 cheese divide the cheesecloth accordingly and use separate mats or boards.
4. Shape the almond curd into a rectangular block and wrap in cheesecloth. Place this on the bamboo mat/wooden cheeseboard, and put the mat/board inside the container. Cover the top, but leave the top ajar for airflow, and place the container in the refrigerator.
5. Check the cheese daily and turn it over. Every second day, unwrap the cheese to evaluate moisture evaporation, and scrape a little cheese from the surface to taste. Wipe away any loose moisture inside the container, and change the bamboo mat or wooden board as needed (if too moist).
6. As the cheese begins to dry and the surface begins to feel firm, remove the cloth and allow the cheese to sit on the bamboo mat or cheeseboard freely. Wash with

light brine or salt very lightly every second or third day. This process will take up to 2 weeks, so be patient and willing to observe.

7. After the cheese is firm enough to cut, store it in light brine with herbs or in an olive oil brine with herbs.

## Storage

Stored in a light brine or in an olive oil brine this cheese will keep for up to 2 months provided you do not cross-contaminate the brine by using unclean tools.

*Almond feta curing at Graze, 2014.*

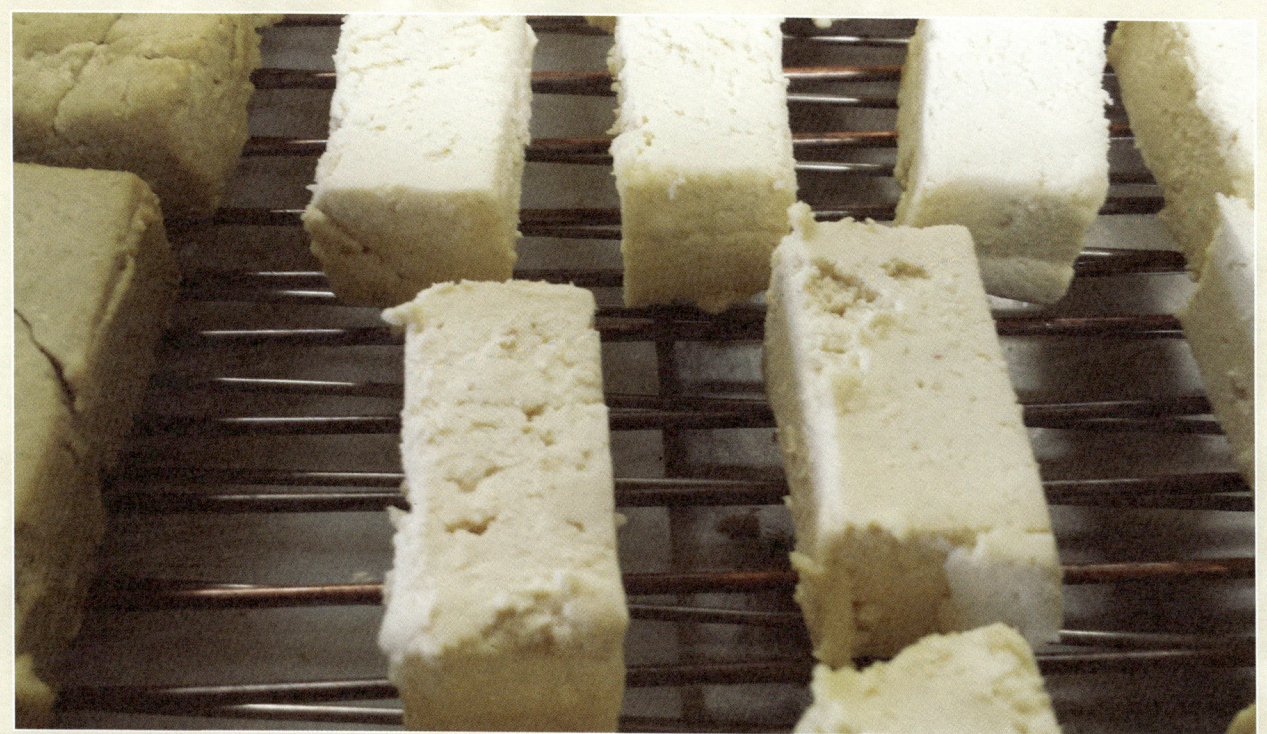

## Tools and Equipment

**Stage 1**

Thick cast saucepan

Measuring cups

Measuring spoons

Knife

Cutting board

Cheesecloth or butter muslin

2 x bamboo mat

Plate (as in dinner plate), or fermenting stones

5 lb weight

Food grade container for fermentation

**Stage 2**

Jars/lids

Spoon or ladle

Thick cast saucepan

Measuring cups

Measuring spoons

Cutting board

Knife

# Fermented Tofu Feta

While it is true that I do not include mention of soy or soy milk in any of my culturing methods, it is not because I dislike soy. Consumption of soy has been the source of fear-mongering. While I will not dig into the misinformation surrounding soy, I will say that I am careful in sourcing my soy products because in North America, 80–90% of soy crops are grown in order to become feed for concentrated animal agriculture operations (CAFO's) and are grown as a mono-crop. My concerns regarding soy are much more about the environmental impact of mono-crop growth and CAFOs than they are about personal health.

In fact, I very much like both tofu and tempeh, and my foray away from dairy began with soy milk. With non-cultured versions of tofu feta being so popular, I thought I would include a method for a fermented tofu feta. It takes longer than a non-fermented tofu, but all culturing processes do. Fermented soy is called chao, and one commercial vegan cheese producer, Field Roast, uses chao in the manufacturing of their cheese analogs and calls one product Chao. This fermentation process occurs at a higher temperature range than the other culturing processes, and thus includes higher amounts of salt as inhibition against pathogens since it is not relying on the addition of microbial culture. Do not reduce the amount of salt in the first stage of this process.

If you decide to make this, be prepared to commit to the time frame. This takes approximately 2 months, but I assure you it is so worth it. Also, because it takes so long, I recommend making a batch 2 to 4 times larger so that you can keep some in storage for yourself.

## Ingredients

**Stage 1 (1 month)**

4 cups water (filtered or rested tap water)

1 lb. firm tofu

1 Tbsp salt

**Stage 2 (brine)**

1½ cups water (filtered or rested tap water)

3 Tbsp salt (I usually use less water in this storage brine and often replace a portion of the brine with preserved lemon juice.)

1 Tbsp sugar

¼ cup rice wine

## Method

This fermentation process is done in two stages. The first stage is the initial fermentation and takes 1 month. The second stage, a secondary curing phase, occurs in brine and takes about 3 weeks.

### Stage 1

1. Wash and clean all surfaces and tools you will be using in this process.
2. Open the firm tofu package, and drain it. You may want to cut the tofu in half.
3. In the saucepan, bring the water and 1 Tbsp salt to a boil.
4. Add the tofu and cook at high temperature for 4 minutes.
5. Remove tofu from the water, place on cheesecloth/muslin and wrap the tofu. Place the wrapped tofu on a plate or in a shallow bowl. Place a plate on top of the tofu and place a heavy weight (I use a 5 lb. fermenting weight) on top, and allow it to press for 1 hour.
6. In a food grade container, place a bamboo mat (or a small cooling rack) on the bottom. Place the cheesecloth/muslin wrapped tofu on top of the bamboo mat, place another bamboo mat on top of the tofu, and place the plate and weight on top of the tofu. Cover the container.
7. Allow the tofu to ferment at 77°F–86°F (25°C–30°C) for about 2 to 3 days. As most households are not this temperature, I recommend doing this in the oven with the oven light on or in a dehydrator at the lowest temperature setting.
8. Check the tofu daily, being sure to wash and sanitize your hands each time before doing so. I usually remove the cheesecloth/muslin after the first day so that it is easier to observe the tofu, but the cloth does help absorb moisture. It is not unusual for the surface of the tofu to begin to turn a little orange and to start developing a funky aroma. You can scrape the orange layer off.

### Stage 2

1. Place the water, salt, and sugar into the saucepan and bring to a boil.
2. Cool the brine to room temperature, and then add the rice wine vinegar.
3. Cut the tofu into 1-inch square cubes, or cubes that resemble feta cubes. Fill the jars with the tofu (yes, it will be a little aromatic or stinky), and then top with brine allowing for ½-inch headspace. Place lids finger tight on the jars.
4. Place the jars in a cool, dark place and allow to ferment for 3 weeks at room temperature, approximately 68°F (18°C–22°C).
5. After this fermentation period is over, you can make a new brine with herbs and garlic and transfer the fermented tofu to the new infusion brine.

## Storage

When fermentation is finished keep the jars in the refrigerator for long-term storage. It will keep for several months.

## Longer-Aged Cheeses

Among the most common queries I receive, whether it be online, from students in my classes, or from Blue Heron customers, is about hard cheese. Can you make a truly hard vegan cheese? How do you make hard vegan cheese? Do you have any hard vegan cheese for sale? Yes, you can make hard vegan cheese. Yes, Blue Heron does sell hard vegan cheese (we release, in small batches, several types that we make, several times a year). How do you make hard vegan cheese? Time. Controlled moisture loss over time is the most important element of achieving a dry, firm cheese that can produce very thin slices and shave or grate in the way that parmesan reggiano or romano do, which is what I often think folks are referencing when they ask the questions.

To achieve a truly hard cheese with pungent flavor and that cheesy—but really it is umami—aroma that many people are seeking takes time. You cannot make it faster by simply adding agar agar and kappa carrageenan and lots of onion powder and other umami rich ingredients. These will give you something pleasant and enjoyable in their own right but do not produce the depth of flavor or textural change that microbial action does over time.

Time is what allows the microbes in the cheese to continue their work, time is what allows moisture to continue to evaporate, and time plus various aging techniques allow a hard cheese to develop its final identifying character, and I

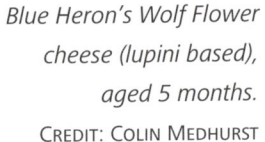

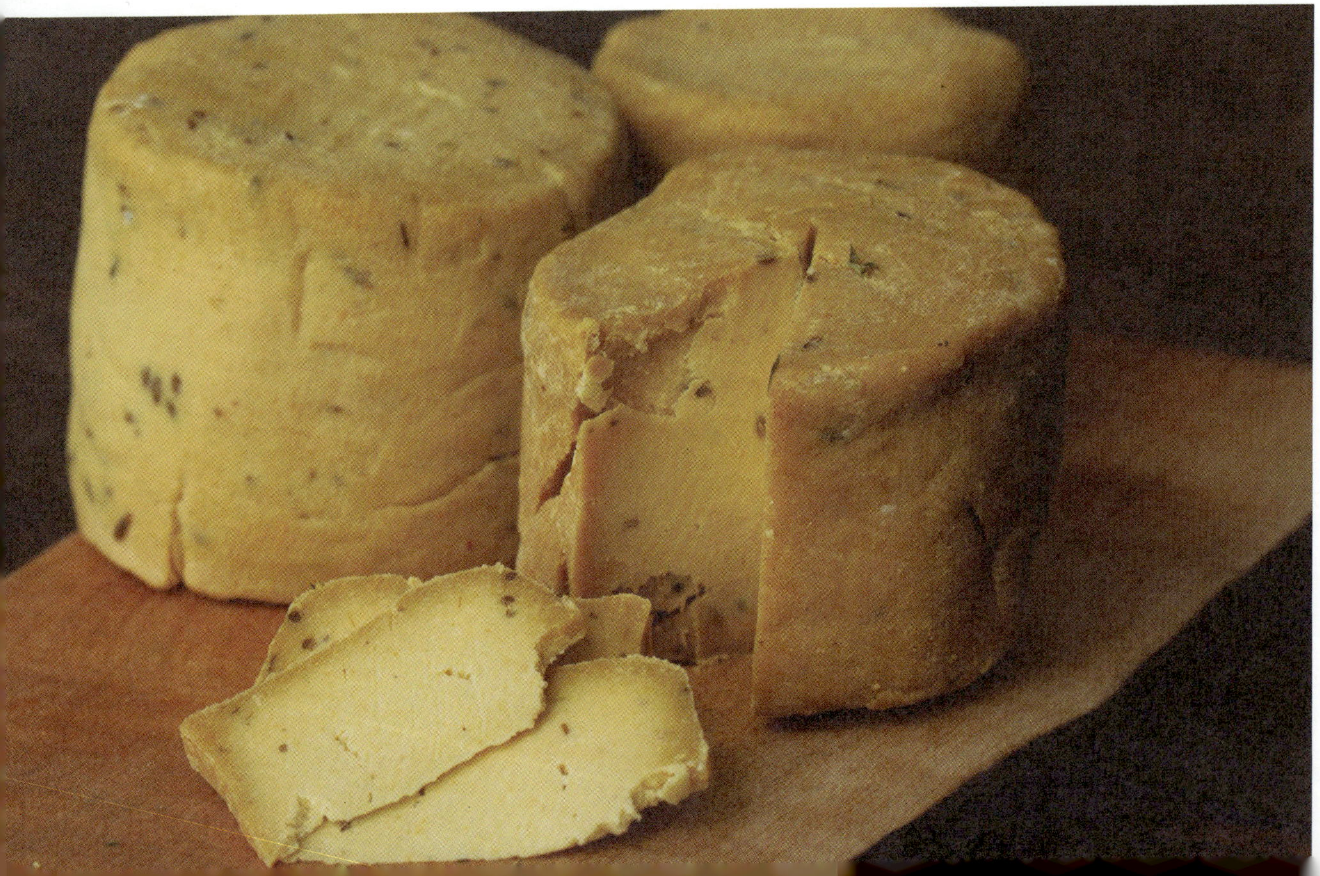

*Blue Heron's Wolf Flower cheese (lupini based), aged 5 months.*
CREDIT: COLIN MEDHURST

do not think that we should be in such a hurry to eliminate this important element. During this time the cheesemaker comes to know all the stages of change and the many nuances that occur during aging and in the process moves closer to being an artisan than a casual DIY experimenter (not to disparage the casual experimenter, not everyone will have the interest or the privilege of time to do more elaborate and time-consuming projects).

In this section, a couple of broad styles of cheese that can be aged to firmness are presented. There are the havarti/gouda-style and the cheddar-style sections, and within each section I include a cultured and aged method and a crossover method (that is the use of a cultured medium with other ingredients such as coconut oil).

I am presenting completely revised methods for the cultured and aged havarti/gouda and cheddar styles due to reader/user feedback that many complications or aspects did not work. While I have had success with the methods I described in the first edition, I have subsequently found in replication that the tweaking and adjusting I did in the execution of the recipes makes the previous methods too complicated for folks to use at home.

In particular, I am removing the use of vegetable or microbial rennet. These digestive enzymes, used regularly in dairy cheesemaking (as alternatives to calf rennet), are used because they break down the casein proteins in dairy. The variety of proteins in the materials we use as vegan cheesemakers are shaped differently than casein proteins, and thus, these enzymes are not particularly helpful. More fortune is had with simply experimenting with culturing times using LAB or using papaya (papain) digestive enzymes.

I am working with Blue Heron production supervisor Lucia Valenzuela, who holds a master's degree in food science, to identify enzymes that may be more effective in working with LAB fermentation in coagulating plant proteins.

I want to thank the folks who took the time to write to me or send me online messages and queries. I hope these revised methods are more

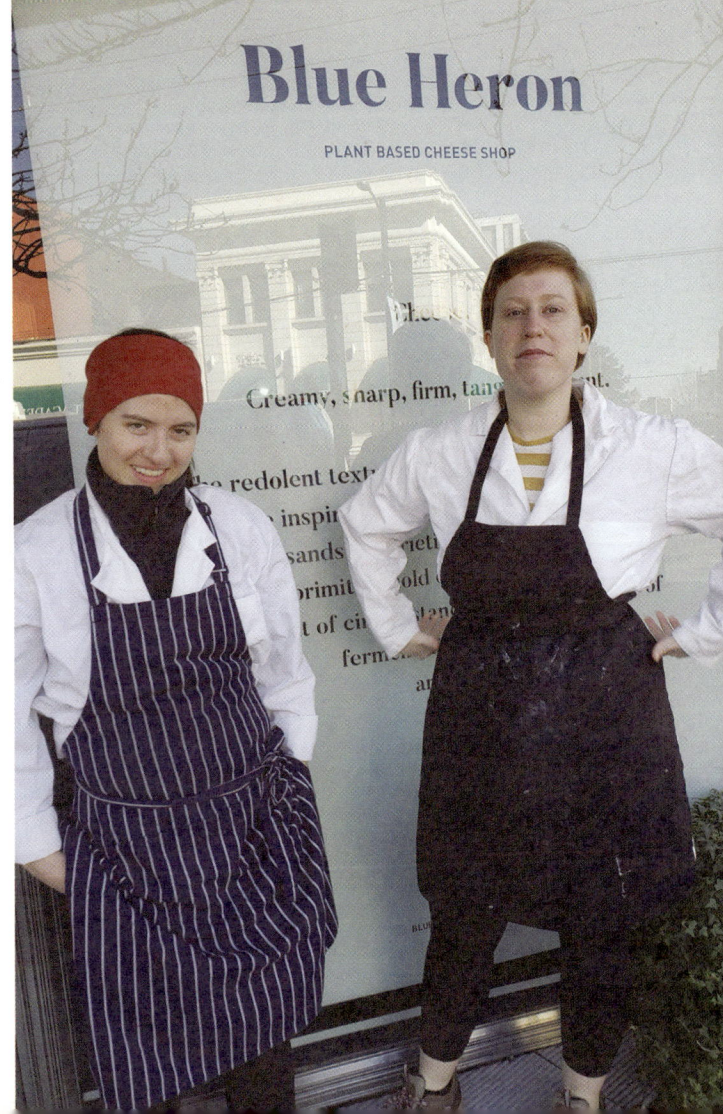

*Left, Lucia, Blue Heron production supervisor, and right, Jolene, Blue Heron assistant operations manager, 2019.*

useful. Aging processes are outlined for cultured and aged cheeses and for the crossover method.

I recommended that folks intending to make these recipes have a secondary refrigerator or some other means of being able to maintain safe and appropriate temperature and humidity levels for long-term aging. The regular household refrigerator is generally not the right tool for aging cheese in. It sits at too low a temperature and the humidity is not right for all types of aging processes. However, more problematic than these considerations is that the refrigerator is shared space for many foods, each carrying its own set of microbes, and for those whose fridge space includes animal products there is an additional risk of cross-contamination. Moreover, with repeated opening of the refrigerator, especially during meal times, the air temperature is not maintained at a consistent temperature. This is not generally problematic for properly stored food, but for a food process that is still active (e.g., aging cheese), it is less than ideal. Refrigeration was designed for the purposes of storing food and prolonging freshness.

Remember that as you proceed into more advanced cheesemaking, great patience is required. Training in observation to recognize the right taste, texture, and appearance is not something that can be taught just by reading a book or even taking a class. Books, instructions, and classes are necessary to support your ongoing experiments, but they cannot teach what something will smell like to you or what something will taste like. You need to develop this ability, and the only way to do so is to keep making cheese.

Get used to a range of aromas and tastes. Learn to recognize that certain kinds of smells and textural changes occur when the temperature gets too high in a fermentation process. Ultimately, it is your palate, your nose, and your ability to recognize what looks and feels correctly aligned with changes in temperature, humidity, and other variables that affect fermenting and culturing that will allow you to progress as a cheesemaker. Batches will fail; results will not always turn out as planned. Success is founded in failure. Do not be afraid to make mistakes and have projects that fail. Learning from failure is the only way we truly succeed.

I recommend keeping a detailed cheese log for your attempts at cheesemaking so that you get used to recording your observations along with dates (date made, date checked, and date finished). This helps to tie your observations to a time frame. You will find sample recording logs in appendix 2. Keeping a log will help you learn how to recognize changes associated with specific variables, both favorable and not. It will help you identify when to make adjustments in subsequent batches, and keeping a log is particularly helpful in keeping track of

Opposite page: *Cheeses made by Chef Emily Davies, Karen's sous chef/student.*

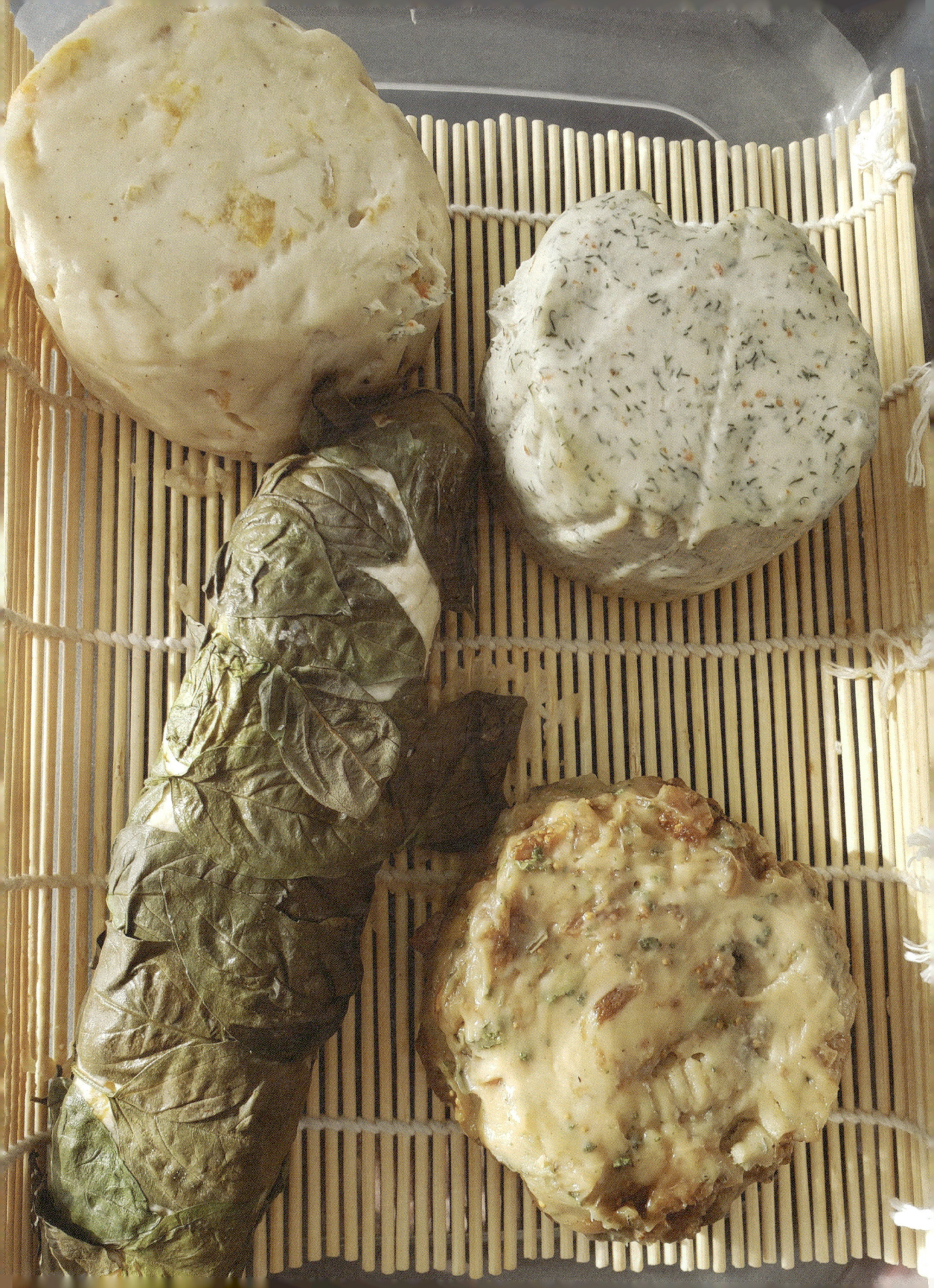

what needs to be done when you are working with projects that require longer aging time and multiple interventions. As we move into some of the longer aging and then mold ripened cheeses, a logbook/tracking sheet will become indispensable.

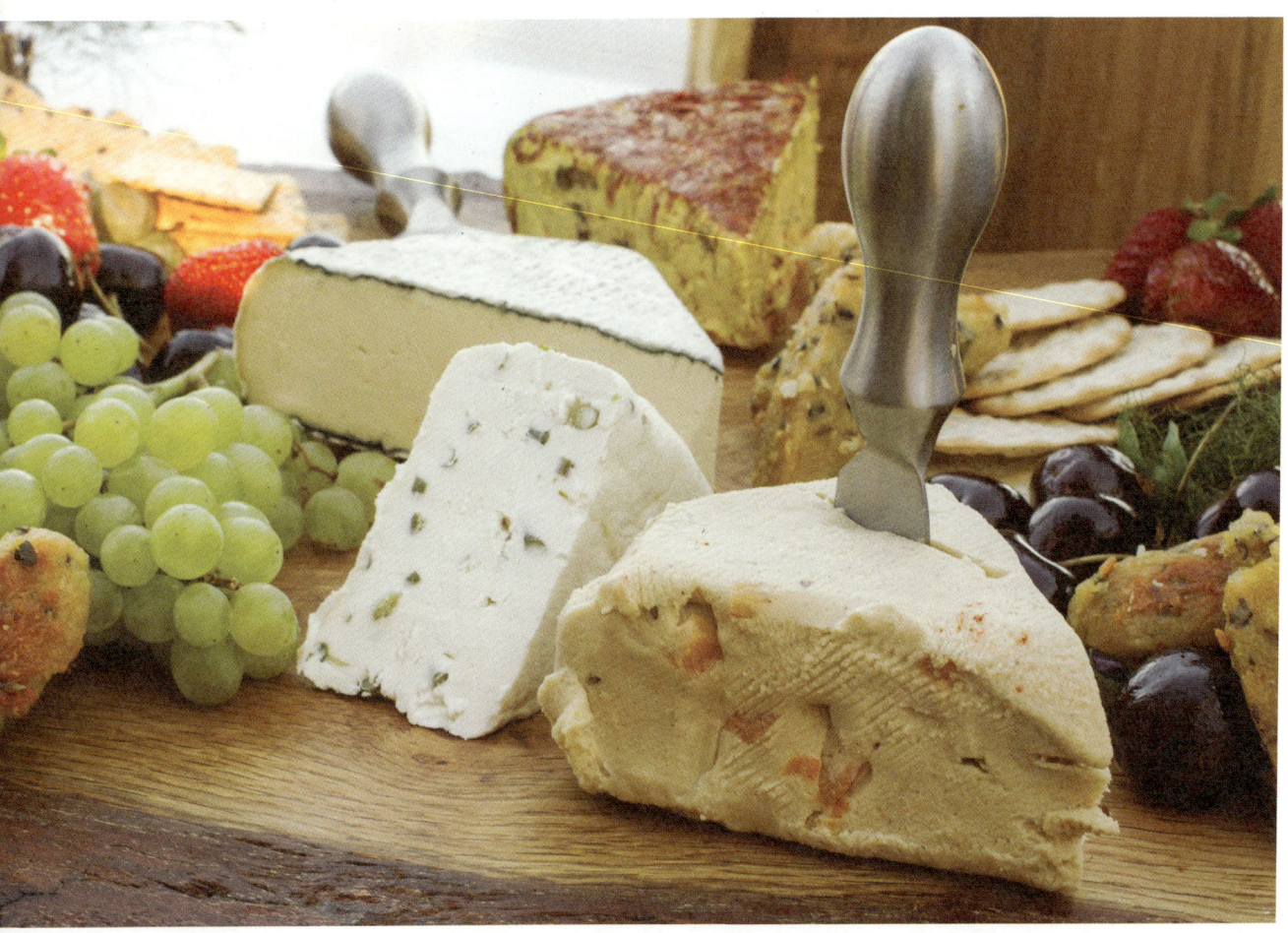

*Blue Heron cheeses at Thrive dinner.*
CREDIT: COLIN MEDHURST

## Cashew and coconut havarti/gouda-style cheeses
### Method 1: cultured and aged

In this method, it is important to understand how I employ the term "curd." If you have made dairy cheese before you will not achieve the same kind of curd with this recipe. The materials you are using are different, the proteins included are different, and most importantly, how these materials behave in culturing is different. This curd also takes longer to achieve than curd making in dairy cheesemaking.

What you will be expecting to see after the culturing period is a mixture that, when cut or tested with a spoon, will appear somewhat clumpy, (not smooth like a blended product). These clumps indicate that protein breakdown has occurred and signify the coagulating of the proteins. With plant based matrices such as the one in the method that follows, the long chain polysaccharide released during soaking and culturing is also part of the formation of the curd structure, which means it is holding in moisture in a way that does not occur in dairy cheesemaking. Moisture removal via evaporation, absorption, surface treatment, and aging is very important to this process.

**Tools and Equipment**

High-speed blender
2 × thick cast 6 L saucepans (one should fit on top of the other)
Measuring cups
Measuring spoons
Spatula
Whisk
Probe thermometer
Container for culturing
Container for holding the cheese in the refrigerator (ripening box)
Cheesecloth or butter muslin
Bamboo mat or wooden board

**Ingredients**

3 cups cashew nuts (can substitute 1 cup of cooked oats, blended and strained for 1 cup of cashews)
1 cup macadamia nuts
2 cups water (filtered or rested tap water)
2 cups coconut milk, full fat, or oat milk
1 tsp calcium chloride
1 tsp salt

starter culture: 2–3 tsp coconut or water kefir or ⅛ tsp TA-061 thermophilic starter

Optional: 2 Tbsp spices or herbs of your choice, for example caraway, cumin, fennel, cracked pepper, dehydrated pepper flakes

**Method**

1. Wash and sanitize all surfaces and tools that you will use.
2. In a high-speed blender add the water, then the almonds and cashews. You may want to start with ½ the amount and gradually add more once you have started blending.
3. Begin blending by pulsing a few times to break the solids down into smaller pieces. Gradually increase speed, and add coconut milk a little at a time. Check the progress frequently, and take your time blending at lower speeds to encourage emulsification of the fluids and solids. Blend until the mixture is very smooth and there is no graininess. This may take some time alternating between higher and lower speeds.
4. Take two 6 L pots and fill one with water and place the other pot on top, essentially forming a double boiler. Place the blended mixture in the empty pot, and begin heating the water at medium to medium-high heat. The heat will transfer to the mixture in the top pot.
5. Heat the mixture in the pot to 185°F (85°C), and maintain that temperature for 10 minutes. Use a probe thermometer to measure and monitor the temperature in order to maintain consistent temperature. Lower heat as needed to ensure that the mixture does not boil.
6. After the mixture has finished heating, remove from heat and begin active cooling via ice bath or very frequent stirring.
7. At 105°F (40.5°C) add the starter culture and stir in. Allow the mixture to sit for 90 minutes. If using the thermophilic culture add it at 120°F (50°C).
8. Transfer the mixture to a food grade container, allow for ⅓ headspace above the surface of the mixture and cover with a lid. Keep the mixture in an even temperature area of your kitchen and try to ensure that the temperature remains between 62°F and 72°F (17°C and 22°C) . Allow the mixture to culture for 24 to 48 hours.
9. During the culturing period, taste, smell, and visually observe the changes every 12 hours. If you have a pH meter, test the pH to ensure that the acidity is dropping fast enough. It should reach 4.6 by 48 hours, if not sooner. After culturing, mix in calcium chloride and let rest for 60 more minutes, and then place it in the refrigerator for 4 hours to overnight to allow this lactic acid curd to set up.

## After the culturing period

1. Wash and sanitize all work surfaces and any tools you will be using.
2. Remove the curd from the refrigerator. Place a fine mesh sieve lined with cheesecloth or butter muslin in a bowl. Use the spatula to scrape the mixture into the cloth. Sprinkle the salt over the surface and fold in.
3. Allow this mixture to drain/lose moisture at room temperature for up to 4 hours. Finish in the refrigerator for 1 to 4 days if needed. Keep the top very lightly covered with cheesecloth. This will not look like a dairy curd. Be sure to taste it and adjust salt if required.
4. After this first stage of moisture loss is finished, set up a bamboo mat or small wooden cheeseboard, place your cheese mold (usually round and perforated with holes to allow moisture to escape) on the mat/board, line it with cheesecloth, add your salted curd to the mold, and press it into place. You may want to make two smaller cheeses, so just be sure to have enough equipment on hand to do so.
5. Lightly cover the top of the cheese with the cheesecloth, and place the bamboo mat/board with the cheese in the mold on top into a container (ripening box) that is large enough to allow for good airflow. Place this in the refrigerator and place a lid lightly on top.
6. Over the next 2 to 5 days, check the cheese to see how it is firming up. Take the cloth off the top, sprinkle a very small amount of salt on top. This helps pull moisture to the surface, and this moisture will evaporate and allow the surface to begin drying. It will also keep the surface hostile to pathogens. Do not salt every day. Wipe away any excess moisture that is in the container, and change the bamboo mat or wooden board if necessary.
7. Depending on how fast moisture is evaporating from the cheese, you may be able to remove the cheese in the cheesecloth from the mold between day 2 and day 5. In any case, once you have removed the cheese from the mold, allow it (in cheesecloth) to continue to age on the bamboo mat or wooden board.
8. Continue to check daily and turn the cheese over each day to allow for moisture to escape from the bottom of the cheese. Lightly salt the bottom of the cheese every second day.

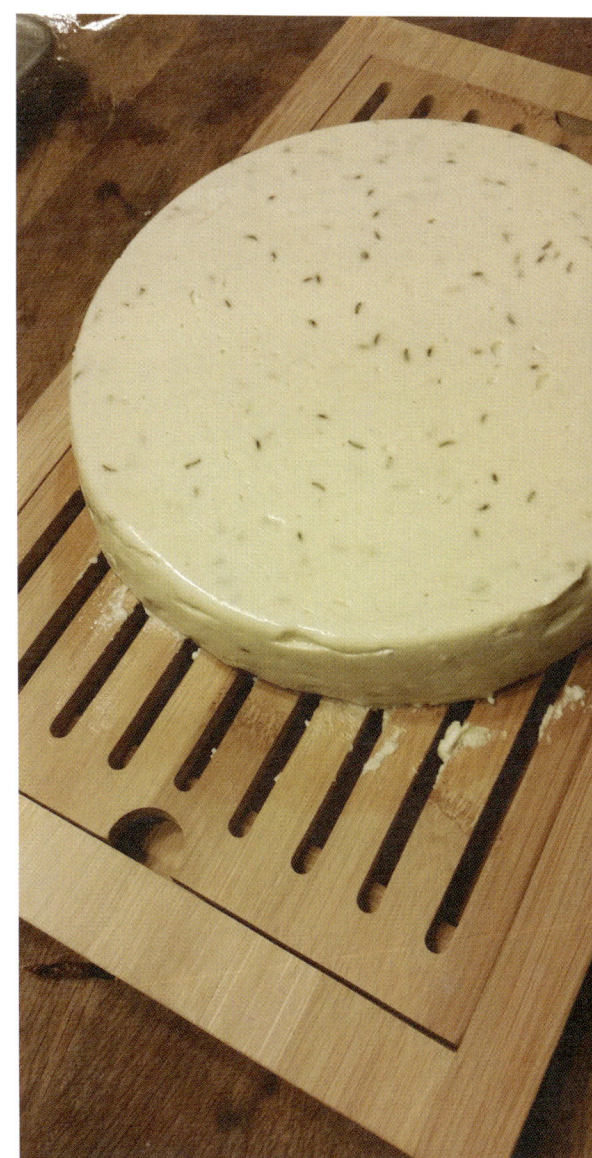

*Freshly set crossover method gouda/havarti-style with cumin.*

9. Once you can handle the cheese without it being too damp or soft, remove the cheesecloth altogether and place the cheese on a fresh bamboo mat/wooden board.
10. Now begins the process of aging and helping the cheese form a natural rind through salting/brining/washing and air-drying. There are multiple ways to achieve this, and you can apply more than one method during an aging process. The method you choose and when you apply it will have an impact on how the cheese will age and on the character it develops. For more in-depth guidance see the section on affinaging in chapter 6.

This cheese will take 6 to 12 weeks to finish depending on the size of the cheese you make (the larger the cheese, the longer it will take to age). It is optimal to age this cheese in a separate refrigerator such as a wine fridge where you can control the temperature and humidity. Optimal temperature is 50°F–55°F (10°C–13°C), and relative humidity about 65–75%. A handy device, a hygrometer, can measure both temperature and humidity.

## Method 2: crossover method

The crossover method involves using the cultured curd made by method 1 above and adding agar agar (or kappa carrageenan), coconut oil (or coconut oil/cacao butter mix) to aid in setting the cheese, allowing you to have a semi-firm cheese in less time than a fully cultured and aged cheese takes.

You can still age these cheeses because you have the acidified culture, but you do need to be mindful that the agar agar and the added fat will reduce the acidity of the cheese, slow down moisture release (agar agar actually holds moisture in), and inhibit microbial activity (they can get entrapped by the fat molecules). The agar agar and added fat, because they are additions to the cultured curd, do not go through the same metabolic (transformative) process that the original mixture does, and the molecular size of the agar agar and the fat are not changed the same way the original mixture is.

**Tools and Equipment**

Thick cast saucepan
Whisk
Probe thermometer
Blender
Measuring cups
Measuring spoons
Spatula

Bamboo mat/wooden board
Cheese mold
Cheesecloth or butter muslin
Container for storage in refrigerator (ripening/aging box)

### Ingredients

1 × batch of curd from method 1 (cultured and aged)
¼ cup coconut oil (cacao butter or a combination of the two), softened
3 cups water (filtered or rested tap water)
2 tsp powdered agar agar (or approximately the same amount of kappa carrageenan)
1 tsp coconut kefir culture
Optional: dried spices or herbs as you wish

### Method

1. Wash and sanitize all work surfaces and any tools you will be using.
2. Remove the curd from the refrigerator and allow it to warm up.
3. In a thick cast saucepan, place the 3 cups of water and then add the agar agar. Whisk continuously as the agar agar heats up over medium to medium-high heat. Agar agar needs to reach 185°F (85°C) and maintain that heat for 5

*Wedge of aged crossover method cumin gouda/havarti-style.*
CREDIT: CATHERINE DOWNES

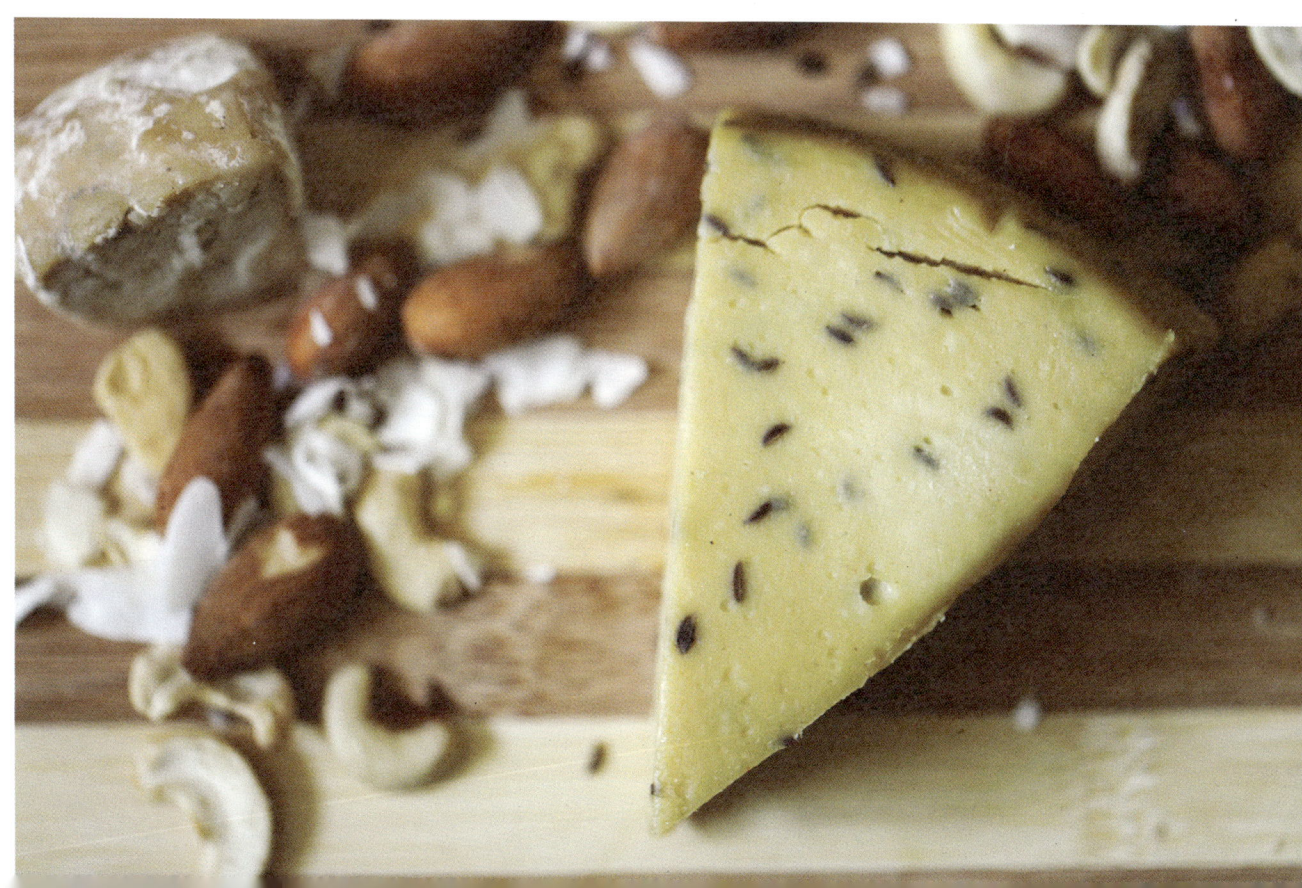

minutes. Use a probe thermometer to check the temperature. If the water/agar agar is thickening too quickly, reduce heat and add a bit more water.

4. Add the batch of curd to the heated agar agar mixture and add the softened coconut oil. Whisk the mixture together, and then remove from heat. Blend at low speed until the mixture is well combined, and then return to the pot.

5. Heat up the mixture over low-medium heat to 185°F (85°C) and stir continuously as it thickens. Heat it for up to 10 minutes. Remove from heat, and cool while actively stirring the mixture. When it reaches 105°F (40.5°C) add the coconut kefir culture, and stir in gently.

6. Set out a bamboo mat or wooden board and place the cheese mold on top of the bamboo mat or wooden board. Line the cheese mold with doubled up cheesecloth or butter muslin and pour the mixture into the mold. Press down lightly and ensure that the top is evenly spread. Sprinkle a little salt over the top, and lightly cover the top with cheesecloth. Allow the cheese to cool to room temperature before placing it in the container/ripening box and in the refrigerator to set.

7. The next day check to see how firmly the cheese has set. It is likely to be a little soft. This is desirable as you will still need to age it to achieve final firmness. Adding too much agar agar can help a cheese set firm but will often lead to a rubbery texture. Too much kappa carrageenan will set but may feel gummy or not as dense as you might like. If the cheese is firm enough to remove from the cheese mold, do so, and set, while still in cheesecloth, on the bamboo mat/wooden board.

8. For further guidance on methods for aging your cheese, refer to the section on affinaging in chapter 6. This cheese should take from 3 weeks to 1.5 months (depending on the size of the cheese) to be fully ready. It can be aged in the home refrigerator or in a separate, dedicated aging space. The surface of the cheese will need close monitoring as it ages, and I recommend using some form of acidity in the washes.

## Cheddar-style cheeses

Like the havarti/gouda-style method, I have also reviewed and overhauled the cheddar process. I have removed the use of vegetable or microbial rennet and probiotic capsules. I am also including two primary methods: cultured/aged and a crossover version. Both versions involve aging in order to achieve full character.

Remember that the curd used for these cheeses will not form like or look like a dairy milk curd. Both methods include the use of calcium chloride, which helps prevent the leaching of calcium from the curd and assists the cheese in firming up. Calcium chloride can be ordered from cheesemaking supply stores, but you can also find it in places that sell pickling supplies. If you purchase crystals, dissolve 2 tsp in ¼ cup water and you have a small amount of ready solution on hand.

## Method 1: cultured and aged

**Tools and Equipment**

2 × thick cast saucepan
Measuring cups
Measuring spoons
Spatula
Blender
Wooden or silicone spoon
Probe thermometer
Container for culturing
Bamboo mat/wooden cheese board
Cheesecloth or butter muslin
Container/ripening box
Cheese mold (one or more)

**Ingredients**

1 cup macadamia nuts
2 cups almonds
2 cups cooked white beans (butter beans, large lima beans, or cannellini, can be canned)
1 cup coconut milk, high fat (or 1 cup coconut cream)
1 Tbsp white miso or chickpea miso
Starter culture: 1 Tbsp coconut kefir starter culture or 2–3 tsp rejuvelac
1 tsp calcium chloride
1 tsp salt

*Microbial action indicated by small bubbles.*

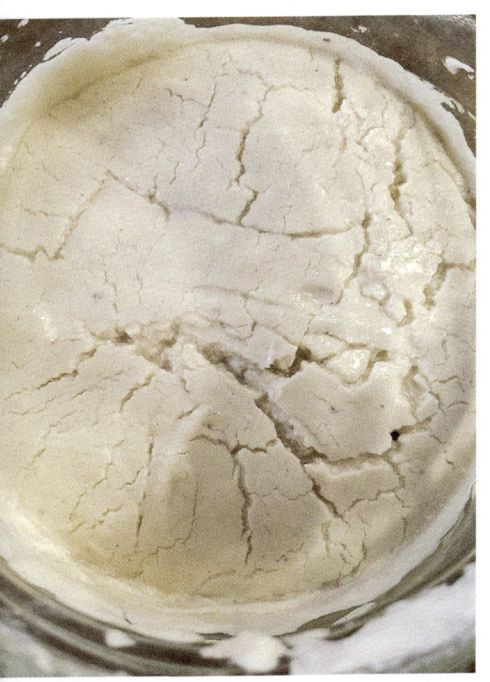

*Coconut kefir cultured lactic acid curd.*

## Method

1. Wash and sanitize all work surfaces and tools you will use.
2. Soak the nuts as per the Soaking Guidelines in chapter 3.
3. After the nuts are soaked and are ready for use, add the coconut milk/cream to the blender, add the almonds/macadamias and pulse several times before gradually increasing the speed. Pulsing allows the harder material to break into smaller pieces making it easier for emulsification to occur.
4. Once the nuts are almost completely blended in, add the cooked white beans and continue blending. If the mixture is getting bound or too thick, add small amounts of water to make blending easier. Gradually increase speed and focus on ensuring that the mixture is well combined and emulsified.
5. Add the miso and blend until the mixture is very smooth.
6. With the two saucepans, fill one ¾ full with water, and place the other on top (this is a double boiler system). Add the blended mixture to the empty pot, and heat the mixture over medium-high or medium heat until it reaches 185°F (85°C). Stir occasionally, and use a probe thermometer to test the temperature.
7. After the mixture reaches temperature, allow it to remain there for 10 minutes, and then remove from the heat and begin active cooling processes (e.g., place on ice bath or stir frequently).
8. When the mixture cools to 105°F (40.5°C), add the starter culture and allow to sit for 90 minutes. Then transfer the mixture to a food grade container for continued culturing and cover with a tight-fitting lid ensuring that there is at least ⅓ headspace above the surface of the mixture.
9. Allow the mixture to culture at room temperature (62°F–72°F/17°C–22°C) for 24 to 48 hours. Check this mixture every 12 hours, and check the curd for appearance, taste, and smell. If you have a pH meter, use it to check the acidity. Acidity after culturing should reach 4.6.

## After the culturing period

1. Wash and sanitize all work surfaces and any tools you will be using.
2. Remove the curd from the refrigerator. Place a fine mesh sieve lined with cheesecloth or butter muslin in a bowl. Use the spatula to scrape the mixture into the cloth. Sprinkle the salt over the surface and fold in.

3. Allow this mixture to drain/lose moisture at room temperature for up to 4 hours, and then finish in the refrigerator overnight if needed. This will not look like a dairy curd. Fold in the calcium chloride. Be sure to taste it and adjust salt if required.
4. After this first stage of moisture loss is finished, set up a bamboo mat or small wooden cheeseboard, place your cheese mold (usually round and perforated with holes to allow for moisture escape) on the mat/board. Line the mold with cheesecloth and add the salted curd to the mold, and press it into place. You may want to make two smaller cheeses, so be sure to have enough equipment on hand to do so.
5. Lightly cover the top of the cheese with the cheesecloth, and place the mold on a bamboo mat/wooden board, and place this into a container (ripening box) that is large enough to allow for good airflow. Place a lid lightly on top and place this in the refrigerator.
6. Over the next 2 to 5 days, check the cheese to see how it is firming up. Take the cloth off the top, and sprinkle a very small amount of salt on top. This helps pull moisture to the surface and this moisture will evaporate and allow the surface to begin drying. It will also keep the surface hostile to pathogens. Do not salt every day. Wipe away any excess moisture that is in the container, and change the bamboo mat or wooden board if necessary.
7. Depending on how fast moisture is evaporating from your cheese, you may be able to remove the cheese in cheesecloth from the mold between day 2 and day 5. In any case, once you have removed the cheese from the mold, allow it (in cheesecloth) to continue to age on the bamboo mat or wooden board.
8. Continue to check daily and turn the cheese over each day to allow for moisture to escape from the bottom of the cheese. Lightly salt the bottom of the cheese every second day or so. With the salting process, it is critical to assess the surface of the cheese to see how quickly it may be drying. It will be tempting to add more salt or salt more often, but resist. Touch the surface of your cheese, check the cheesecloth or aging mats for dampness, change them so that fresh ones can absorb more moisture. Too much salt or too much salt applied too frequently can lead to an overly salty cheese but also a cheese that will crack and pull apart because the surface dries more rapidly than moisture is lost from the inside of the cheese. As the cheese ages, you will need to salt the surface less often, so use observation to guide you.
9. Once you can handle the cheese without it being too damp or soft, remove the cheesecloth altogether and place the cheese on a fresh bamboo mat/wooden board.

10. Now begins the process of aging and helping the cheese form a natural rind through salting, brining, washing, and air-drying. See the section on affinaging in chapter 6 for further information on how to proceed.

This cheese will take 2 to 4 months to finish depending on the size of the cheese you make (the larger the cheese, the longer it will take to age). It is optimal to age this cheese in a separate refrigerator such as a wine fridge, where you can control the temperature and humidity. Optimal temperature would be 10°C–13°C (50°F–55°F), and relative humidity about 65–75%. A handy device, a hygrometer, can measure both temperature and humidity.

## Method 2: crossover method

### Tools and Equipment

2 × thick cast saucepan
Measuring cups
Measuring spoons
Spatula
Blender
Wooden or silicone spoon
Probe thermometer
Container for culturing
Bamboo mat/wooden cheese board
Cheesecloth or butter muslin
Container/ripening box
Cheese mold (one or more)

### Ingredients

1 × batch of curd (not aged) from method 1 (cultured and aged)
½ cup coconut oil, softened (or half and half coconut oil and cacao butter)
1 tsp powdered annatto (or several drops of liquid annatto)*
3 cups water (filtered or rested tap water)
2 tsp powdered agar agar (or approximately the same amount of kappa carrageenan)
Salt (sparingly)
½ tsp citric acid

Optional: dried spices or herbs as you wish

Optional: 1 Tbsp white miso to boost the umami as this is a shorter aging cheese than the previous method

\* Annatto is a food coloring derived from the seeds of the achiote tree and imparts an orangish color. Annatto or achiote finds use in many Mexican, Central and South American dishes. You can order liquid annatto from cheesemaking supply shops, or you can find powdered annatto at Mexican or South American grocer

### Method

1. Wash and sanitize all work surfaces and any tools you will be using.
2. Remove the curd from the refrigerator, and allow it to warm up.
3. In a thick cast saucepan, place the 3 cups of water and add the agar agar. Whisk continuously as the agar agar heats up over medium to medium-high heat. Agar agar needs to reach 85°C (185°F) and maintain that heat for 5 minutes. Use a probe thermometer to check the temperature. If the water/agar agar is thickening too quickly, reduce heat and add a bit more water.
4. Once the agar agar is activated, add the curd to the saucepan as well as the softened oil, annatto, and the miso (if you choose to add it) and stir in vigorously to ensure that the mixture is well combined. I recommend blending at low speed after the mixture has been combined and then returning it to the pot and heating it to 185°F (85°C) and maintaining that temperature for 10 minutes.
5. Once the mixture has heated up, add the citric acid. This helps to lower the pH, which is important for prolonging shelf life during aging. Stir until well combined.

    Alternatively, you can remove the mixture from heat and cool until it reaches 105°F (40.5°C) and add 1–2 tsp starter culture (rejuvelac or coconut kefir).
6. Set out a bamboo mat or wooden board and a cheese mold. Line the mold with doubled up cheesecloth or butter muslin, and pour the mixture into it. Press down lightly and ensure that the top is evenly spread. Sprinkle a little salt over the top, and lightly cover the top with cheesecloth. Place the mold on top of the mat/board. Allow the cheese to cool to room temperature before placing in the container/ripening box and setting in the refrigerator to set.

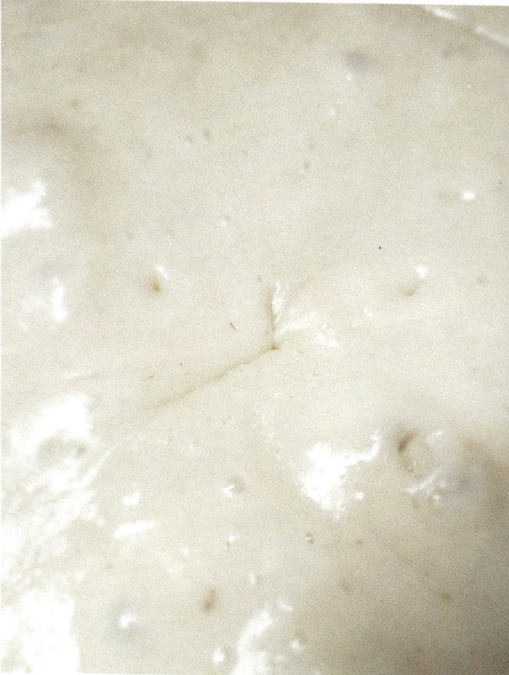

*Cultured curd with coconut oil and agar agar on heat.*

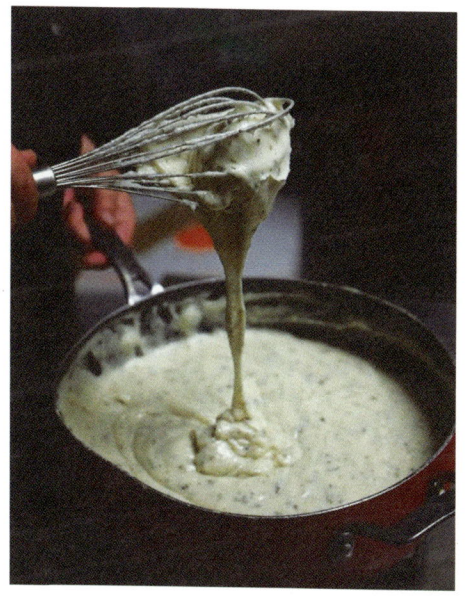

*Whisking/stirring the cultured curd with agar agar and coconut oil mixture.*
CREDIT: ANDRE SHEPPERD, DREMOND STUDIO

7. The next day check how firmly the cheese has set. It is likely to be a little soft. This is desirable as you will still need to age the cheese to achieve final firmness. Adding too much agar agar can help a cheese set firm but will often lead to a rubbery texture. Too much kappa carrageenan will set but may feel gummy or not as dense as you might like. If the cheese is firm enough to remove from the cheese mold, do so, and set, while still in cheesecloth, on the bamboo mat/wooden board.

8. For further guidance on methods for aging your cheese, refer to the section on affinaging in Chapter 6. This cheese should take from 3 weeks to 1.5 months (depending on the size of the cheese) to be fully ready and can be aged in the home refrigerator or in a separate, dedicated aging space. The surface of the cheese will need close monitoring as it ages, and I recommend using some form of acidity in the washes.

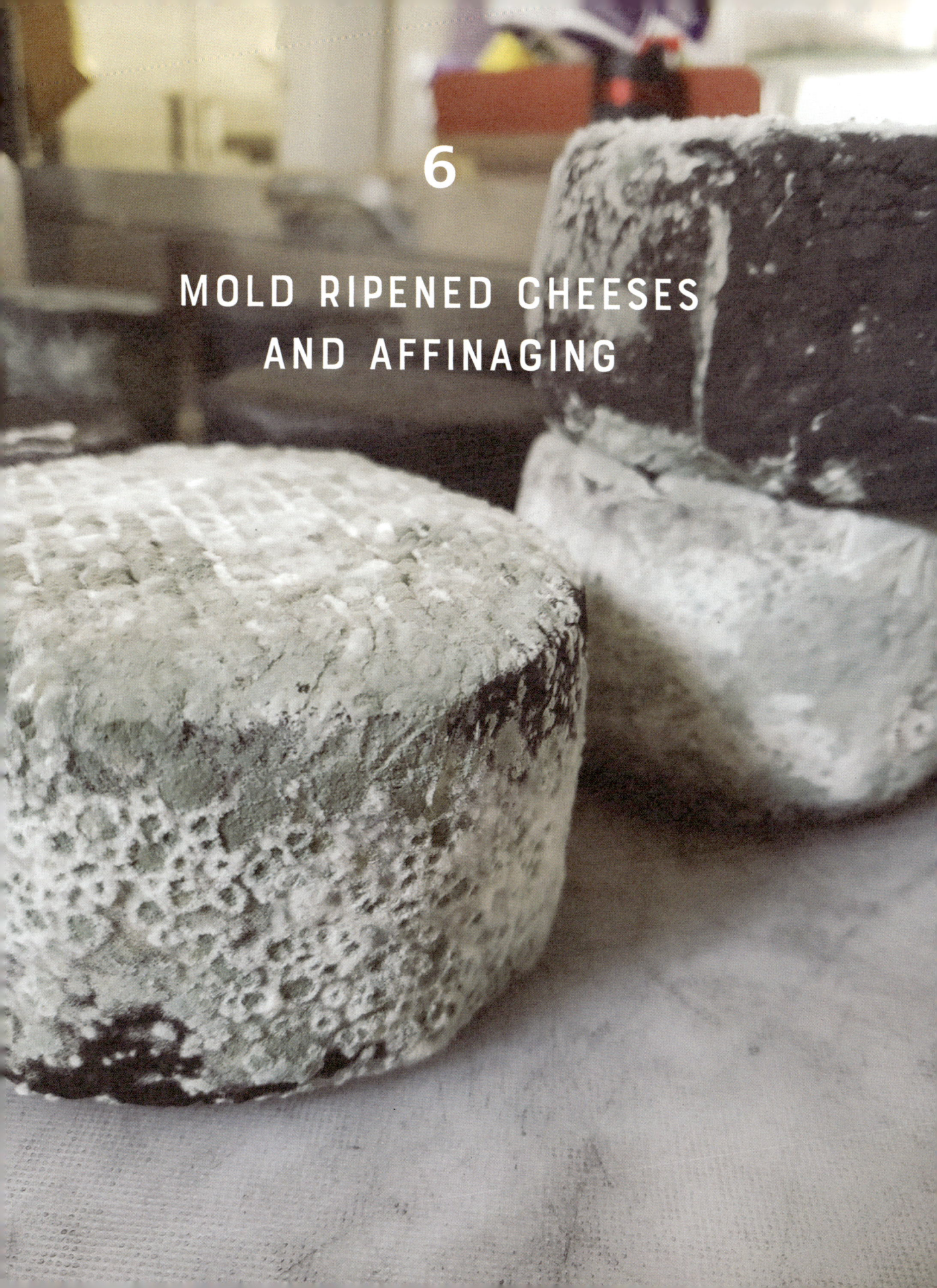

# 6
# MOLD RIPENED CHEESES AND AFFINAGING

Though infrequently released at this time, the blue cheeses and white mold ripened cheeses I make for Blue Heron sell so quickly we rarely get to advertise that they are available. Though admittedly more polarizing, the demand we receive for blue cheese is almost in line with the folks seeking true hard vegan cheese. Blue and white mold ripened cheeses and combinations of the two are my favorite types of cheese to make, albeit the most particular and fussy. They offer the most degree of challenge, and require a commitment to observation and an understanding of the principles and materials more than simply following a recipe.

While there is an ever increasing number of small scale artisan vegan cheesemakers making versions of blue cheese and white mold ripened cheeses,[6] these types of cheeses using real cheesemaking molds are not yet being made by the larger scale vegan cheese companies, but this will change soon.

There are multiple reasons for the slowness of the commercial sector to take on production of the blue cheese and white mold ripened cheese, firstly, the fact that they are fussy, as I mentioned above, and secondly, that they take more time than the non-cultured cheeze-type products and therefore are more costly in terms of the amount of space they occupy during aging time. For the home DIYer, these cheeses are no less challenging. I say this not to put you off, but a number of methods floating around out there do not fully represent the various factors one should consider when embarking on making either a white mold or blue mold cheese.

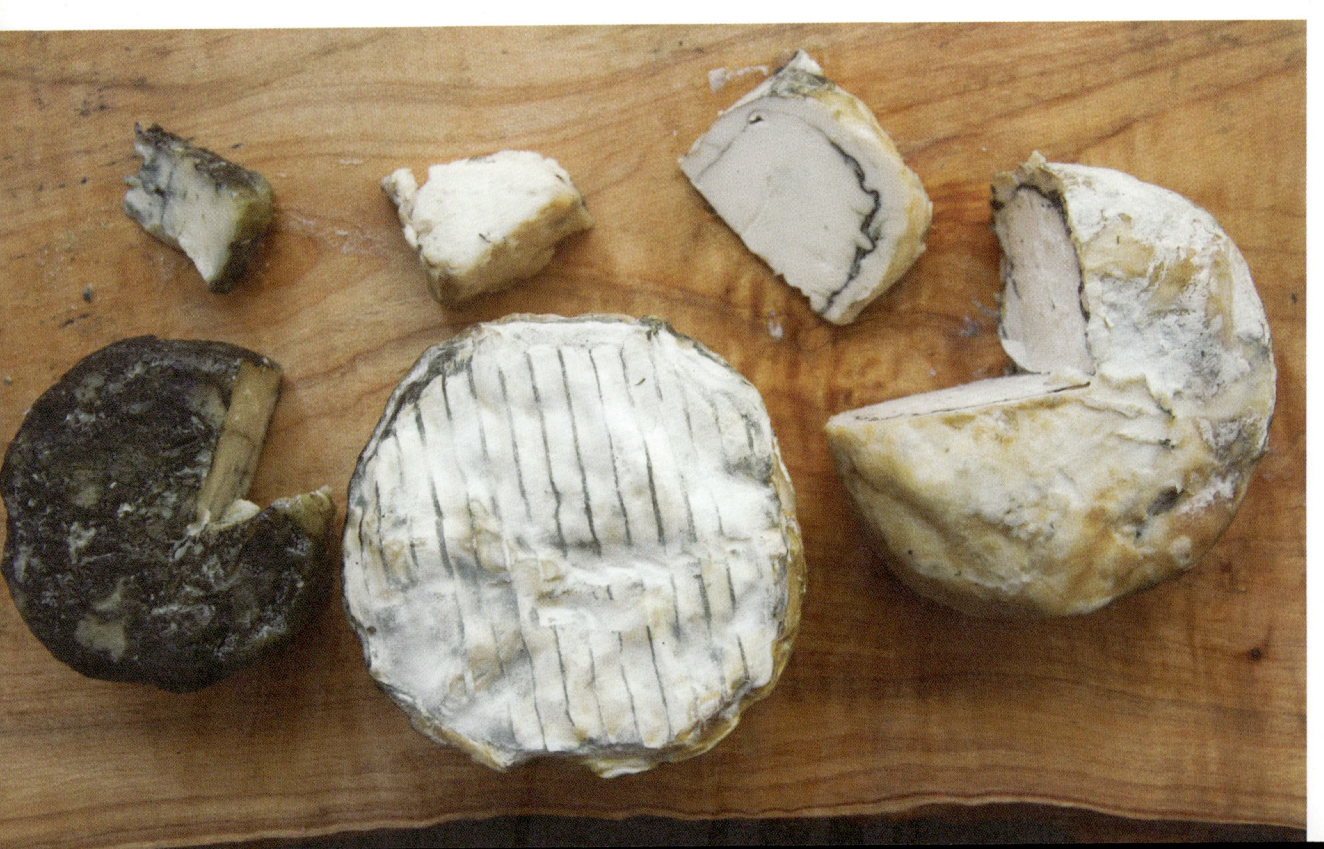

*A variety of Blue Heron mold ripened cheeses.*
Credit: Colin Medhurst

## Before You Start

First, make sure you have the appropriate equipment to complete the aging processes and that you have a space other than your home refrigerator for these cheeses. You will be working with mold spores, and this means the potential for these spores to get into and populate your refrigerator and other foods is highly likely. Blue mold, in particular, is very aggressive and can thrive in a variety of environments.

Equipment that will be helpful includes a small refrigerator or wine fridge that you can dedicate to cheesemaking. Even though these will still not be set up with the appropriate temperature and humidity controls, there are ways to work with and around them. The most important thing about using them is that they keep the mold ripened cheeses separate from other foods and allow you to manipulate the environment specifically for the cheeses. Additionally, an ice chest or even a cooler (the type one might use going camping) can be useful and a good way to do a small scale test project before you commit to an entirely separate refrigerator.

Measuring pH (acidity/alkalinity) is important, and I recommend that you obtain a pH meter. Affordable meters can be found online, and knowing how to use one is indispensable when learning how to identify the types of conditions that affect your projects and the changes they undergo. I reference pH a lot in the following sections on method, and there is no other way to measure precise pH than with a meter.

In the sections that follow, I focus on the important principles that you need to understand, and the related methods are less about precise sorts of cheese such as roquefort or gorgonzola, which do not technically apply within the vegan cheese sector, in any case, because of very specific requirements for making those types of cheese. These methods are the basis for making an undefined type of blue cheese and an undefined white mold ripened cheese. Using these two methods and with the principles in hand, you can begin experimenting with your own variations.

## White Mold Ripened Cheese

In the dairy cheesemaking world, white mold ripened cheeses include brie, camembert, cambozola (which also includes blue mold), valençay (a French goat cheese), and a large number of local and regional types. More generally, the use of white mold is referred to as bloomy rind or surface ripened cheese. Of all the types of cheese ripening processes in the dairy realm, bloomy rind cheeses are considered to have the most complex process. This is because the molds used (desired molds) grow well only under very specific conditions, variation of which can cause the demise of your project, and then, once you have achieved the mold rind you seek, another set of conditions must be met and maintained in order to allow the cheese to develop its flavor and texture.

While in dairy cheesemaking there are two types of curds used for bloomy rind cheeses (lactic-set or rennet-set), I focus on only the slow acid building lactic-set curd that has been the general focus of the cultured cheese section of this book. With this type of curd, you end up with a firmer style of white mold ripened cheese, but it will have good aroma and flavor. Before diving into method, let me unpack a little bit of what happens when you are working with white molds in cheesemaking.

Both blue and white mold cheeses are lower acidity cheeses than the cultured cheeses that have been covered so far. They may start at a low pH (high acidity), but gradually this changes upward, and it is during this move from low pH (high acidity) to higher pH (low acidity) that mold can grow. Lactic-set curds (as you have been making with the other cultured cheeses in this book) are high in moisture. This high moisture allows acidity to continue building slowly during the draining phase of the cheese, and during this time bacteria are continuing to metabolize the sugars and produce acidity, and they are also creating the food needed for the molds.

The pH level, salt content, temperature, and humidity/moisture level are very important conditions during the process of converting the lactic-set curd into a bloomy rind cheese.

Having a pH meter on hand is very important because you need to measure the pH changes and determine when to add salt to the surface and when to move the cheese into different conditions at different stages of its development. It is particularly important to be diligent in following the process as outlined because white mold cheeses are high alkaline cheeses with high moisture content and are at greater risk of growing pathogenic bacteria (that were either already present or arrive from contamination).

Outlined here are the general phases of a white mold cheese process and some of the key principles involved. This is not a full deep dive into all of the science (as some of this would be changed by different types of plant-based mediums being cultured, for instance, coconut milk versus almond milk) but it does give you the key principles involved in what is happening and why it matters.

Phase 1 can be considered the curd creation phase. This is when you make the lactic-set curd. This is the phase during which mesophilic starter cultures acidify the medium creating lactic acid and other by-products, some of which will become food for the mold spores.

Phase 2 is the draining phase, which, in the case of this plant-based method, will occur after the culturing period (phase 1 is longer in the plant-based method than in a dairy method). This draining phase will refer to what is technically a second draining phase, in that it happens once the cheeses are formed and in their molds (being shaped).

The draining phase is very important as white molds do not grow in an environment that is too wet. Draining should take 1 to 2 days at a temperature of 62.6°F (17°C) with a relative humidity of 80–85% (which can be measured using a hygrometer). Ensuring that you measure the conditions and maintain a constant environment is important. This means draining cannot occur in the home refrigerator, and you will need a separate area to do this.

Phase 3 is ripening. Ripening in cheesemaking can be a bit confusing as it can refer to the initial acidification phase in curd making that is done over heat, or it can refer to the period of time following draining during which the cheeses are put into an environment that will encourage a particular activity to happen. In this case, after draining is finished, the cheeses are moved into an environment with a temperature range of 50°F–55°F (10°C–13°C) and a relative humidity of 95%. With both the draining and ripening phases requiring temperature and humidity conditions well outside the household refrigerator, it should be clear by now that ensuring you have appropriate equipment to make this cheese is the necessary first step.

During the ripening phase, the cheeses will be quite soft but should be turned daily. Be sure to use gloved or sanitized hands to prevent brown or black mildew fingerprints from showing up. The pH of the surface should be tested (scrape a little off and mix with water before measuring with a pH meter), and while the pH of the surface is 4.6–4.7, the surface should be salted.

Salt for the cheese should be about 1–2% of its weight. Weigh the cheese, and then calculate the amount of salt required by multiplying the weight by 0.01 or 0.02. The number you end up with indicates the number of grams of salt you use. For

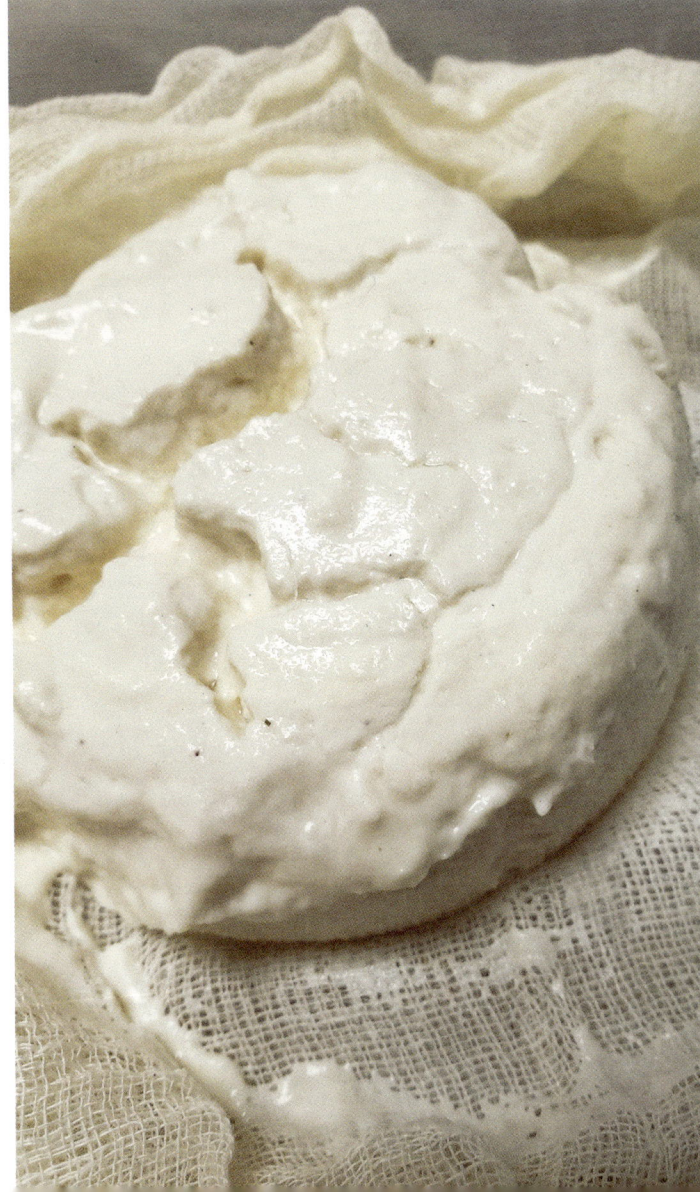

*Delicate inoculated macadamia, oat, cashew camembert.*

instance, if the cheese round you are preparing to salt is 150 grams and you multiply that by 0.01, the amount of salt you use is 1.5 grams.

This ripening phase continues with daily turning and with temperature and humidity levels maintained. A shiny slick beginning to form on the surface of the cheese is a sign that yeasts are beginning to grow and metabolize sugars, which precedes the growth of mold. As the yeasts work metabolizing sugars, the pH of the surface begins to rise.

The mold will begin to appear as white patches and as it grows will unite into what you will recognize from brie or camembert. Once you have a good surface cover of white mold, the pH should be 7.0 (neutral) at the surface, and about 6.0 in the center.

The final phase of ripening occurs at a much lower temperature, 38°F (3°C), but still with a humidity of 95%. While the previous phases are much warmer than a household refrigerator, this is cooler than a typical home refrigerator and with much higher humidity, so once again, you need to do this in an environment in which you can control both factors. If you are doing this in a converted refrigerator, keep in mind that refrigerators are designed for keeping food cold and delaying decomposition for as long as possible, and this means the temperature and the humidity are different than the conditions that are ideal for ripening cheese and aging cheese over longer periods of time. Units designed specifically for aging cheese allow for a slightly higher temperature and greater humidity.

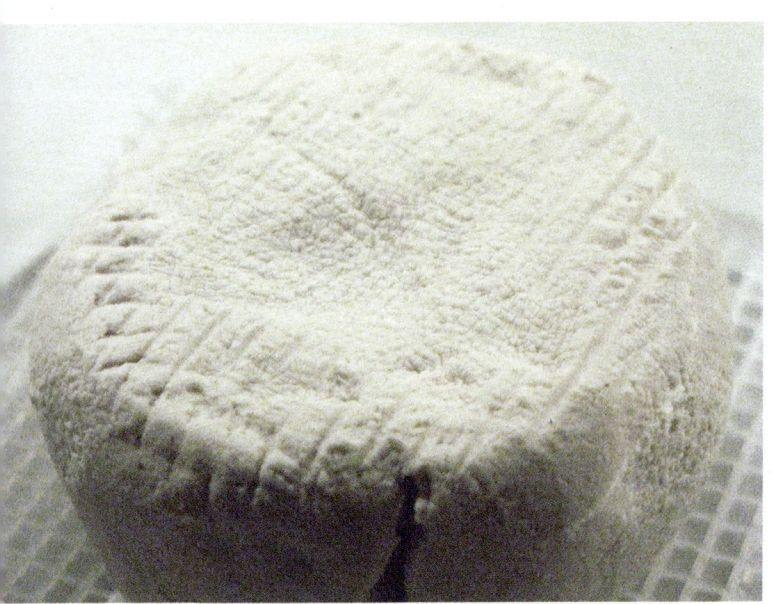

Above: *Very early stages of white mold blossoming.*

Right: *Young white mold blossom.*

Aging your cheese in a refrigerator will have its own impact on the development of the cheese. This means you will have to monitor humidity closely, and should it begin to drop below 90% you can amend conditions by placing a clean, never used, damp sponge or two into the space to increase ambient humidity.

White mold responds very well to the use of ripening paper, a paper designed specifically for cheeses, and you can find ripening paper at a number of cheesemaking supply stores online. It allows for oxygen exchange and prevents drying. The white mold you should work with is HP6 direct-set *P. candidum* from Danisco Choozit. It is a freeze-dried mold culture. Follow instructions given next for activating it in small batches prior to use. Follow manufacturer's instructions for storage.

The cheese will take approximately 3 weeks to finish from phase 2 depending on the size.

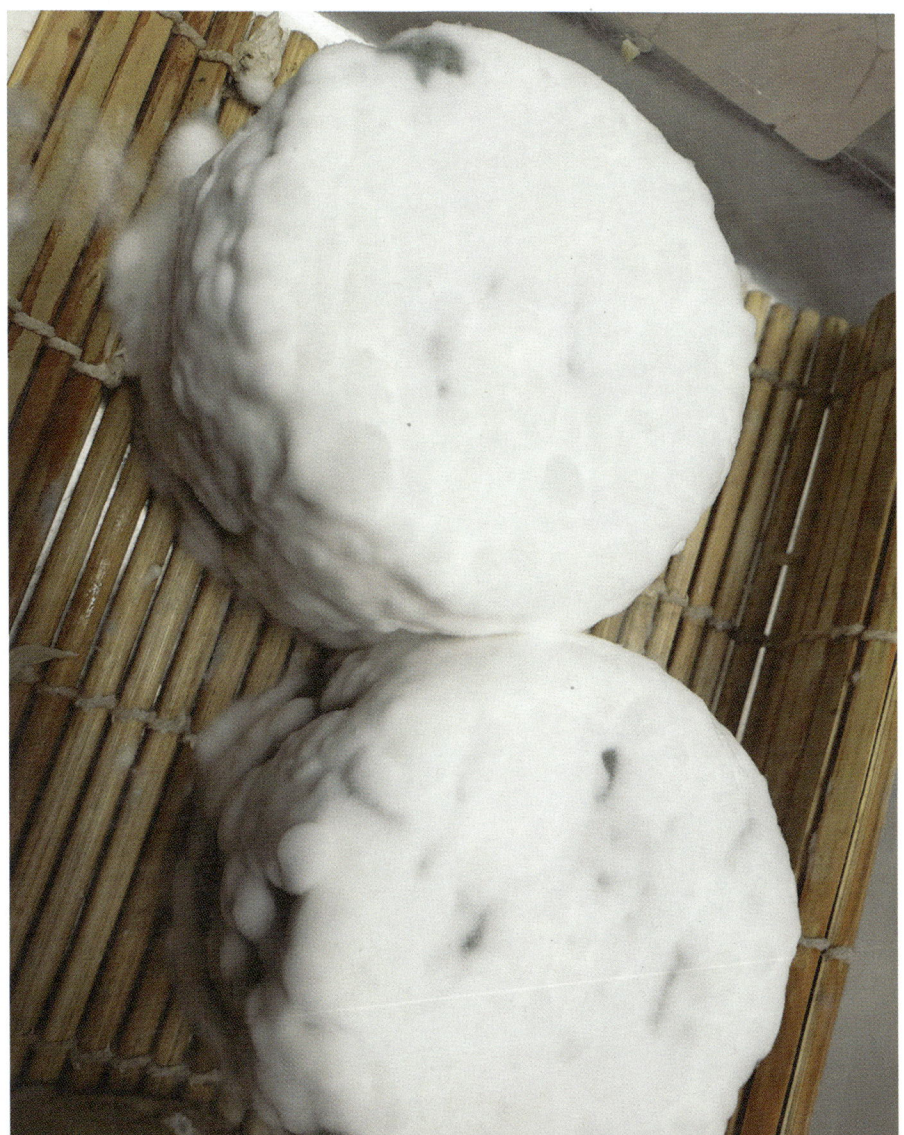

*White mold growth on surface (mold spores were sprayed on).*

## Tools and Equipment

Dedicated refrigerator or large cooler/icebox in which you can control humidity and temperature

1L jar, sanitized, for mold rehydration

pH meter

Probe thermometer

High-speed blender

2 × thick cast saucepans

Slow cooker or Instapot

Measuring cups

Measuring spoons

Scales (for weighing salt)

Spatula

Wooden or silicone spoons

Open-ended cheese molds or stainless steel cold hoops/cold forming rings

Bamboo mats or wooden cheeseboards

Cheesecloth or butter muslin

Ripening paper

Container for culturing period

Container to serve as a ripening box

## Ingredients

1.5 L high fat coconut milk (or ½ oat milk and ½ coconut cream)

3 cups macadamia nuts

3 cups cashew nuts

½ cup oats

4 cups water for blending (filtered or rested tap water)

starter culture: 3 tsp coconut kefir culture or 100MM direct-set mesophilic culture from Danisco Choozit

ripening culture: ⅛ tsp reactivated *P. candidum* (HP6) from Danisco Choozit starter culture (either the MM 100 direct-set mesophilic culture, Danisco Choozit, or the coconut kefir)

½ tsp calcium chloride

salt (amount to be calculated as a percentage of weight per cheese round after curd is drained and shaped into individual rounds)

## Method

This method employs a direct inoculation approach, including mold spores into the mixture at the same time the starter culture is added.

1. Activate the *P. candidum* (*Penicillium candidum* is the ripening mold culture that will create the white bloomy rind). Make a solution of ½ tsp salt (non-iodized), ½ tsp sugar, a scant 1 L of water and add to a clean and sanitized jar; then add ⅛ tsp *P. candidum* spores from the packet. Allow the spores to activate in solution for 16 hours prior to use. Make sure the jar is covered and left at room temperature during rehydration of the spores.
2. Wash and sanitize all surfaces and tools you will be working with.
3. Add ½ the coconut milk to the high-speed blender. Then add ½ of the nuts and oats, and begin pulsing to break the materials down. Starting from lowest setting, gradually increase speed and add 2 cups of water over the course of blending. Keep blending until the mixture is very smooth and creamy in appearance. Repeat this process with the remaining coconut milk and nuts and oats. You want to end up with a matrix (blended nuts/oats/coconut milk/water) of about 3–3.5 L.
4. Fill one pot with water and place on the stovetop, place the other pot atop the first pot (it should fit just inside), and using the spatula scrape the mixture into the empty pot (both batches). Warm the matrix over medium to medium-high heat to 95°F (35°C). Use a probe thermometer to check the temperature. Add the starter culture (either the MM 100 direct-set mesophilic culture, Danisco Choozit, or the coconut kefir) at the same time as adding the ⅛ tsp of activated ripening culture (*P. candidum*). Do not stir. Just allow the cultures to rest for 2 to 3 minutes.
5. Gently stir the matrix for 3 to 5 minutes while maintaining heat at 95°F (35°C).
6. Allow the mixture to ripen for 3 to 4 hours. Use the pH meter to check pH level. It should read between 6.0 and 6.2 by 4 hours.
7. Add the calcium chloride and stir in gently. Continue to maintain heat at 95°F (35°C) for another 2 hours.
8. In dairy cheesemaking, this is where you would expect to find a soft curd that you would then cut. This is not the case in a plant-based version. As the plant proteins involved are not structured the same as the casein proteins of dairy, they do not behave the same way in this process, and generally they need more time to break down in the lactic acid fermentation process. Remove the mixture from the heat and place in a food grade container with headroom for gas exchange and airflow. Cover the container and allow the mixture to culture/ferment at a warm temperature between 77°F and 95°F (25°C and 35°C).
9. If the batch is small, this could be done in a slow cooker on low heat or in an Instapot on the lowest heat setting. If you use one of these devices for the

culturing period, put the mixture directly into the pot and make sure the pot is covered. Allow this to culture overnight.
10. Transfer the mixture to a food grade container, and during the process, assess the thickness of the mixture. If it is still quite loose, cover the container and continue to culture at room temperature, 64°F–72°F (18°C–22°C), for another 24 hours.
11. After the culturing period, place the container in the refrigerator for up to 8 hours. I find this helps the curd set up and makes it easier to place into the cheese molds later.

**After the culturing period**

1. Set up bamboo mat/aging mat/wooden board, place a cheese mold or stainless steel ring mold on top, and then place double layered cheesecloth or butter muslin inside the ring mold.
2. Gently scoop the curd into the mold and fill to just under the top. Place the cheese on mat/board inside a large, well cleaned and sanitized cooler or container that can be closed and used for the first stage of post-culturing drying. During this time, the goal is for the cheese to continue to lose a lot of moisture, as white mold does not grow well in an overly wet environment. The cheese will spend 1 to 2 days in this box/cooler at a temperature of 62°F (17°C) and at 80–85% humidity. Open the container once or twice a day to allow gas to escape and open up the airflow. Check the temperature, the humidity, and pH.
3. After this phase, the cheese will still be delicate but needs to be transferred to the first stage of ripening and held at 50°F–55°F (10°C–13°C) with a relative humidity of 95%. This should be done in a refrigerator or container where you can control temperature and humidity. You can remove the mold at this stage if it seems the cheese will hold its shape, but if it seems too loose for that, leave the mold on. When the mold has been removed, begin gently turning the cheese daily. Use gloved or sanitized hands to avoid having brown/black mildew fingerprints appear on your cheese.
4. Observe the cheese daily, checking temperature and humidity. During this time, the yeasts on the surface will be metabolizing sugars and producing food for the mold spores. A shiny, slick surface means mold will appear soon. Test the surface pH of the cheese, and once it has reached 4.6–4.7, begin salting it lightly. I either apply small amounts of dry salt (calculated by determining the weight of the individual cheese and multiplying that by 0.01 or 0.02) or wash using a light brine. It is easier to control salt level with the dry salt method than the brine wash, but it is more delicate work to apply. Apply salt lightly every 2 to 3 days for the first week.

5. Continue to turn the cheese daily as the mold grows (it will still be in this 50°F–55°F (10°C–13°C) and 95% humidity environment). Observe for patches and excess moisture coming from the cheese. Wipe up excess moisture and change out the bamboo mat/aging mat/cheeseboard. This stage of ripening can take more than a week. Be patient.
6. Once the cheese has a thorough cover of white mold on all surfaces, it can be moved to the second stage of ripening, which occurs at low temperature, 38°F (3°C), with relative humidity of 95%. Humidity at this low temperature can be tricky to sustain, so you can use a clean, never used, sponge dampened and placed inside the ripening area to increase ambient humidity. During this final stage of ripening, which is really intended to allow flavor and texture to develop, you can wrap the individual cheese in ripening paper designed specifically for white mold cheeses (this kind of paper can be found at cheesemaking supply shops). The paper allows airflow/oxygen, helps to prevent drying out, and increases humidity at the surface of the cheese, which promotes mold growth.
7. This process will take at least 3 weeks, and requires your diligent attention to ensure a safe cheese is made. Once the cheese is ready or finished, surface pH should be about 7.0 pH and core pH 6.0.
8. Store the cheese wrapped in the ripening paper (which is also called cheese paper) away from other foods that may contaminate it. It keeps for 3 to 4

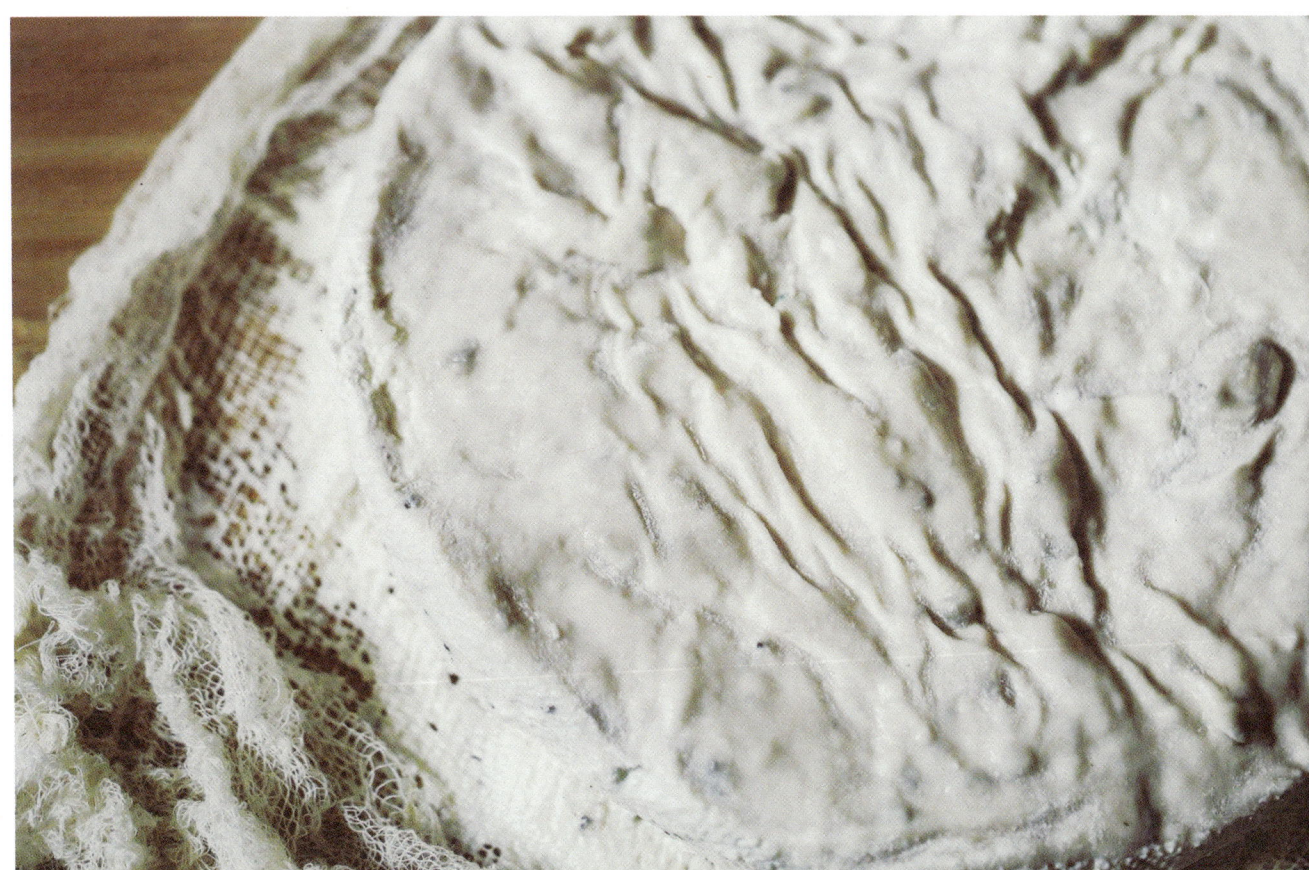

*White mold growing on cheese surface.*
CREDIT: CATHERINE DOWNES

weeks after being determined to be ready, but, remember, this is a living cheese, the microbes will continue to slowly do their work, and the cheese will continue to change over this time.

## Blue Cheese Method

Blue cheeses are likely the most polarizing of all cheeses, like coriander (cilantro) is among herbs. The robust pungent aroma and piquant flavor can either win committed fans or confirm serious opponents. There is not an in-between. No one hears someone declare, "I kind of like blue cheese." It is generally love or hate.

I fall into the love category. While my history of dairy cheese consumption is limited and confined to a period of time a very long time ago (I have been vegetarian and then vegan the majority of my life now), my appreciation for the process of making blue cheese and getting familiar with the molds and what they do and what they produce in the way of smell, taste, and texture, finds me deeply attached to them.

I love the pungent aroma, and now, from experience, I know how to recognize through smell what has occurred in a particular cheese's development (too much heat early, not enough humidity at certain times, new matrix to feed on, et cetera). Now, when I go to take a slice of a blue cheese test batch, my stomach grumbles and my mouth begins watering just upon smelling it. I am devoted.

Blue cheeses pose the most degree of challenge to both a commercial vegan cheesemaker and the home-based vegan cheesemaker. Like the white mold cheeses, blue cheese requires specific conditions that are not suited to the home refrigerator. The mold, *Penicillium roqueforti* (*P. roqueforti*), responsible for the iconic blue veins/mottling of dairy favorites like stilton, gorgonzola, roquefort, Danish blue, and so forth, is aggressive and spore producing and will readily jump to other cheeses or foods in its environment.

And since spore production is part of the active phase of a blue cheese ripening, those spores can move easily through an environment with little trouble. Making blue cheese requires the capacity to keep the project segregated from other foods. It also requires that you are diligent with respect to cleaning and sanitizing equipment you use before, during the ripening and aging process, and after.

*P. roqueforti* produces a range of colors, which is important to know especially if you are new to working with molds. Colors can range from light blue to green, and different shades of gray. Different strains of *P. roqueforti* exist, and each behaves differently and has a unique impact on a cheese. It loves high fat and salty environments, grows well in low oxygen, and is very good at breaking down fats (lipolysis) and proteins (proteolysis).

The breakdown of fats to fatty acids by the mold produces methyl ketones from the free fatty acids, and these are responsible for the characteristic aromas associated with blue cheeses. This means, then, that the profile of fatty acids present in the matrix being cultured is important as these will inform the overall flavor and aroma.

Salt is incredibly important in the making of blue cheese, and it is not possible to make a low salt blue cheese made with real *P. roqueforti*. The mold grows well in an environment with a salt concentration of about 13% and ends up with a 2–5% salt content inside the cheese. As the NaCl (sodium chloride) moves toward the inside of the cheese (from washes/brining/salting processes), it changes the way the mold grows.

Instead of seeing a spread of fuzzy mold, the mycelia, growing, the mold is triggered to grow more conidia, or spores. This will appear as flat patches of gray, green, or blue, and when you touch them, spores will be released (this will look like a fine dust). It is important to know that the colors you see indicate what is happening. Conidia (spores) present as blue-green. The mycelia usually form a thick mat that can appear as dark blue/blackish, feels rubbery, and will often slip off the surface of the cheese.

Obtaining the desired pockets of blue mold internally or thin veins within the cheese requires piercing the cheese or breaking up the cheese into large pieces of curd containing mold and reshaping the cheese. Both of these methods oxygenate the interior of the cheese, and create physical space for the mold to grow inside.

The starter (lactic acid) culture also affects how the blue mold forms and behaves. A culture that has yeasts which also produce gas, ($CO_2$), are not only important in terms of how they metabolize sugars and provide food for the

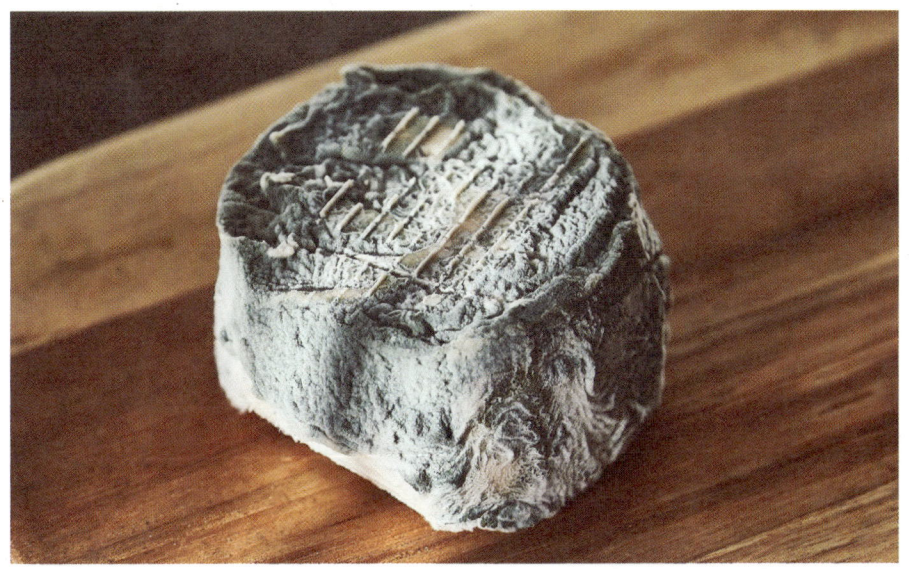

*Young blue cheese with mycelia mat forming on surface before being pierced and washed.* CREDIT: ANDRE SHEPPERD, DREMOND STUDIO

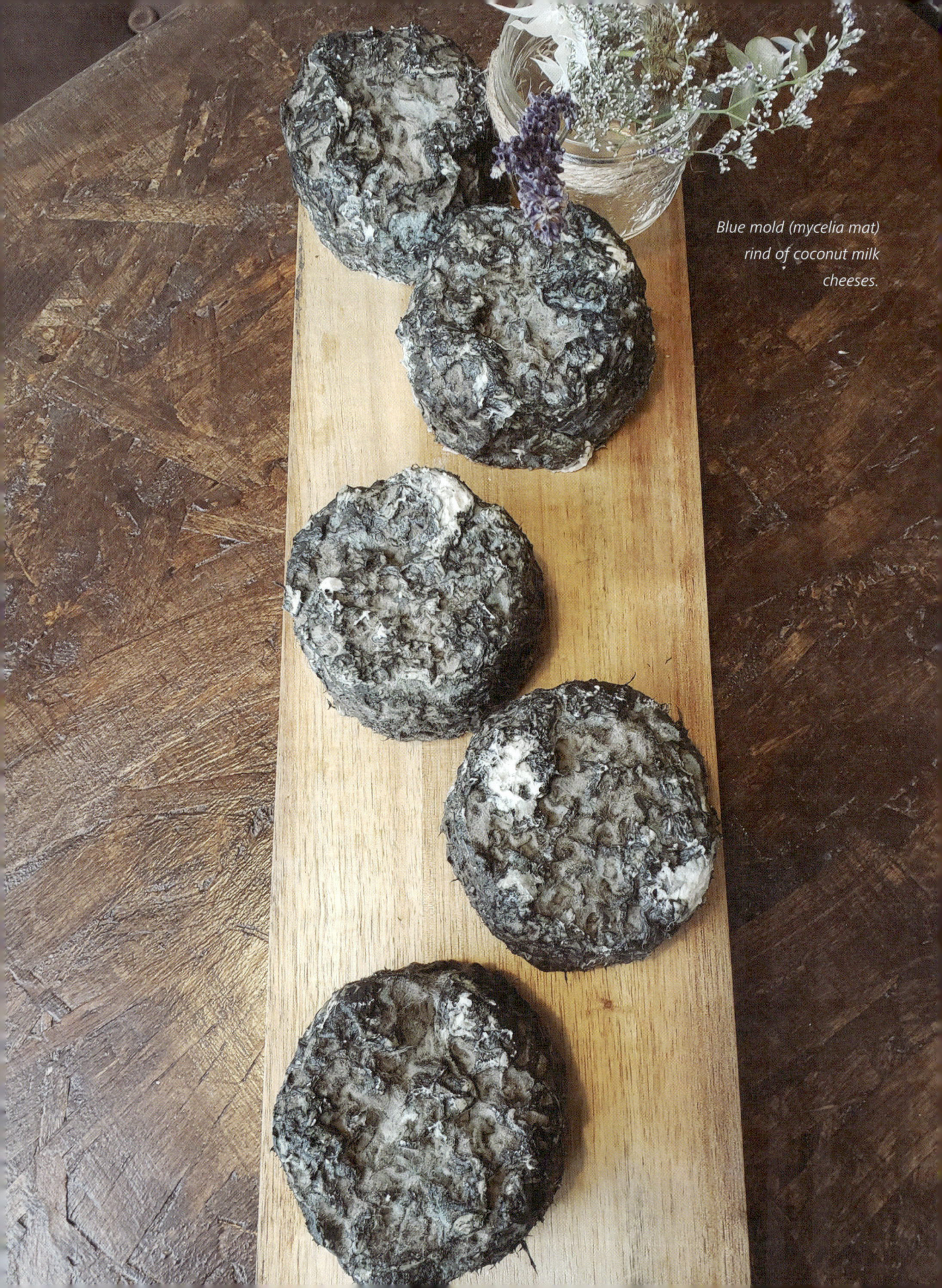
*Blue mold (mycelia mat) rind of coconut milk cheeses.*

mold, but the gas produced creates air pockets in the curd, which will become places for the mold to grow. Ensuring that the inside of the cheese gets oxygenated is important to the development of blue veins and pockets, and the piercing of the cheese is done at particular stages of its development in order to achieve this. If piercing does not occur, mold will not grow internally, particularly in dense, wet curds, and you will end up with only a blue mold mat surface.

Blue cheeses are typically made from uncooked, unpressed curd, and the type of lactic-set curds that are presented in this book can be inoculated with blue

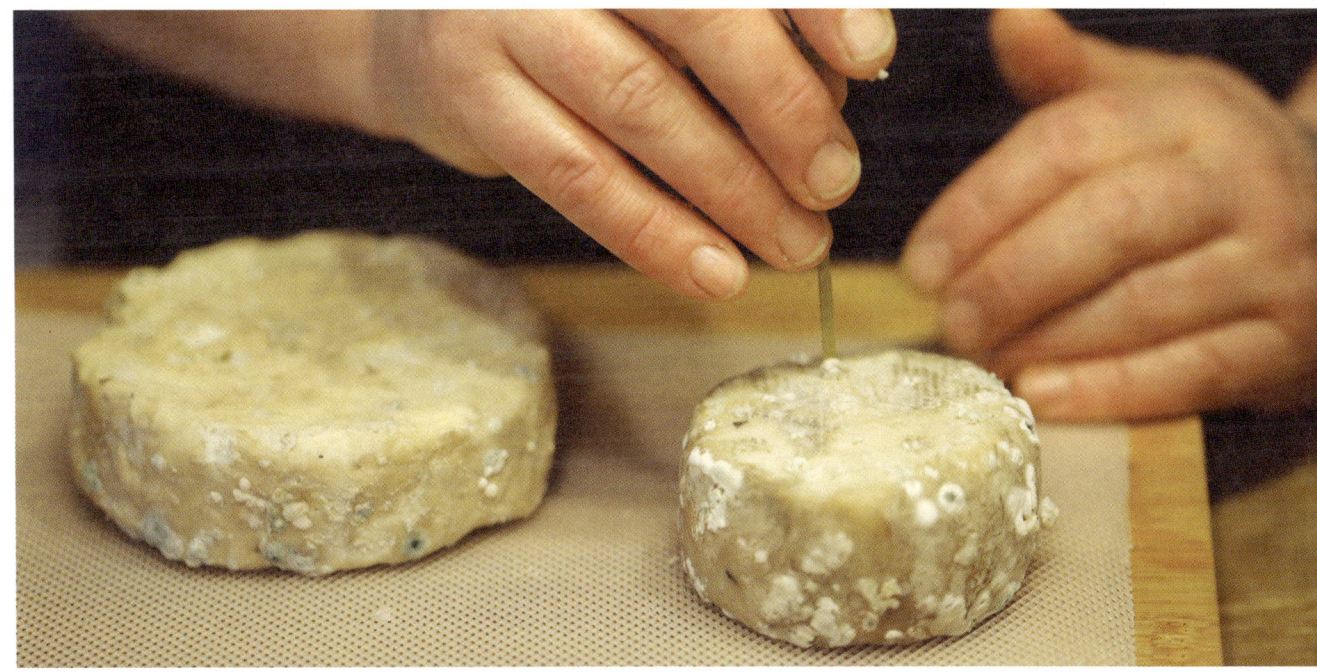

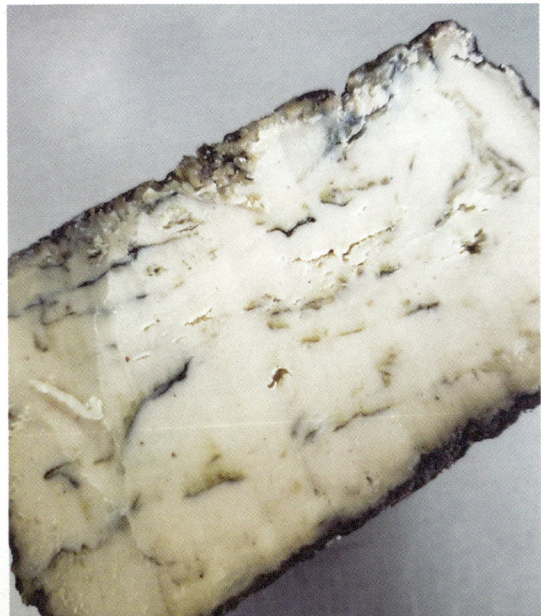

Above: *Author piercing young blue cheeses to increase oxygen and encourage mold growth inside, which results in veins developing.* CREDIT: CATHERINE DOWNES

Left: *Small fine veins marking Blue Heron's Ardea Blue coconut milk blue cheese. These veins are greenish when the cheese is first cut and turn bluish as it is oxygenated (exposed to air).*

mold to make a blue, cheese. I outline two processes for making blue cheese. One roughly follows a roqueforti method. The other is roughly based on the idea of a stirred or milled curd approach from the dairy cheesemaking world. Although informed by these methods, I've developed these processes based on what my best results have been, working with plant-based mediums. The blue mold you should work with is PRB6 by Danisco Choozit. It is a liquid form of *P. roqueforti*. You will need very small amounts of this mold, so please follow instructions on the package for appropriate storage of excess.

PRB6 strain is a fast growing, blue-green appearing mold and produces very strong blue cheese flavor. You will be able to mitigate the strength by using tiny amounts of the mold, using salt to control its growth, and measuring pH regularly as well as tasting frequently during its development to ensure the cheese is evolving the way you want it to. Be patient, and accept that you may have one or two or maybe more failures with this process as you get used to working with the mold. Before embarking on this process, please ensure that you have the right equipment in place.

## Tools and Equipment

Refrigerator/wine fridge exclusively for ripening and storage
Large, cleaned and sanitized cooler for early stage ripening
Container for culturing period
2 × thick cast pots (appropriate for the size of the batch you are preparing)
2 or 3 × wooden or silicone spoons
Spatula
High-speed blender
Measuring cups
Measuring spoons
Scales (for weighing salt)
pH meter
Hygrometer
Probe thermometer
Knitting needle, 3.5 mm (for piercing)
Bamboo mat/aging mat/wooden cheeseboard
Foil paper
Cheesecloth or butter muslin

## Ingredients

4 L matrix composed of:
    2 L high fat coconut milk

500 mL homemade almond or oat milk (Almond adds a nice level of sharpness as the cheese ages.)

6 cups cashew or macadamia nuts soaked according to the Soaking Guidelines in chapter 3. Alternatively, you can substitute almonds for half the amount of nuts.

4 cups water (filtered or rested tap water)

starter culture: 2 Tbsp rejuvelac or 2 Tbsp coconut kefir

ripening culture: ½ drop PRB6 *P. roqueforti*

calcium chloride: ¼ tsp diluted in ½ Tbsp water (to be used in wash during affinaging)

Salt 11.2 g

## Method 1: heat stimulated lactic-set curd

1. Wash and sanitize all work surfaces and all equipment and tools you plan to work with.
2. Fill one pot with water and set on the stovetop and place the other pot inside it.
3. Make the matrix. You will likely need to do this in two batches. Place ½ of the fluid ingredients into the blender, followed by ½ of the nuts. Begin pulsing to gradually combine the wet ingredients with the solids. Gradually increase the speed, and occasionally pause to observe how the matrix is forming. Blend at increasing speeds until the mixture is very smooth. Repeat until all of the wet and solid components have been blended together.
4. Scrape the blended mixture into the top saucepot and begin heating the mixture over medium heat. Heat the matrix to 89°F–90°F (32°C) and use a probe thermometer to measure the temperature. Heat for 30 minutes.
5. Add the starter culture and the tiny amount of PRB6 to the matrix and allow the drops of culture to rest on the surface of the mixture for 2 to 5 minutes. Gently stir the mixture for 3 to 5 minutes.
6. In-pot ripening: maintain the temperature at 89°F–90°F (32°C) for 30 to 35 minutes. Do not stir.
7. Add the calcium chloride and gently stir. Do not overstir. Continue to maintain the mixture at 89°F–90°F (32°C) for 3 hours. Use the probe thermometer to check the temperature and adjust the heat accordingly to ensure heat stability.
8. Here we depart from traditional dairy methodology as the plant matrix will require more time exposed to the cultures in order to form a lactic-set curd. Transfer the mixture to a food-grade container to allow the culture to continue to work. Ensure the container is large enough to accommodate ⅓ headspace for gas exchange and airflow. Cover the container and leave the mixture to culture in an ambient temperature of about 68°F (20°C) for 24 to 36 hours.

9. During the culturing phase, check the mixture every 12 hours. Observe the changes in appearance, aroma, and taste. Measure the pH. It should be dropping to 4.8–4.6.
10. After the culturing phase, place the mixture in the refrigerator for up to 4 hours to allow it to set up before beginning the next stage.

**After the culturing period**

1. Ensure that you have a ripening container large enough for the cheese and with enough space that you are able to control temperature and humidity with ease. Make sure that it is cleaned and sanitized and away from other cheese projects or foods.
2. Lay out the bamboo mat/aging mat/small wooden cheeseboard. Place the stainless steel ring mold or cheese mold on the mat/board, and line the mold with cheesecloth or butter muslin.
3. Sprinkle the salt over the curd and gently fold in; then add the curd to the mold. Do not press down. You want to allow pockets to form. This will be necessary for mold development.
4. Place the cheese inside the ripening box and ensure the temperature is 68°F–73°F (20°C–23°C) with a humidity of 90%. Check the starting pH, and record. Allow the cheese to lose moisture for 2 to 3 days in these conditions. By day 3 the pH should be 4.8–4.6.
5. For the first two days sprinkle salt over the cheese (if it is ready to remove from the mold, do so and leave the cheese on the mat. Maintain a temperature of 72°F (22°C) for the first day and gradually decrease to 68°F (20°C).
6. Move the cheese to the next stage of ripening/affinaging. This should be in a separate fridge/wine fridge. The temperature should be between 50°F and 55°F (10°C and 13°C), and relative humidity should be 90%. Turn the cheese daily for the next 8 to 10 days.
7. On day 10, with a clean and sanitized 3.5 mm knitting needle, pierce the surface of the cheese vertically, with 3–4 holes per square inch. Continue to turn the cheese daily, and wipe away any excess moisture draining away from it. Make sure to smell and taste the cheese to observe changes as it develops. Salting should be every 3 to 4 days at this point.
8. 14 days after the first piercing, you should pierce the cheese again. This cheese ages for 60 to 75 days, but the time will depend on the size. If the cheese is very small, the aging time will likely be significantly less than this, so this requires extra attention to observing the changes. During this time you should be seeing blue-green spots and patches forming. When the mold first appears, it is usually only in one or two spots, like pinpricks, and then

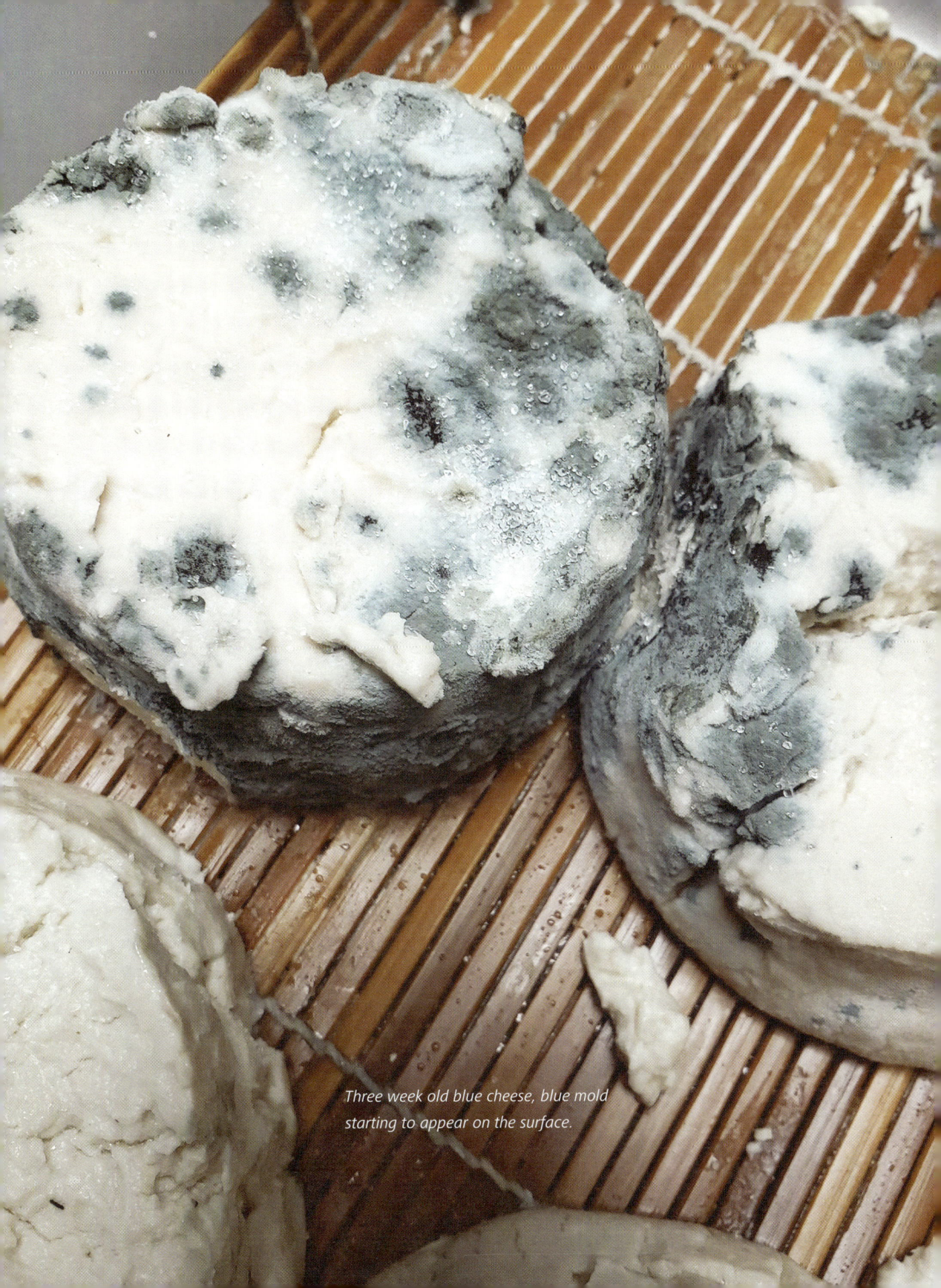

*Three week old blue cheese, blue mold starting to appear on the surface.*

it gradually starts to appear in more spots on the surface of the cheese. This is indicative of the different rates at which surface yeast metabolizes sugars (which the mold feeds on). Once the mold begins to take hold, its proteolytic and lipolytic abilities create new by-products, including the methyl ketones that create aroma, and you should start being able to smell the cheese at this stage.

9. The cheese requires regular monitoring during this time. I suggest making a log for recording (see appendix 2). If a sticky surface forms on the cheese, scrape it off and use a light-medium salt brine to wash the cheese.
10. Once the cheese has reached the level of blueness that you desire, wrap it in foil paper (cheesemaking supply stores carry this) and store it in a separate container and at a temperature range of 38°F–40°F (3°C–4°C). It can keep for 2 to 3 months, but you will need to make sure that it is kept separate from other cheeses and foods. If you have a vacuum sealer at home, vacuum seal the blue cheese for longer storage.

## Method 2: broken curd method

This method is quite a bit different than method 1 in that it uses a lactic-set curd that you make using one of the methods outlined previously in this book (coconut milk kefir curd, cashew curd, or almond curd) without the PRB6. The PRB6 is added after a few other steps are completed. For lack of a better term, I refer to this as a broken curd method because we will be taking a curd that has already been made, drained, and is on the way to becoming an entirely different cheese and inoculating it with the blue mold. I have used this approach numerous times now and used different types of lactic-set curd to great success (after many repeated efforts).

The best curds to work with have a fair amount of fat, so high fat coconut milk can be very helpful when you are making the lactic-set curd even if you want to use another component like almond, oat, or something else suggested in the cultured cheese section.

### Tools and Equipment

Bamboo mat/aging mat/small wooden cheese board
Bowl for mixing the curd
Cheese molds, closed bottom or open ended, preferably ones made for cheesemaking with perforations
Foil paper
Knitting needle, 3.5 mm, cleaned and sanitized
Large cooler/ice chest for ripening

Measuring cups
Measuring spoons
pH meter
Separate refrigerator for secondary ripening
Spatula

**Ingredients**

6 cups lactic-set curd (such as coconut kefir curd, cashew curd, or a combined curd. Select the curd based on amount of fat as blue mold likes high fat.)
1 tsp salt
1 tiny drop of PRB6
¼ tsp calcium chloride diluted in ½ Tbsp water (to be used in wash during affinaging)

**Method**

1. Wash and sanitize all work surfaces, equipment, and tools you will work with.
2. In the bowl, add the lactic-set curd of your choice and break it up with your hands. The curd should have already been made a few days ahead of time, finished its culturing period, and have gone through the first draining process. This means that the curd should be thick, clumpy, and not too loose. I sometimes use plain curd that has already been aging into a plain, unflavored cheese, break the chunks of cheese up before inoculating it. There is enough moisture in the curd to still allow bacterial culture in it to continue to metabolize sugars, and breaking up the cheese means that when reforming in molds, there will be more air pockets for the mold to grow in.
3. Sprinkle the salt over the curd, let it rest for a few minutes, and then gently fold the curd (you don't want to stir or mix with a heavy hand).
4. Add the droplet of PRB6 to the curd and again gently fold into the curd or place 1 larger drop of PRB6 into ¼ cup water and into a spray bottle, and spray the curd with the inoculated water. The starting pH of the curd should be around 4.6–4.5.
5. Lay out the bamboo mat/aging mat/small wooden cheeseboard. Lay doubled up cheesecloth or butter muslin on top and then the cheese molds for shaping. Line the cheese molds with cheesecloth or butter muslin. Place the salted and inoculated curd inside the cloth in the molds. Do not press down heavily.
6. Place the cheese on the mat/board into the ripening box and allow the cheese to ripen for 2 days at 72°F (22°C) and relative humidity of 80–90%. On

each of the 2 days, sprinkle a small amount (less than ¼ tsp per cheese) of salt over the top surface.

7. Begin the second stage of ripening in a secondary fridge or wine fridge at a temperature of 50°F–55°F (10°C–13°C) with a relative humidity of 90%. Turn the cheese daily, with periodic salting or salt brine washing every few days. At day 10, pierce the surface vertically with a clean and sanitized 3.5 mm knitting needle, with 3–4 holes per square inch. Maintain the same ambient conditions and repeat turning of the cheese and monitoring temperature, humidity, and pH. Observe the surface for blue-green mold growth, which will begin to appear in spots likely even before day 10. Maintaining humidity during this growth phase is important as the mold thrives in humidity.

8. On day 14 pierce the cheese again. With blue mold cheeses the acidity changes from the inside to the outside of the cheese (the opposite of white mold cheeses), and as bacteria from the lactic acid consume sugar, the mold will consume the by-products. Oxygenating the interior will allow airflow and create more pockets for the mold to grow in. There should be a good amount of surface growth at this time, and you will need to decide whether you want to have a full surface cover of blue mold. If you do want a heavier mold covering on the surface (this is the growth of the mycelium mat), you will need to lightly dry salt or light brine wash the surface at least once a week during the early weeks of aging. Once the mold has begun to bloom and spread, you need to lightly wash the cheese to prevent the mold growing to the point of spore production and to encourage an even surface cover.

    Once the mycelium mat is thick, it is easy to wash, and it will darken in color to a dark blue/blackish blue. It is important to avoid allowing the mold to produce spores as the spores will spread throughout your environment and will "jump" to other projects.

    Mold on the surface that is light blue-gray or greenish (the color differentiation indicates what species of mold is at work) and powdery indicates that spore production is active. When you wash the surface, do so with a wet cloth and gently rub the surface. Avoid brushing so that you do not "dust" off spores.

    The cheese should be fairly aromatic at this point, and flavor testing will be important to help you avoid the soapy or overly piquant flavor that can occur with rapid blue mold development.

9. If you want to avoid a full mold surface, you will need to do regular washing or brushing of the surface. This means that if your cheese is in a high humidity environment, which will encourage mold development, you need to pierce the cheese regularly to aerate it and allow internal mold growth, while controlling mold growth on the surface. This is where you can use

the calcium chloride solution to wash the surface. Not only will calcium chloride help the surface knit together, it can help with acidification of the surface. Acidification of the surface declines during aging.

However, the biggest impact on reducing mold growth on the surface is from reducing the humidity from 80–90% to 55–60%. This can be done in a number of ways, including opening up the ripening container for up to 1 hour at a time to let excess moisture evaporate, or adding dry, never used sponges or humidity absorbing pads to the ripening/affinaging box.

10. Some time after day 20 to 25 (depending on size of the cheese, more days for larger cheeses, fewer days for smaller cheeses), wrap the cheese in foil paper and move the cheese to a storage temperature of 37°F (3°C). Blue cheeses typically age between 60 and 75 days, but this, again, depends on size.

With respect to blue cheese, it is important to note that despite all written directions around aging the cheese, it is only experience and learning the principles that allow you to be able to read the cheese, as dairy cheesemaker Gianaclis Caldwell refers to it. Reading the cheese means that you will be able to make the appropriate adaptive changes in method and process based on what you are observing from the cheese. Is the surface sticky? Is it too dry? Is the mold becoming

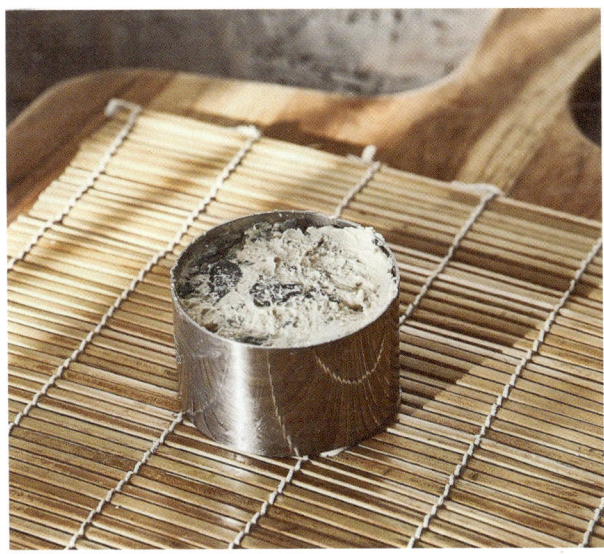

*Blue cheese, broken curd method. Cheese is allowed to develop significant blue mold on the surface and lose some moisture. It is then is broken apart and recombined when pressed into a mold.* CREDIT: ANDRE SHEPPERD, DREMOND STUDIO

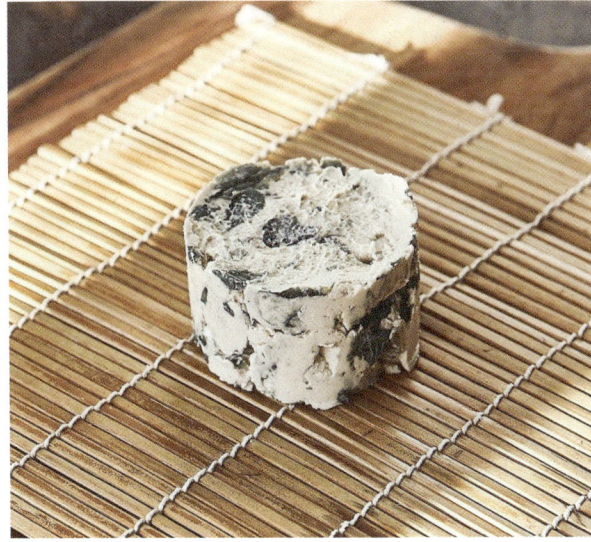

*Fresh broken blue cheese on bamboo mat, ready to age.* CREDIT: ANDRE SHEPPERD, DREMOND STUDIO

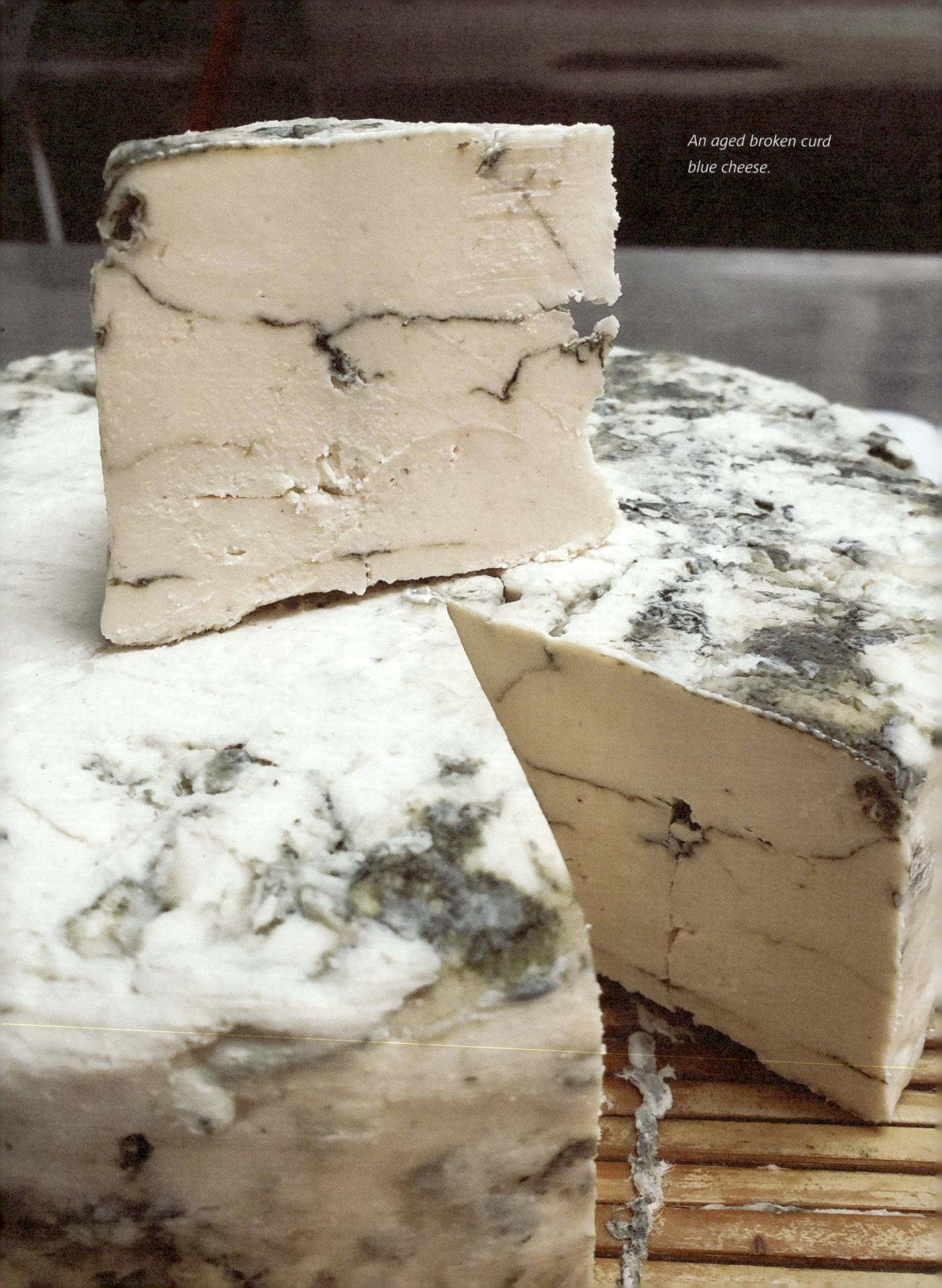

*An aged broken curd blue cheese.*

hairy? Are the veins not developing? All of the observations indicate specific microbiological and biochemical changes, and once you know what principles are at play and what each observation means, you will be able to be flexible in guiding the cheese to its final character development. This is, in many ways, the empirical method in pure form.

Have fun and be attentive and observant. Record your processes and the data of temperature, time, and pH, and practice good food safety handling practices. Most importantly, be patient.

## Affinaging

Though I reference aging, affinaging, and related processes in each of the hands-on methods, it is worth diving a little bit deeper into some of the ways by which you can help your cheese experiments evolve.

Affinaging refers to techniques and methods used to refine a cheese during its aging process. To affinage a cheese is not to do one single thing. Rather, it may involve several processes over a period of time. This can be as simple as flipping and turning the cheese each day or using infused washes to add additional flavor to the cheese via surface treatment.

All forms of affinaging a cheese involve controlling moisture loss and pH, usually oriented around the specific characteristics you want to develop in the cheese. If you want the cheese to become very firm, focus on helping it lose moisture over a long period of time. However, this must be controlled so moisture is not lost too fast or the cheese will end up too dry and crumbly. If you want the soft cheese to hold a shape better, still focus on controlling moisture loss but over a shorter duration and with a different humidity requirement.

Flavor can be developed by using different substances (wine, cocoa, grape leaves, etc.) to treat the surface, by cold smoking the cheese, or by soaking the cheese in brine. Whatever the action you choose, it should be selected on the basis of what works best for the cheese at different stages of the aging/curing process. In many ways affinaging is where the art meets the science in the craft of cheesemaking.

A note before you start aging up your cheeses: if you have several cheese projects that you want to age simultaneously, it will be necessary to ensure that they all require similar conditions, and if you are aging any white or blue mold cheeses, they will need to be kept separate from the other projects.

### *Salt: dry salting, brining (soaking), washing*

Salt is an incredibly important and useful ingredient in cheesemaking. It enhances flavor, it can inhibit unwelcome microbes, and it is a key component of many aging processes as it can leach moisture away. Much of aging cheese is about controlling the loss of moisture over a time frame. Salt is used in applications of dry salting, in washes used to treat the surface, and in brining, a process in which cheese is immersed in a brine solution.

Keep in mind that blue and white molds (the ones used in cheesemaking) can grow in salty environments, and with blue, the addition of salt is important in its development. Keep mold ripened cheeses away from other cheeses. Most undesirable molds (usually brought in via other foods) do not grow–or do not grow well in a salt rich environment. So during aging, especially when the cheese is still quite moist, it is important to observe the surface for any unwelcome or unintended growth.

## Dry salting

All aging methods work in conjunction with dry aging (air-drying), in other words, relying on the ambient temperature and humidity of the air to assist in curing the surface of the cheese. Generally, you begin aging a soft cheese into a firmer cheese using dry salting (sprinkling salt directly over the surface) and air drying.

Air drying/dry aging relies on good airflow around the surface of the cheese and requires enough room for air movement as well as evaporation of moisture. Venting is important in dry-aging, or having a means to ensure flow is adequate, for instance, using a fan in a dedicated aging space to increase airflow.

Dry aging and dry salting generally begin just before the cheese comes out of the mold. It begins during the draining phase, but once the cheese is out of the mold and is in just cheesecloth or by itself on an aging mat (bamboo mats are also aging mats), attention needs to be focused on the aging of the cheese.

Moisture absorption is achieved through the use of bamboo mats, cheese aging mats (white mesh plastic mats) or wooden boards (not treated with wood stain or other sorts of chemicals), upon which the cheese rests. Moisture removal should happen evenly, so pressing, and flipping/turning cheeses encourage even moisture loss.

During aging, it is important that the surface of the cheese is even, smooth, and without large cracks or divots. Unless you are making blue cheese, you want to avoid having any spaces where unwelcome molds and bacteria can grow. Maintaining surface integrity is essential, as the development of a rind protects the cheese inside when you are aging for long periods of time. Uneven surfaces mean that there are fissures and cracks where moisture can accumulate and provide a nutrient rich breeding ground for unwelcome microbes.

Typically, you will ripen, or cure, the cheese (for projects aiming past 30 days these should be done in a dedicated environment separate from your home refrigerator) between 50°F and 55°F (10°C and 13°C), with relative humidity anywhere from 65–95% depending on what cheese you are making and what your goals are for the cheese. The number of days you keep the cheese in aging will, again, depend on what kind of cheese you are making. Harder cheeses take longer, softer styles of cheese less.

## Brining

It should be noted that salting/brining/washing along with air-drying are used to develop what is known as a natural rind (no wax). As the cheese begins to form a dry surface, or natural rind, and as long as you have not committed to something like dry or fresh herb treatments of the cheese surface, you can consider building flavor through washing the cheese surface with either a plain salt brine or a brine that is flavored (e.g., beer, wine, preserved lemon–there are so many alternatives).

Brines can be used in a number of ways: as a treatment for washing the cheese surface as it ages, as a vector to deliver flavor, or even as a way to store the cheese. You can alternate washing the cheese with brine and with a flavored brine. Some basic approaches are presented in this section, but, first, here are some guidelines for making brines and what applications suit each type best.

### Brine solutions

Brine is salt dissolved in water. Use filtered water or rested tap water. Heat brine solutions to 165.2 °F (74°C) and then allow to cool fully before using. Heating the brine allows the salt to fully dissolve and not just sink to the bottom.

Store brine in jars with plastic (non-reactive/non-metallic lids) for future use, or make smaller batches, but keep the ratio of salt to water the same. You can use brines in a spray bottle to apply to the cheese or you can soak cheesecloth in brine to wash the cheese. This is not the same as washing the cheese with a bacterial culture. Washing the surface of the cheese with a bacterial culture introduces more living microbes to the surface of the cheese. These microbes are metabolically active producing acids and other by-products and changing the surface pH as well as making other chemical changes in the cheese.

The ratio of salt to water is important. Light brine is 10% salt by weight; medium brine is 20% salt by weight; and saturated brine is 25% salt by weight. The amount of salt to be added to make a small batch is calculated as follows: water weighs about 1 gram per 1 milliliter, so if you want to make a 500 mL batch of light brine, you multiply 500 by 0.10, which would mean that you add 50 grams of salt to the 500 mL of water.

My preferred method of using brine is as a wash because when soaking cheeses in a brine it is harder to control the amount of salt the cheese ends up with.

## Making and Using Brines

| | |
|---|---|
| **Light brine: 10%**<br>13 oz (368.54 g) salt<br>1 tsp calcium chloride<br>1 gal (3.78 L) water<br><br>You may also use brine from preserved foods such as preserved lemon brine, olive brine, sour pickle brine. These brines will also infuse flavor into your cheese. | **Uses**<br>• as a wash for young cheeses that are just forming a rind<br>• for frequent use over a long period of aging for most types of cheese<br>• for infusing flavors into the cheese by creating flavored brines<br>• as a storage brine for cheeses like mozzarella or feta |
| **Medium brine: 20%**<br>26 oz (737g) salt<br>1 tsp calcium chloride<br>1 gal (3.78 L) water | • as a wash or soak for cheeses that have a rind dry enough for you to handle the cheese, especially for cheeses that you intend to age for a long period of time |
| **Saturated brine: 25%**<br>32 oz (907.18g) salt<br>1 tsp calcium chloride<br>1 gal (3.78 L) water | • for soaking cheeses that age for a long time. Soaking time: 20 minutes<br>• combine with other ingredients for infusing flavor into cheeses |

Ultimately, dry-salting is the best option for controlling the amount of salt your cheese ends up with.

### Washing

Washing is very much as it sounds: using a brine, plain or flavored, to wash the surface of the cheese. I use soaked cheesecloth or a spray bottle of brine to wet the surface of a cheese. After you wash the cheese, you need to return it to drying. Allow the cheese to dry fully between washing sessions. As the surface begins to harden, reduce the frequency of the washes and the saturation of the brine you are using. Remember that as your cheese loses moisture and firms up, salt will concentrate, as it does not evaporate. So be patient and be prepared for the cheese to take longer than you may want to age fully.

If you pre-make a batch of brine, portion out the amount you will use at one time so that you do not cross-contaminate the full batch.

With washing you can add a number of other components to introduce layers of flavor. Make the brine first. Then add the flavor component. You can heat this brine mixture if you like, cool, then use. Here are some suggestions for additions for flavoring.

- Wines (including port/sherry)
- Preserved Lemon/Olive/Pickle brines
- Beer

- Teas (Be mindful that the tannins can accumulate on the cheese surface and impart some bitterness. If you use tea in the brine, add a small amount of something sweet to balance the tannins.)
- Hot sauces
- Coffee (Similar to tea, tannins can impart bitterness, but the addition of a sweet component in the coffee brine can mitigate this. Also, with coffee, you will end up with an amplification of whatever dominant flavor notes the coffee itself presents.)
- Herb pastes (dried or fresh herbs made into a paste and rubbed over the surface of the cheese)

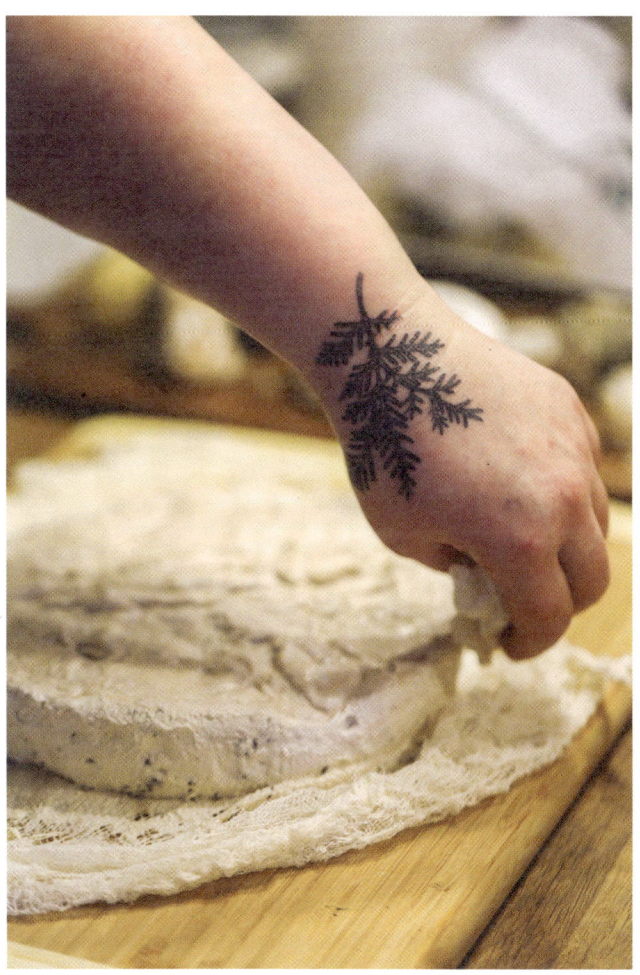

Author washing cheese with a light (10%) brine.
CREDIT: CATHERINE DOWNES

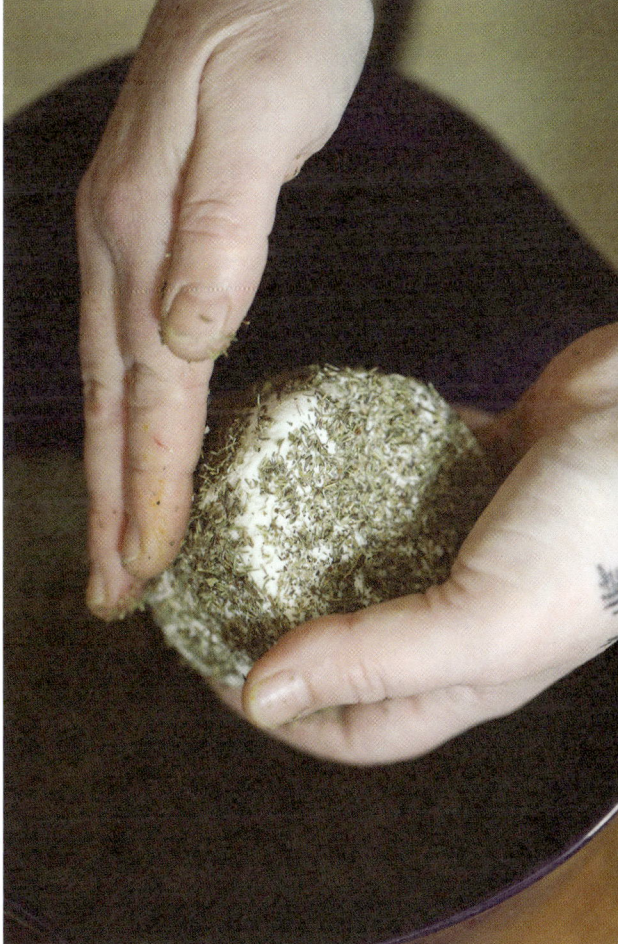

Author applying dry herbs to the surface of the cheese.
CREDIT: CATHERINE DOWNES

### Oil curing/leaf wrapping/bandaging

Oil curing, leaf wrapping, and bandaging are slightly more involved affinaging methods and may incorporate brine and washing methods.

Oil curing should only be done on low moisture cheeses with a fully dry rind. Oil curing can be a great way to protect the moisture content of the interior of a cheese, but can potentially trap pathogens at the surface of the cheese, so be sure that food safety handling procedures throughout the process are diligently followed. Smoked oil is a wonderful surface treatment, as are other culinary infused oils. Be mindful to purchase, rather than make your own infused oil, to avoid food safety risks.

Once the cheese surface no longer has damp patches, using cheesecloth dipped in oil, rub a little salt onto the surface of the cheese. Allow the cheese to dry between oil treatments during aging. I have made olive oil and cacao pastes to cure cheeses I have experimented with and have been very happy with the results.

Leaf wrapping and bandaging are similar but use, obviously, different materials. Leaf wrapping is one of my particular favorites, especially for select, limited release specialty cheeses. Both methods are meant to protect the surface of a cheese from intrusive surface growths, control moisture loss, and assist in infusing flavor. Leaves also behave like cheesecloth in the sense that they are natural materials, porous (good for airflow), and will dry/cure with the surface of the cheese, forming a protective rind. Leaves and cheesecloth bandaging can be used on soft to firm cheeses.

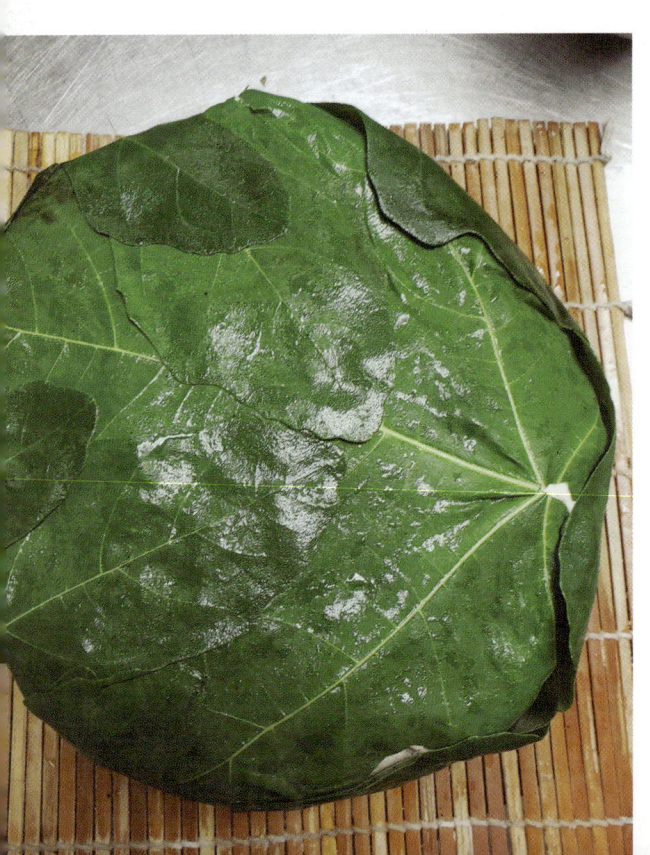

*Freshly poached/blanched fig leaves wrapped around a 3 week old cheese will serve as a natural cheese paper, allowing air to pass through, infusing the cheese with flavor and protecting it.*

Leaves that you use must not be toxic, of course. Be very certain of this before using leaves. I count fresh basil, mint, and sage among leaves. Using these on the surface of a cheese is visually appealing, and they will impart flavor. You can also use leaves such as brined grape leaves or unbrined leaves like fig, maple leaf or chestnut.

If you do use leaves such as fig, maple leaf, chestnut, or unbrined grape leaf, poach them first. Bring water to a boil, place the leaves in the water, and poach for 90 seconds. Remove from the water, and lay out on a drying rack to lose some moisture (avoid letting them dry out completely). Lightly salt the surface of the cheese. Then wrap the damp leaves around the cheese, gently rubbing the leaf onto the surface and making sure that there are no air pockets. Place the leaf wrapped cheese on an aging mat to dry at regular affinaging/storage temperatures.

Leaf wrapped cheese can be rubbed down with wine washes or smoked for added layers of flavor.

Cheesecloth bandaging protects from pathogens and prevents moisture loss like leaves do, but is not edible. Dampen cheesecloth in a brine, plain or flavored, and wrap strips of the cheesecloth around the cheese. Bandaging will hold a cheese together as it ages and as the cheese dries you can peel the cheesecloth off. This method can be helpful for adding moisture when an environment has a humidity level that is too low and is encouraging moisture loss too rapidly.

*Blue Heron's summer seasonal cheese highlighting locally grown wild berries and edible herbs, leaves, and flowers, Sunshine Coast.*
CREDIT: COLIN MEDHURST

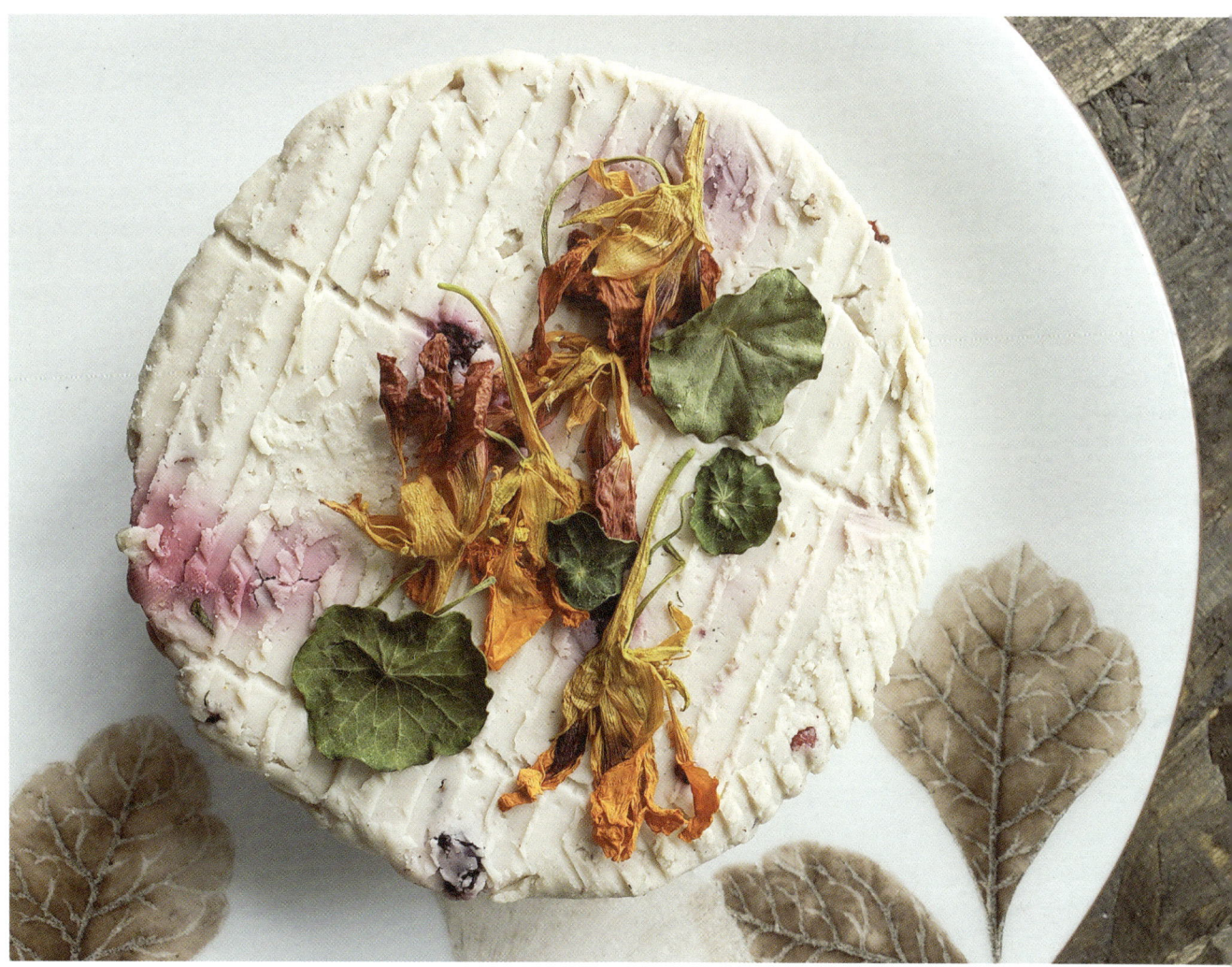

### Cold smoking

I am frequently asked about how to smoke cheese or how to help a cheese acquire a smoky flavor. Certainly there are many easy ways to achieve a smoky cheese. Liquid smoke (seek a high quality one intended for adding to foods) added to the curd or rubbed on the surface, smoked tea like Lapsang Souchong, smoked spices such as smoked paprika or ancho, and a smoked oil all work well, but my preferred method is to actually smoke the cheese over wood smoke.

Cold smoking avoids direct heat and wet smoke, making it safe for smoking cheese. Smoking cheese over heat causes the fat to leach out and raises concerns with regard to food safety. If you have a smoking gun or a small smoking unit, you can easily smoke your own cheese safely. If you have a smoking gun, make sure you maintain a container with a lid that is used only for smoking. Repeated use for smoking cheese will leave that container forever carrying the scent of smoke.

Place the cheese inside the container and place the lid on top. Make sure the container has an access port (hole) to put the nozzle into. Follow the instructions that come with the smoking gun to light the wood chips that will produce the smoke.

Smoking times should be at least 10 minutes, and during that time you should ensure that the container is not leaking smoke. I like to keep smoking sessions short and repeat them frequently, layering flavor. If you are advanced in the art of cold smoking and possess an enclosed smoker, you will already be skilled enough to adapt it to smoking cheese.

---

6. White mold: Conscious Cultures from Pittsburgh, PA, USA; New Roots, Switzerland; Blue mold: Reine from Ventura, CA, USA; Strictly Roots, London, UK.

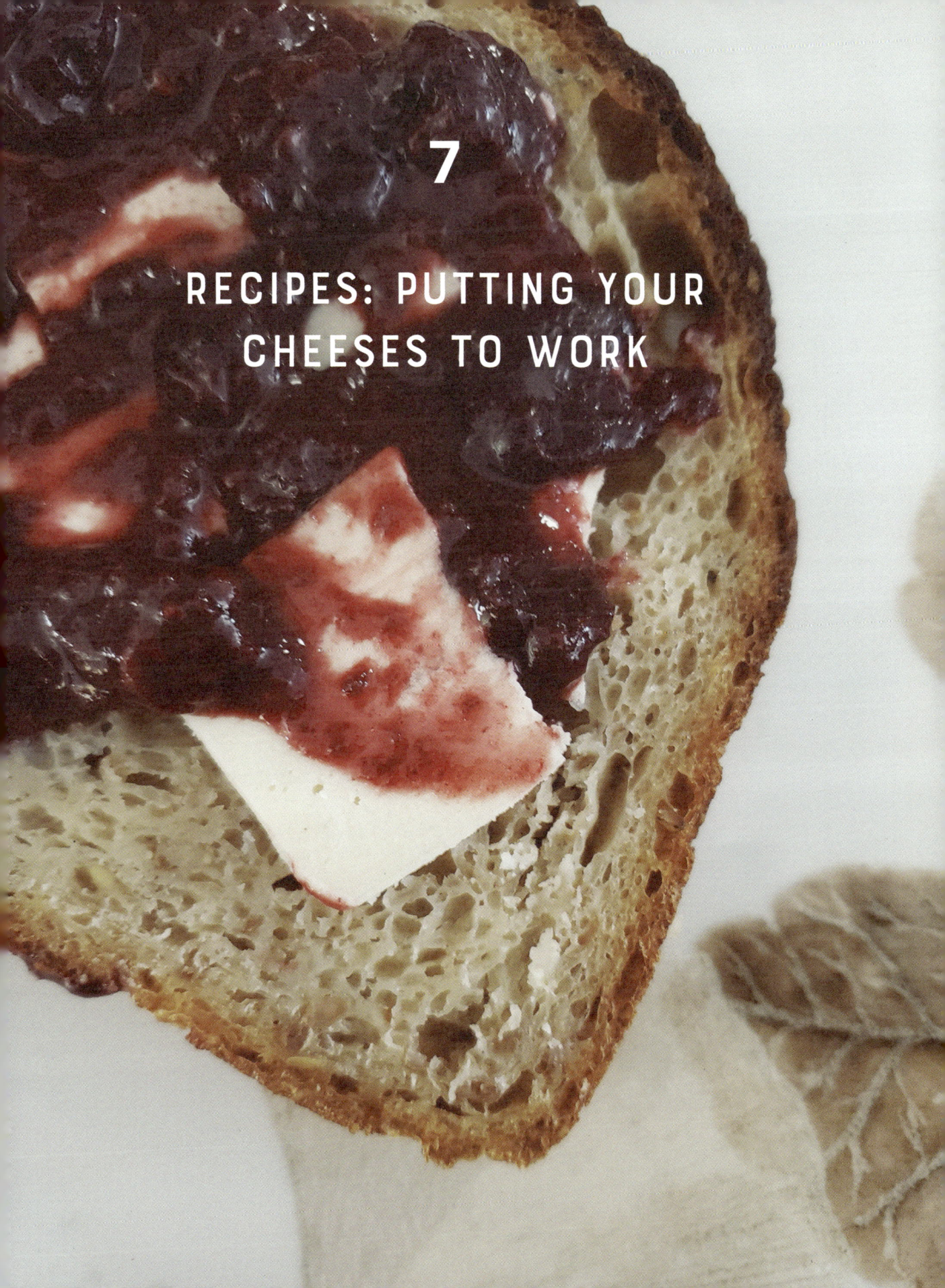

# 7

## RECIPES: PUTTING YOUR CHEESES TO WORK

My first true love is being a chef. I think that all chefs, at the core, are empirically inclined. Leaving aside the adrenaline rush of a high paced service, I think that those who strive to lead or work with a kitchen team in bringing thoughtfully prepared dishes to people, are deeply curious. The work it takes to understand a multitude of ingredients individually and how they work together in different circumstances (cooking/fermenting/preserving) requires intense observation by all the senses, and requires a commitment to replication in an effort to seek optimal outcomes, and many failures occur along the way to achieving, first, that one glorious moment and then achieving consistent results. Vegan cheesemaking amplifies all of this.

I am often asked "what can I do with this?" in reference to either the cheeses I sell or the ones I teach folks to make in my classes. So, it seemed necessary to add a section with recipes that put your cheese efforts to use. There is a range of recipes providing you with simple ways to use by-products of your cheesemaking efforts (e.g., cultured butter, kefir-yogurt, sour cream) and to use your cheeses beyond just eating them on their own. Most of these recipes I have developed, and some have been developed by chef friends and members of the Blue Heron team.

You will not find recipes for "bowls of food." I assume you can all make one of those; inspired by your own preferences. You can use any of the cheeses that you make with this book to enhance your bowls or make cheesy dressings.

Have fun, do not fear failure, be adventurous, and eat good food with good people.

# More Cultured Foods (that are not cheese)

## Cultured "Butter"

This is not a churned butter, but it works reasonably well in baking (has not been tested in croissant making yet!) and cooking recipes and is delicious on really good sourdough bread with a little fresh fruit or fruit compote, which is my favorite way to enjoy it. I have used it in making pie crust and scones as well as sautéing and even in making a vegan beurre blanc. Emulsification is key with this recipe as it does not employ the use of a stabilizer such as lecithin, so remember, slow and low is best!

### Tools and Equipment

High-speed blender or food processor
Silicone mold (whatever shape you like)
Measuring cups
Spatula
Measuring spoons
Container for storing set butter

### Ingredients

½ cup olive oil (not extra virgin)
½ cup coconut oil, softened (unscented if you prefer)
¼ cup cacao butter, softened
¼ cup coconut cream (or drained high fat coconut milk)
1 cup coconut kefir, drained, or ½ cup cultured cashew curd or ½ cup almond ricotta whey (post draining material)
¼ tsp salt

### Method

1. Wash and sanitize all work surfaces and tools you will work with.
2. Ensure that the coconut kefir (or cultured cashew or almond ricotta whey) is at room temperature or very close to it before starting, likewise the coconut cream or milk. Emulsification works best when ingredients are at the same temperature.
3. Place the oils in the blender and begin emulsifying on low speed. Avoid blending at high speed as this will cause separation. Blend until the oils are well combined and the mixture appears buttery in color.
4. Slowly add the cultured element (drained coconut kefir/cultured cashew/almond ricotta whey). Maintain low speed to ensure that emulsification occurs. Observe how the materials are binding to one another. If there is clumping and liquid separation, it likely means that one of the higher fat ingredients such as the coconut oil or coconut cream were too cold when added.

5. Add the salt last. Continue emulsifying. Taste and adjust the salt according to your preference. You may also add herbs or dried garlic or other flavoring components at this stage.
6. Once the mixture is well combined, pour it into a silicone mold and place the mold in the refrigerator to cool and set. Allow the mixture to set for at least 4 hours; I usually let it set overnight.

### Storage

This "butter" can keep for up to 60 days properly stored or in the freezer for longer. Keep it wrapped in wax paper, parchment, or foil paper (butter paper) inside a closed container after removing from the silicone mold.

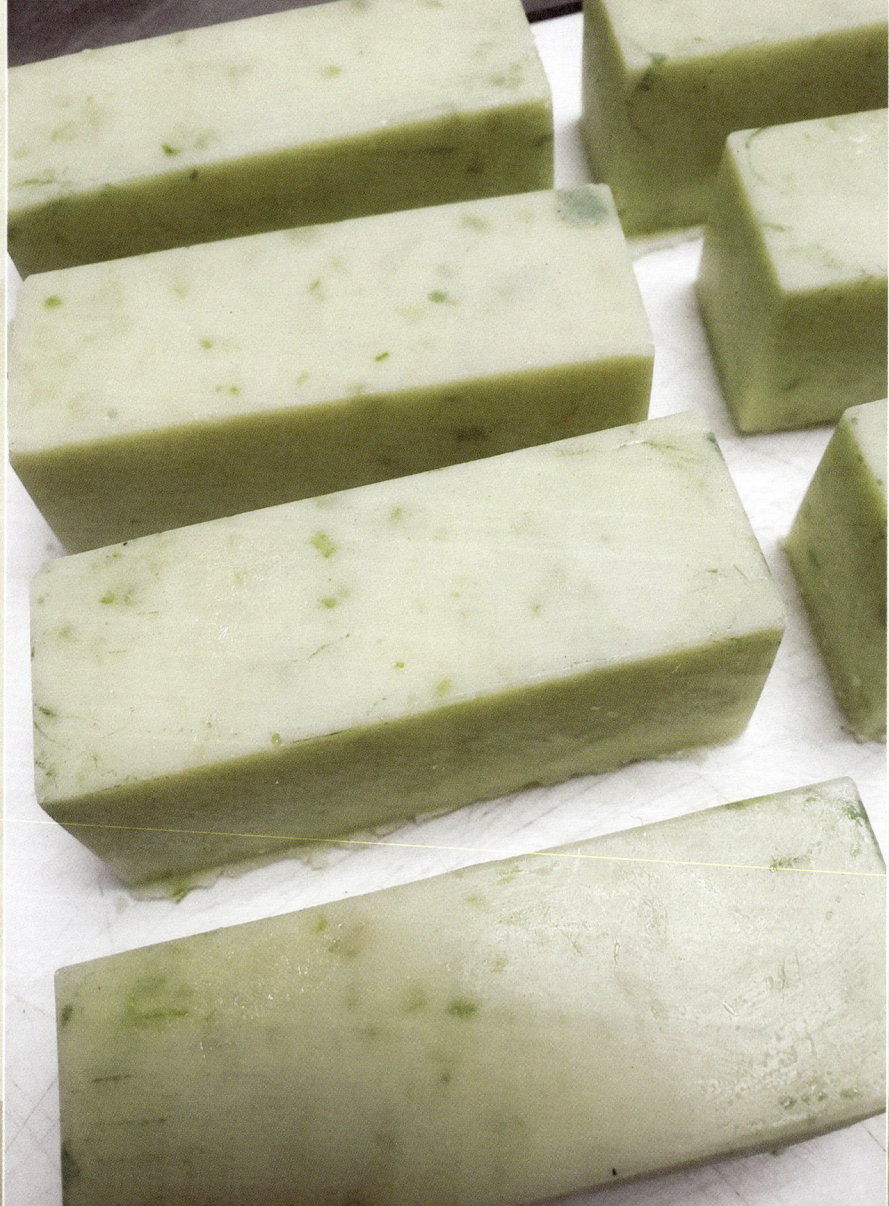

*Cultured butter using cultured coconut kefir that has been drained and emulsified at low speed with coconut oil, olive oil, and cacao butter.*

# Coconut Milk Yogurt

Traditional yogurt cultures are thermophilic, which means that the bacteria involved perform their metabolic functions optimally at higher temperatures than mesophilic cultures, which prefer a temperature range of 62°F–72°F (18°C–22°C). Thermophilic bacteria activate at a higher temperature, and use of thermophilic bacteria means that the culturing period occurs over heat, usually at 105°F (40.5°C).

A common error many folks make is to use mesophilic cultures such as kefir culture with higher heat as found in a yogurt maker or yogurt setting on an Instapot or crockpot. This extra heat destabilizes the microbial culture and produces results that are not very pleasant (too sour, sulphuric aroma, for example).

Two of the signature strains of bacteria found in traditional thermophilic yogurt cultures are *Lactobacillus bulgaricus* and *Streptococcus thermophilus*, and in the US and Europe, dairy yogurt products must contain these two strains (in addition to requiring a certain number of these and other bacteria in the culture set to be present) in order to be considered a yogurt.

Typically in a yogurt process, the dairy milk is heated up, cooled to a certain temperature, the culture is added, and then the mixture is placed in a container that is kept over low heat for a set amount of time. Here I offer two methods using dairy-free yogurt culture sets (thermophilic cultures), one made with coconut milk and mirroring the dairy yogurt process, the other a yogurt made with a combination of oats, cashew, and coconut.

### Tools and Equipment

Stainless steel thick cast pot
Food grade container with tight-fitting lid (large enough for the batch you wish to make)
Measuring cups
Measuring spoons
Jar with lid or other food grade container with a tight-fitting lid for storage
Probe thermometer
Spatula

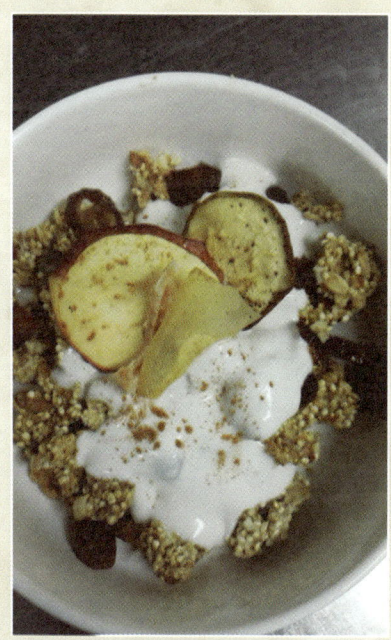

*Coconut milk yogurt over warmed muesli with dehydrated apples and cinnamon.*

### Ingredients

3 cups full or high fat (18–30%) coconut milk
(or substitute 1 cup of full coconut cream for 1 cup of high fat coconut milk)

⅛ tsp–¼ tsp dairy-free yogurt culture*

* Dairy-free yogurt cultures such as Yo-Mix Vegetal 7 from www.thecheesemaker.com, coconut milk yogurt starter from www.holykraut.biz, and a vegan yogurt starter from either www.culturesforhealth.com or www.yogourmet.com are available. Each of these dairy-free yogurt starters contains different species of microbes, but most of them do contain Lactobacillus bulgaricus and Streptococcus thermophilus. They each produce slightly different results. When purchasing dairy-free yogurt cultures be sure to find the list of microbes included. It should be listed on the package or in the online listing.
**Note: if you use thermophilic (yoghurt cultures, and not kefir cultures), you can use a yoghurt maker or the yoghurt setting on a crock pot or Instapot

## Method

1. Wash and sanitize all work surfaces and tools that you will use.
2. Place the coconut milk (and coconut cream if you choose to use it) in a thick cast stainless steel pot. Heat the coconut milk to 185°F (85°C). Be sure to avoid letting the coconut milk boil. Use the probe thermometer to measure the temperature.
3. Once the coconut milk reaches 185°F (85°C) allow it to remain at that temperature for approximately 30 minutes.
4. Remove coconut milk from heat, and using an active cooling process (either ice bath or frequent stirring) cool the coconut milk to 105°F (40.5°C), and then add the starter culture. Gently stir it in.
5. Place the mixture into a food grade container large enough to allow for ⅓ headspace for gas exchange. Cover with a tight-fitting lid. Allow to ferment/culture at 105°F (40.5°C) for 12 to 30 hours. The longer you culture, the more acidic and thicker the yogurt will become. You won't really notice the thickening of the yogurt until you rest it in the refrigerator after the culturing period is over. The temperature at which you culture it will determine how fast the acidity develops and the degree of tang your yogurt develops.
6. When the culturing is finished, put it in a jar with a tight-fitting lid, and store it.

## Storage

Stored in a jar with a tight-fitting lid and in the refrigerator, the yogurt will keep for up to 30 days, provided it is not cross-contaminated.

Note: You can use some of the yogurt to make a new batch of yogurt (back slopping), but please note that depending on which yogurt culture you use, you may get variable results doing this and that when you are using direct-set cultures as many freeze-dried cultures are, you can only do this so many times before you will need to make a new batch of yogurt with fresh culture.

### Ways to use this yogurt

With yogurt parfaits

On granola

In cultured vegan cheesecakes

In smoothies

As a sour cream (after draining for at least 1 hour)

However you wish

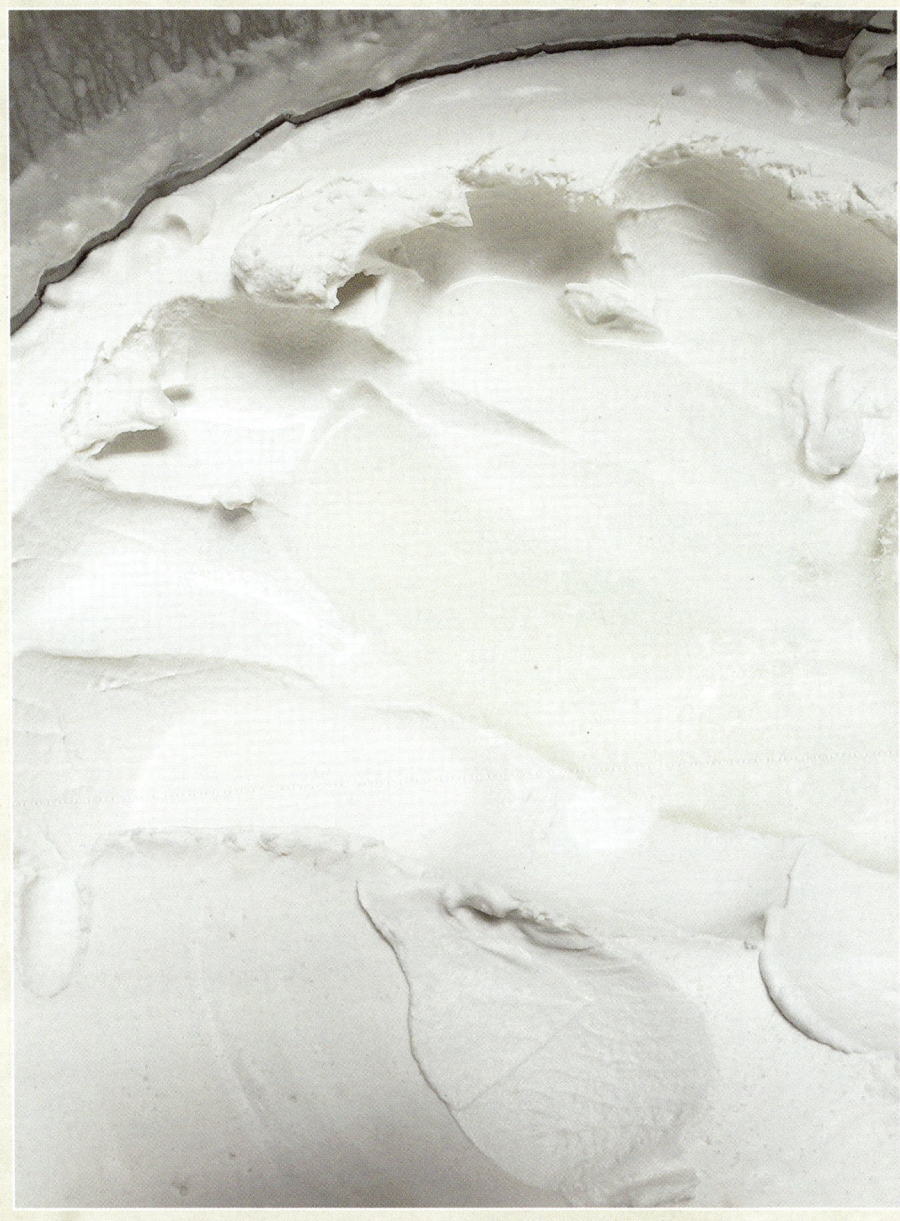

*Coconut milk yogurt, cultured 30 hours, and after refrigeration.*

# Oats, Cashew, and Coconut Yogurt

This method is a fusion approach that combines a little bit of method from cheesemaking and the use of a thermophilic culture in addition to the yogurt culture set.

## Tools and Equipment

High-speed blender
Thick cast pot
Spatula/spoon
Probe thermometer
Measuring cups
Measuring spoons
Cheesecloth/nutmilk bag
Fine mesh sieve
Bowl
Jar or food grade container for culturing
Yogurt maker/Instapot, dehydrator, crockpot, or oven with oven light on

## Ingredients

½ cup rolled oats, cooked, rinsed
½ cup high fat coconut milk
1 cup cashews, rinsed
4 cups water (filtered or rested tap water)
1 tsp maple syrup
⅛ tsp thermophilic culture Danisco TA 061 (This culture will have slow building acidity and provides a soft, buttery flavor.)
⅛ tsp yogurt culture

## Method

1. Prior to preparing any food in your kitchen, always wash your equipment with hot soapy water, air dry, then sanitize your equipment, and, of course, wash your hands.
2. In a blender, add the oats and rinsed cashews, and some of the water. On low speed, pulse several times to help the material incorporate. Gradually increase the speed, adding small amounts of the water as you go. Observe the texture of the mixture as you blend, and avoid going to high speed right away. Add enough water to achieve a thick, creamy consistency.
3. Run the mixture through a nut milk bag or cheesecloth or a cheesecloth-lined sieve. You may also blend the oats first, strain them, and then blend the strained mixture with the cashews and coconut milk. This will eliminate some of the bigger pieces of fiber and grit. You can save the matter that is retained in the cloth/sieve for use in a sauce or baking or even add it to a cheese you are making.

    Note that oats absorb a lot of moisture and release long chain polysaccharides, which will make the mixture very thick when it cools. So, make sure that the mixture does not begin to set up thick after blending.
4. Place the strained mixture in a thick cast pot (or double boiler setup) and put the heat on low. Using a probe thermometer, heat the mixture to 185°F (85°C) and maintain this temperature for 10 minutes.
5. Sprinkle the TA 061 culture over the top of the mixture and allow to rehydrate/activate for 30 minutes. You can bring the temperature down a bit if the mixture is getting too thick.

Note that TA 061 is used in cheesemaking as a secondary lactic acid forming culture. It contains, as one of its microbial community, *Streptococcus thermophilus*, which activates better under warmer temperatures than mesophilic cultures do. It builds acid slowly, but along with other members of this culture, it also builds a round flavor with soft, buttery/cheesy notes (umami).

6. After you have allowed the culture to begin the acidification of the mixture, remove the mixture from the heat and cool the mixture to about 105°F (40.5°C). Add the yogurt culture and gently stir into the mixture. Add the maple syrup at this stage as well. This will help the microbes "latch" onto the mixture, providing them with a food source that is easily metabolized.
7. Place the culture in a container, which is then covered, and incubate at 95°F–105°F (35°C–40.5°C) in a yogurt maker, Instapot (yogurt setting), crockpot, oven with oven light on, or dehydrator. It is important that the heat is maintained evenly during the culturing/fermentation phase.
8. Check the yogurt at 12 hours and again at 30 hours. Typically, it will be done between 12 and 30 hours, and sometimes sooner, depending on how active the cultures are. Refrigerate after the culturing period is over.
9. IMPORTANT: This yogurt tastes best when it is left to rest in the refrigerator for at least 2 to 4 days after the culturing period.

This process will give you a very thick yogurt with a complex flavor. It will be good for any savory applications in which you want to use a yogurt. It does take a few days longer in refrigeration to develop optimal flavor than the coconut-milk-only yogurt does, so be patient.

## Storage

Stored in a jar with a tight fitting lid and in the refrigerator, the yogurt will keep for up to 30 days, provided it is not cross-contaminated.

## Sour Cream/Crème Fraîche

This recipe combines two of the cultured curds presented earlier in this book, cultured cashew curd and coconut kefir. While the coconut milk yogurt or the oat, cashew, coconut yogurt recipes can serve as sour cream when drained, this recipe allows you to have a thicker, more heat resistant soured cream or crème fraîche for use with foods like baked potatoes, on top of soups, as a garnish for dishes that require a fatty/acidic component. This recipe takes a little less time than the yogurt recipes.

**Tools and Equipment**
- Blender
- Large bowl
- Measuring cups
- Measuring spoons
- Whisk
- Spatula
- Jar with lid for storage
- Sieve
- Cheesecloth
- Storage Container

### Ingredients

1 cup cashew nuts (or macadamia nuts, or oats blended, then strained)
cashew curd (or alternative curd)
1 cup coconut kefir, drained
½ tsp salt

### Method

1. Wash and sanitize all work surfaces and tools you will use.
2. Rinse nuts, drain, then add to blender.
3. Add coconut kefir to blender, then pulse the nuts and kefir together, being careful to not proceed to high speed right away.
4. Add salt and pulse together.
5. Use spatula to scrape mixture into cheesecloth-lined sieve and allow to drain/express moisture for up to 30 minutes.
6. Place mixture in a jar with a lid for storage. Be sure to leave space for gas exchange as the coconut kefir microbes will continue to culture.

### Storage

Store in the refrigerator. It will keep for up to 30 days.

*Crème fraîche, can be used as a light sour cream, as a garnish on dishes, in making dips, or served with jam and warm scones.*

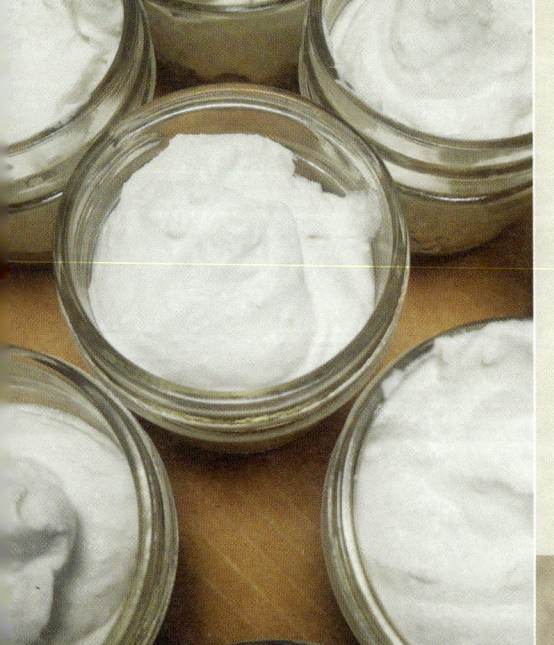

**Ways to use this sour cream/crème fraîche**

| On baked potatoes | In savory pastry |
| Add to creamy pasta sauces | As a pasta filling |
| As a garnish | However you wish |

## Something Sweet

The recipes in this section allow you to use cultured curds or even the completed cheeses in dessert recipes. Since I am not particularly fond of very sweet recipes (when I am catering and must make desserts, I do so under duress) please note that these may tend toward sweet-savory, and sweet-tart flavors. My preference when working with desserts is to add a sweeter component as a supporting element. If you wish, you may add more sweetness to these recipes.

## Coeur à la Crème with Syrah Infused Cherries

This dessert takes 2 days, aside from the time it takes to make the cheeses for this. However, once you have the cheese curd ready, this is actually a very easy dessert to make and brings a high presentation score for a dessert table at a social gathering or presented at the dinner table. This is a lovely dessert for mid to late summer when cherries are at their ripest and best. Depending on the type of cherry you use (Bing, Rainier, or sour), the flavor profile will differ, but each brings its own charm.

I recommend making the cherry mixture first and setting it aside while you prepare the coeur à la crème, which will take at least 12 hours to drain and set.

### Tools and Equipment

- Heart shaped mold (cheese mold or baking mold)
- Cheesecloth
- 2 x bowl
- Bamboo mat
- Baking sheet
- Measuring cups
- Measuring spoons
- Scales
- Spatula
- Thick cast skillet or sauté pan
- Container for storing cherries
- Saucepan (pot)
- Whisk
- Hand mixer/stand mixer or blender (for whipped cream)
- Measuring cups
- Measuring spoons

NOTE: you may use a food processor to combine all of the cheese components before folding in whipped cream.

### Ingredients:

**Coeur à la crème:**

170 g (6 oz) freshly made cultured cashew or almond curd (or any combined cultured curd that you have made), drained for a minimum of 2 hours

114 g (4 oz) coconut kefir cheese (approximately 1–2 weeks old)

⅔ cup coconut cream, chilled minimum 1 hour

1 Tbsp powdered sugar (If you can find a vegan confectioners' sugar, use that.)

Optional: ⅛ cup cacao butter, softened. This can give you a slightly firmer set.

**Syrah infused cherries:**

½ cup sugar

1 Tbsp maple syrup (or brown rice syrup)

¼ cup water (filtered or rested tap water)

½ cup Syrah (you may substitute another wine if you wish)

2 whole cloves

2 black peppercorns

1 small stick of cinnamon

1 black cardamom pod

½ vanilla bean, scraped and seeds set aside or ¼ tsp vanilla powder or ½ tsp vanilla extract

3 cups cherries, washed, pitted, and rough chopped or hand torn (if you desire, you may choose to cut them neatly in half, after pitting)

Optional: Fresh tarragon, for garnish

Optional: Cracked black pepper, for garnish

## Method: Coeur à la Crème

1. Wash and sanitize all work surfaces and tools you will use.
2. In one bowl, whisk together the cultured cashew (or almond) curd and the coconut kefir cheese, along with the softened cacao butter if you choose to use it. Whisk until the ingredients are well combined.
3. In a second bowl, add the chilled coconut cream and the sugar. Whisk until it forms soft peaks. You can hand whisk or use a hand mixer. The small amount would not whisk well in a stand mixer.
4. Fold the whipped cream mixture into the cheese mixture in stages. I do a little at time over three additions. Be gentle and employ a folding motion rather than heavy stirring motion.
5. On a baking sheet, place a bamboo mat and place the coeur à la crème mold on the mat. Line the mold with cheesecloth that has been soaked in cold water and hand wrung until all excess moisture is gone.
6. Place the mixture into the cheesecloth-lined mold and fold the cheesecloth gently overtop. Refrigerate overnight.

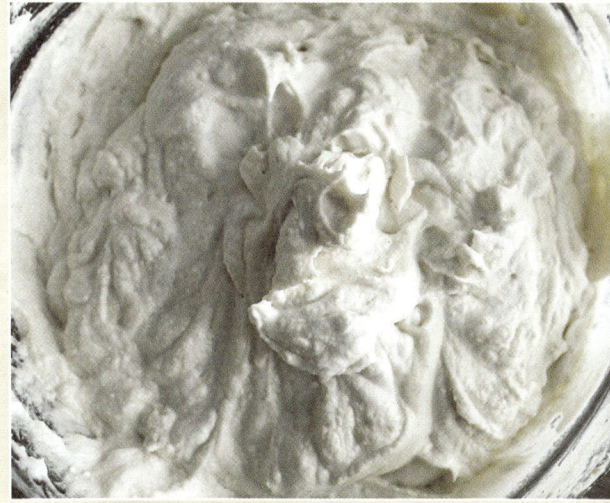

*Coeur à la Crème mixture after the whipped cream has been folded in.*

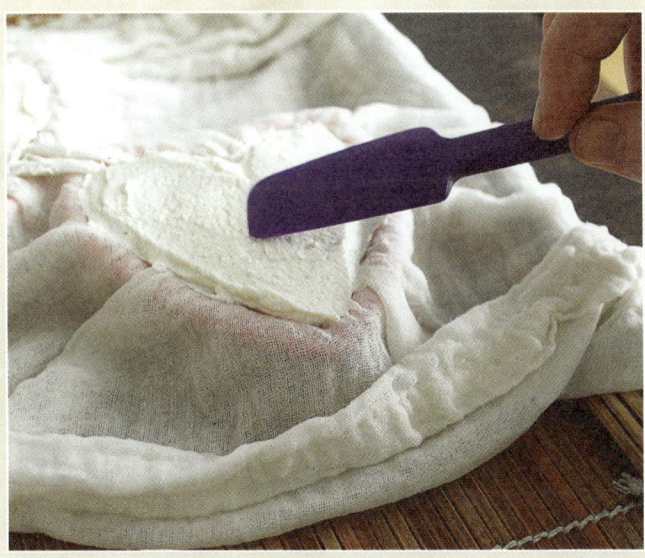

*Mixture placed in coeur à la crème molds.*

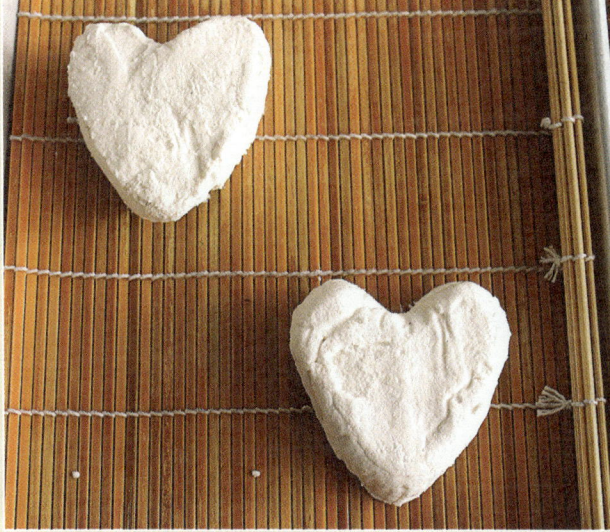

*Hearts removed from molds and cheesecloth, resting on bamboo mat.*

### Method: Syrah infused cherries

1. Wash and sanitize all work surfaces and tools you will use.
2. In a thick cast skillet or sauté pan, add the sugar, maple syrup, Syrah, and ¼ cup water. Heat over medium-high heat and stir the sugar into the mixture. Gently move the pan, and cook the mixture for about 4 minutes, until the maple syrup is combined into the water and sugar.
3. Add the spices and cook for a further 3 minutes, or until sugar is fully dissolved.
4. Add the cherries and cook for 2 minutes, reduce heat, and cook over low heat for 1 hour. I like to allow the infusion to develop over a long period of time, so I will often do this over 3 to 4 hours over very low heat.
5. When finished, remove from heat, cool to room temperature, and put into a container for storage.

### To serve:

On a chilled serving dish, place the Coeur à la Crème (removed from the refrigerator and the cheesecloth). Spoon the cherry mixture around the heart shape. Garnish with fresh tarragon and cracked black pepper if you wish.

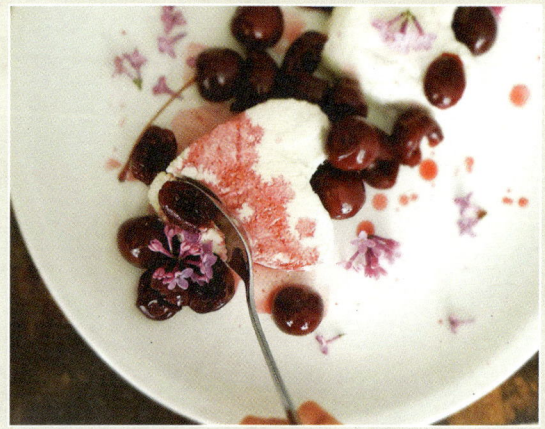

Above: *Coeur à la Crème served with Syrah infused cherries and garnished with flowers.*

Below: *Close-up of Coeur à la Crème with Syrah infused cherries.*

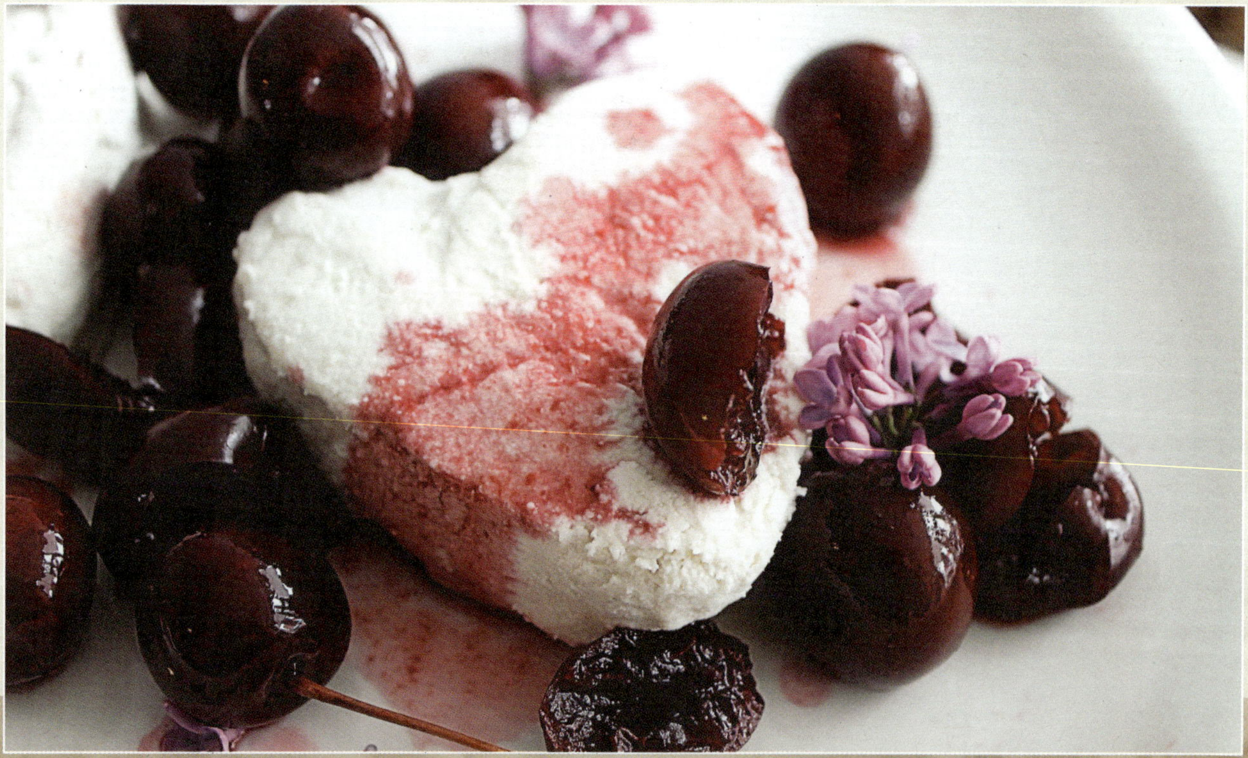

# Almond Ricotta Mocha Mousse

This coffee and chocolate mousse is ideal for a light dessert after dinner. It should be made ahead of time so that the mousse has time to rest before serving. It is also very easy to adapt this recipe to make a vegan panna cotta. You may amend coffee and chocolate amounts to skew the flavor profile in your preferred coffee versus chocolate direction. I like to serve this with a crispy element such as a sable, a thin sweetish crisp, or even a chocolate coffee bean streusel.

**Tools and Equipment**

High-speed blender
2 x bowls
Measuring Cups
Measuring Spoons
Whisk
Thick cast saucepan
Spatula
Storage container
Optional: piping bag

## Ingredients

2 cups of almond ricotta, drained 1 hour
1 cup coconut cream, chilled
¼ cup powdered sugar (or vegan confectioners' sugar if you can find it)
1 Tbsp melted dark chocolate, or 2 tsp cacao powder
1 tsp agar agar powder
¼ cup coffee

## Method

1. Puree almond ricotta with the cacao powder or melted chocolate until smooth, scoop into a bowl, (because you are folding in in step 4 and 5) and set aside.
2. In a separate bowl whisk together the sugar and coconut cream until soft peaks form. Set aside in the refrigerator.
3. In a thick cast saucepan, add ¼ cup coffee and the 1 tsp agar agar powder. Heat the mixture over medium-high heat until it reaches 185°F (85°C), and allow it to remain at this heat for 5 minutes.
4. Add the coffee/agar agar mixture to the ricotta and fold in.
5. Add the whipped cream to the ricotta mixture over 3 stages, folding in each time.
6. If desired, place the mousse into a piping bag and pipe into sundae glasses (I chill mine first). Place the glasses in the refrigerator.

## Storage

The mousse can be left in a container in the refrigerator to set up and once set it will keep for up to 7 days.

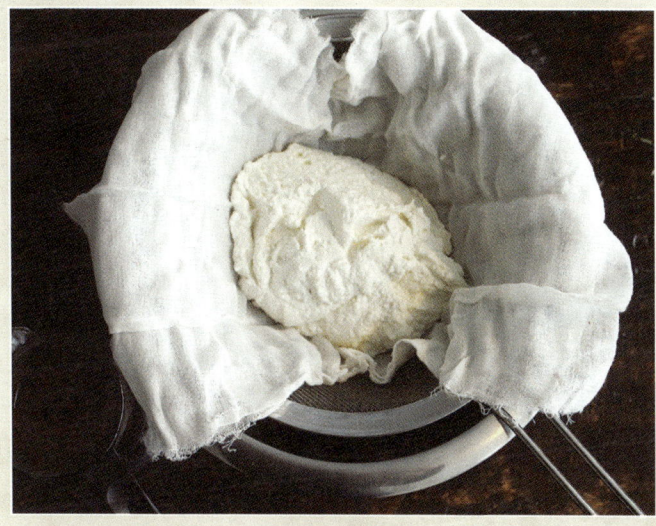
*Almond ricotta draining.*

**Ways to use this mousse**

As a garnish for other desserts

As a crepe filling with fresh fruit

As part of a cookie recipe

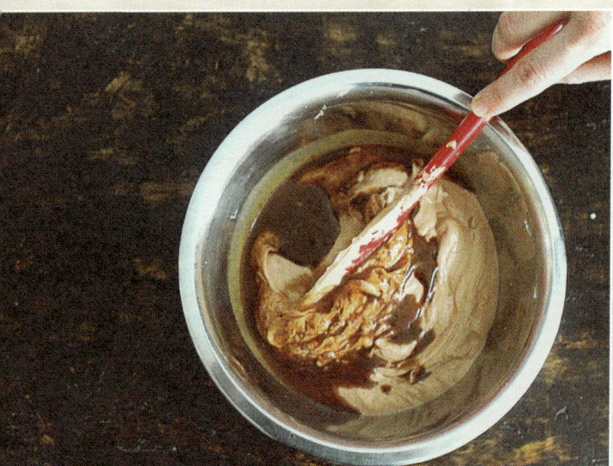

Folding cold coffee into chocolate and ricotta blended mixture.

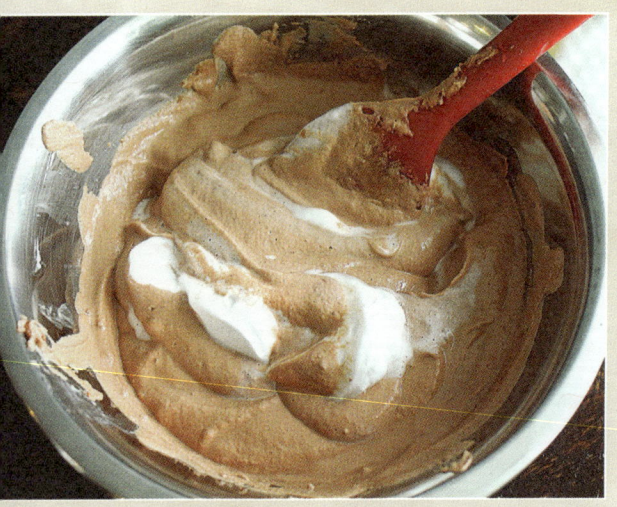

Folding in whipped cream.

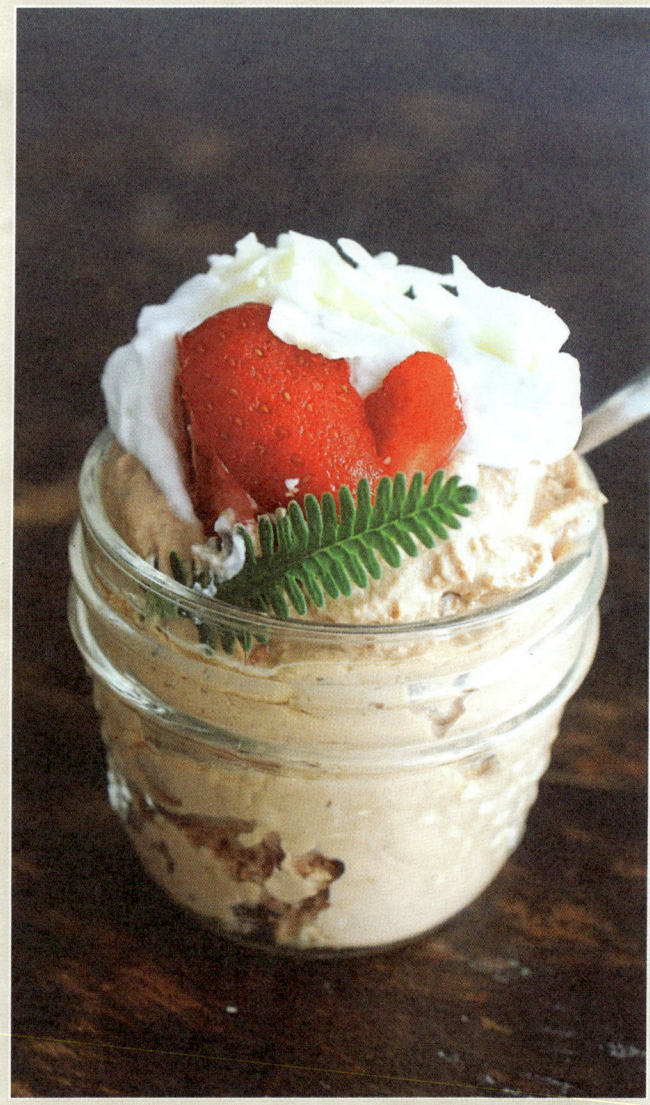

Almond ricotta mocha mousse in mason jar.

# Unbaked Lemon Cheesecake with Blueberry Bay Compote

Would this even be a vegan recipe section without an unbaked vegan cheesecake recipe? Possibly not. Unbaked vegan cheesecake-type desserts have become mainstream. They are generally easy to make and easy to adjust in different ways for texture and flavor. I have made hundreds of this kind of dessert, but one of my all-time favorites remains a lemon one.

I make batches of the blueberry compote every year for use in catering and just for my own use. I love adding herbal components to fruit compotes and generally prefer compotes over jams because more of the fruit flavor can shine through. If you do not want to use bay leaf, you can substitute fresh basil, sage, or thyme for the bay.

## Ingredients

**Crust:**
2 cups rolled oats, toasted until golden brown
2 Tbsp poppy seeds
2 Tbsp coconut oil or cocao butter softened
1 Tbsp water
pinch of salt
Optional: 1 tsp fresh thyme leaves

**Cheesecake filling:**
2 cups cultured cashew cheese, aged 2–3 weeks (You can use younger cultured curd; you just need to drain it in cheesecloth for a few hours first.)
½ cup drained coconut kefir curd
2 Tbsp maple syrup or ¼ cup chopped dates
½ cup coconut oil softened
Juice and zest of 2 large lemons (I like a lot of lemon juice, so you can reduce this if you like.)
¼ tsp vanilla powder

**Blueberry-bay compote:**
½ kg (1.1 lb.) fresh blueberries, washed, drained
2 cups sugar
1 tsp lemon juice
1 bay leaf
4 Tbsp gin

## Tools and Equipment

Baking sheet
High-speed blender
2 x bowl
Measuring cups
Measuring spoons
Springform pan
Parchment
2 x spatula
Thick caste saucepan (for softening coconut oil)
Saucepan (for compote)
Sheet pan (for toasting toasting oats)
Jar or container for compote

## Method: Crust

1. Wash and sanitize all of the work surfaces and tools you will work with.
2. Toast oats and poppy seeds at 275°F (135°C) for 15 minutes or until golden brown. Do not let them burn. Remove from the oven and allow them to cool.
3. Add the oats, poppy seeds, and salt to a high-speed blender and pulse several times before blending on low speed. Blend until the oats are almost a flour. If you want to add thyme, do so at this stage and pulse a few times to incorporate it.
4. Place the blended mixture in a bowl and with clean hands massage the oil into the mixture. Sprinkle 1 Tbsp water over the mixture and continue working until the mixture clumps together.
5. In a springform pan, place a round of parchment on the bottom. Press the crust mixture onto the bottom of the pan very firmly. If you want a thinner crust, just put some of the mixture aside and freeze it. Place the crust in the oven and toast it at 325°F (162.78°C) for 10 to 20 minutes. Remove from the heat and allow to cool fully before putting the cheesecake filling on top.

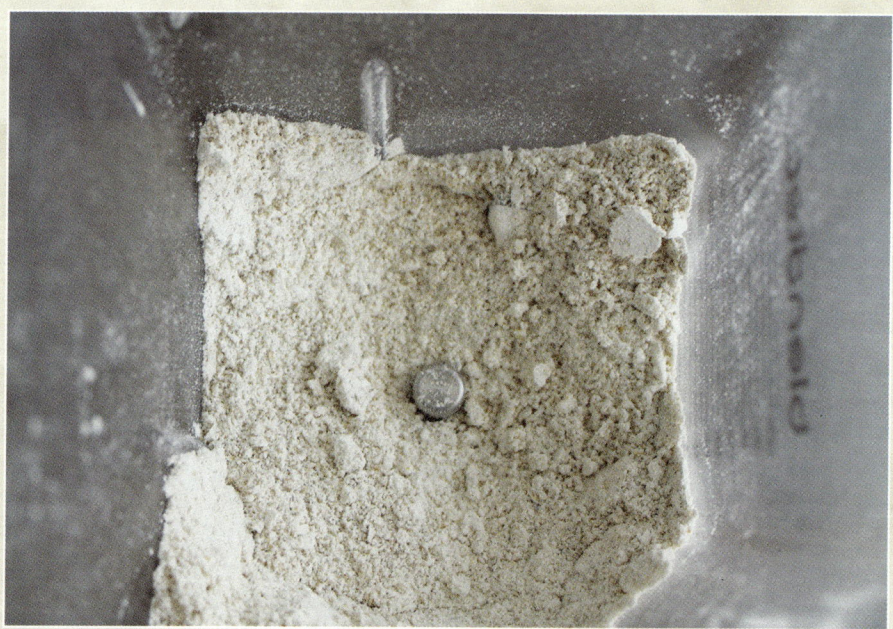

*Desired texture of blended dry ingredients for crust.*

## Method: Cheesecake filling

1. Wash and sanitize all work surfaces and tools you will work with.
2. In a high-speed blender add the cheese, coconut kefir curd, and maple syrup (or dates). Start at low speed and pulse a few times to allow the mixture to begin incorporating. Increase to low speed, and blend at low speed allowing the mixture to emulsify.
3. Add vanilla powder, lemon juice and zest, and blend until well combined.
4. Add the softened coconut oil and blend until very smooth and well combined.
5. Pour the mixture over the cooled crust, and smooth the surface with a spatula, or gently wiggle the springform pan until the mixture smooths out. You can put some preserved lemon zest on top, if you like.
6. Place the cheesecake in the refrigerator and let it rest overnight.

## Storage

This cheesecake will keep in the refrigerator for up to 10 days. It will also freeze well and can be kept frozen for up to 5 days.

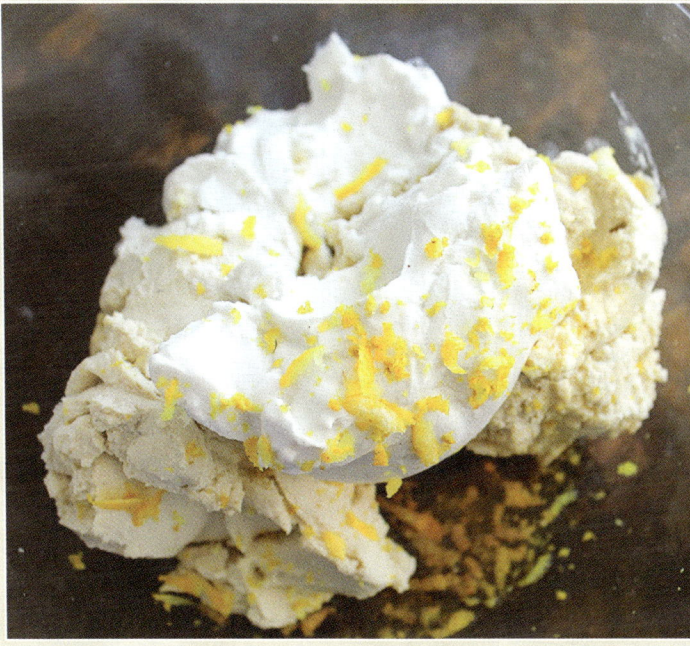

*Pre-measured coconut and cashew curd with grated lemon zest in bowl.*

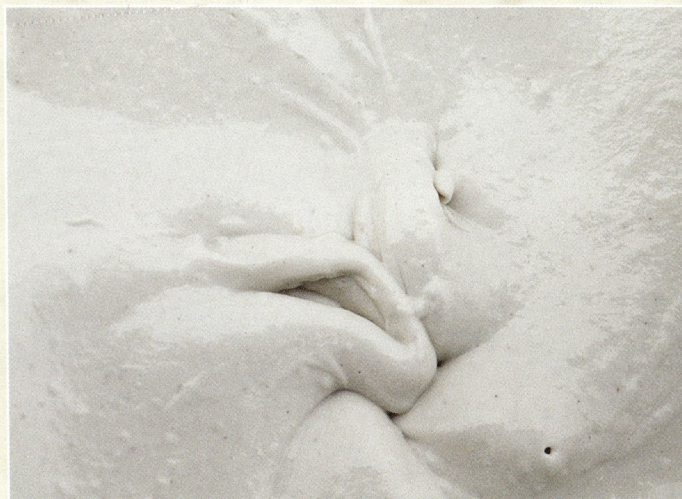

*Ingredients emulsifying at low speed.*

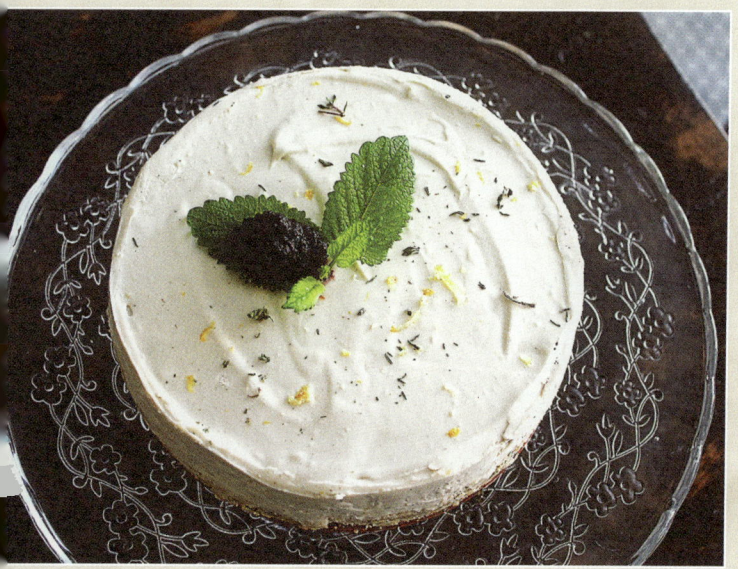

*Chilled, lemon-thyme unbaked cheesecake garnished with blueberry-bay compote.*

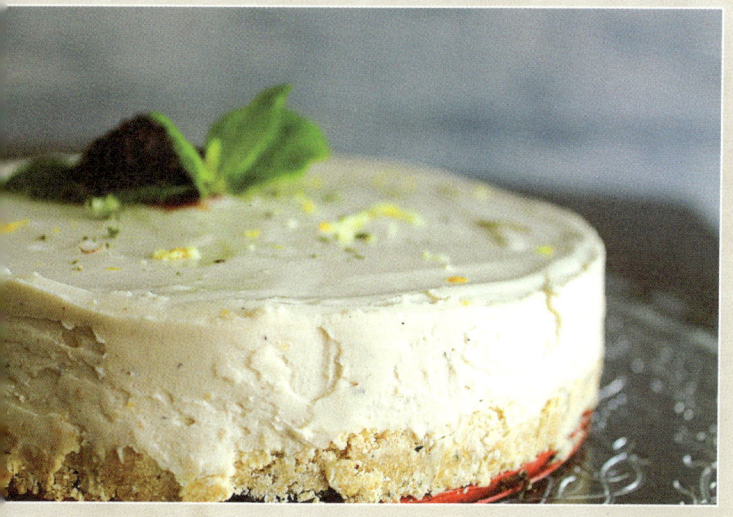

*Close-up of garnished lemon-thyme unbaked cheesecake.*

## Method: Blueberry-bay compote

1. Wash and sanitize all of the work surfaces and tools that you will use.
2. In a bowl, place the blueberries and add the sugar. Allow the sugar to macerate the blueberries for 1 hour. This will encourage the release of the blueberries' juice.
3. In a thick cast saucepan, add the gin and the bay leaf, and heat over medium heat for 10 minutes. Add the macerated blueberries, and bring the mixture to a boil. Allow it to cook for 15 minutes at a boil.
4. Reduce the heat, and allow the mixture to continue to cook for up to 4 hours over medium-low heat until it thickens but does not become jammy. Add the lemon juice, and allow to cook for another 30 minutes.
5. Remove from the heat, and allow it to cool. The mixture should be thick, but still loose, and the blueberries should not be completely broken down.
5. Place in a jar or container and store covered in the refrigerator until ready to serve..

## Storage

Stored properly in a covered jar or container in the refrigerator the compote will keep for up to 6 months.

# Pear Tarte Tatin, Sort of (But Not Really)

This is sort of a cross between a tarte tatin and a tome de cantal (cheese curd tart). This is a great lightly savory dessert, which can be paired with fresh herbs or a little black pepper. This is a great dessert for late summer and throughout the fall and winter, and though I use pears in this one, you may substitute apricots, nectarines, peaches, plums, or apples for the pears.

## Ingredients

**Crust:**

1½ cups flour

1 tsp salt

7 Tbsp cultured butter, cubed and chilled

¼ cup ice cold water

1 tsp apple cider vinegar

**Cheese curd filling:**

1 cup almond ricotta, drained, or cultured cashew curd

½ cup powdered sugar or vegan confectioners' sugar

¼ cup oat milk

¼ cup canned white beans

1½ tsp vanilla extract

1 tsp psyllium powder

½ tsp agar agar powder

¼ tsp kala namak (Himalayan or Indian black volcanic salt)

1 tsp rose water

Optional: 1 black cardamom pod

**Caramelized pears:**

2 medium-large semi-firm (not overly ripe) pears
(I like Comice pears, but really, any will do.)

¼ cup sugar

2–3 Tbsp cultured butter

## Tools and Equipment

2 x bowls

Food wrap

Blender

Sieve

Knife

Measuring cups

Measuring spoons

Spatula

Cutting board

Tart pan

Thick cast sauté pan

Cast iron skillet (9- or 10-inch)

Foil or parchment

## Method: Crust

1. Wash and sanitize all work surfaces and tools that you will use.
2. Combine flour and salt in a bowl; using your (washed) hands, rub the butter into the flour mixture until you have achieved approximately pea-sized lumps.

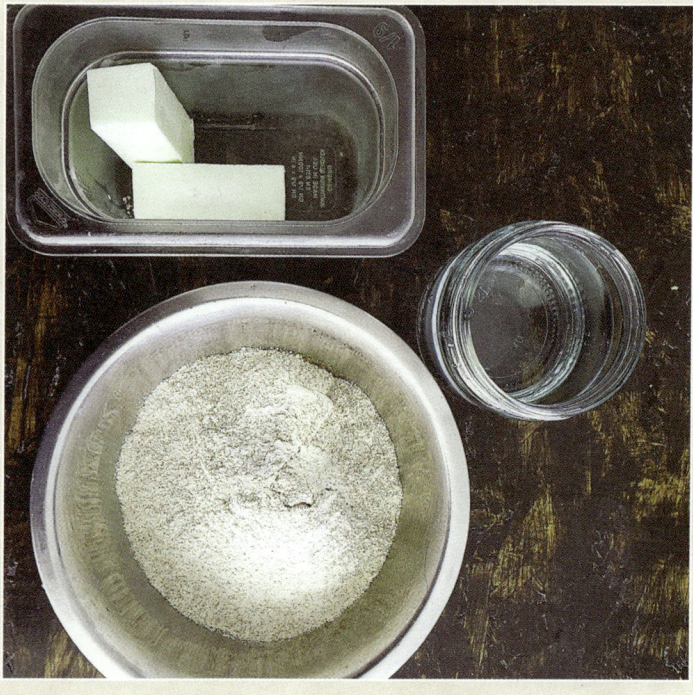

*Crust components ready to work (vinegar is in the water).*

3. Make a well in the flour/butter mixture and add the ice cold water along with the apple cider vinegar (add the apple cider vinegar to the water first).
4. Combine this mixture into a dough. Wrap in food wrap or plastic wrap and refrigerate for 1 hour. During this hour you can make the caramelized pears and the custard (cheese curd) filling.

## Method: Cheese curd filling

1. Wash and sanitize all work surfaces and tools that you will use.
2. At low speed in a blender, blend all of the ingredients together at once. You may need to increase speed to ensure that the beans end up smooth. Taste to adjust flavor as you see fit. I often include black cardamom in this mixture, so if you wish to, you may do the same.
3. After the mixture is blended, place it in a sieve to strain out excess moisture.

## Method: Caramelized pears

1. Wash and sanitize all work surfaces and tools that you will use.
2. Wash the pears, then cut in half. Remove the stems and seeds. Slice the pears into 1½-inch thick long slices.
3. In a thick cast sauté pan, heat the butter until it has melted, add the pear slices, and sauté over medium heat. As the pears begin to soften, add the sugar, sprinkling it over the pears. Continue cooking until the pears begin to caramelize. Do not cook them all the way through. Remove them just as they begin to brown.

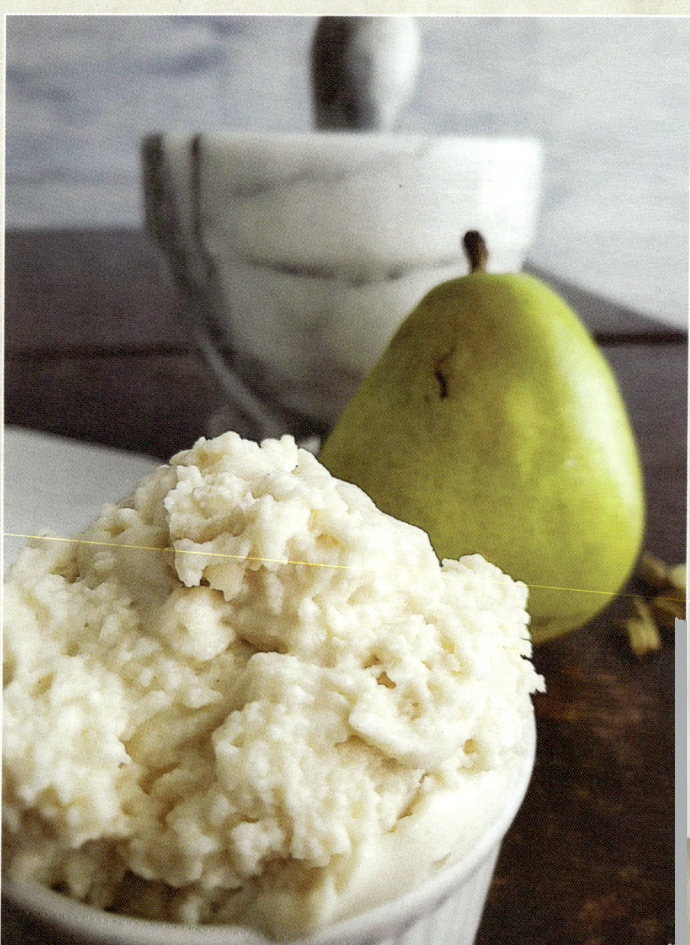

*Close-up of almond ricotta ready for use.*

## Method: Putting the tarte tatin together for baking

A tarte tatin is basically an upside down pie with the crust on top and the fruit on the bottom. I like to bake mine in a well-seasoned cast iron skillet, but you can do this in a springform pan or tart pan.

1. In the well-seasoned 9- or 10-inch cast iron skillet, rub the skillet bottom with a little coconut oil, and place the pears in concentric circles so that they form an even covering of the bottom of the pan. Pour any pan juices from the pears over the pears.
2. Spoon the cheese curd custard overtop the pears but not right to the edges. Leave about ¼-nch space between the outer edge of the pears and where the curd circle ends. Make this layer about 1 inch thick. If there is extra curd custard, save it for garnish.
3. Remove the crust dough from the refrigerator, break the chilled crumb crust over the top of the layered cheese curd filling and pears, and pat down gently. Preheat oven to 400°F–425°F (about 220°C). Place the skillet in the center of the oven, and bake for 10 minutes at this temperature. Reduce heat to 375°F (190°C) and continue to bake for another 20 to 30 minutes. Cover the top of the pastry with foil or parchment to protect from overbrowning.
4. Remove from heat, and allow to rest for 20 to 30 minutes before inverting the pan (placing an appropriately sized plate over the top of the pan and turning the pan over). Rest a few more minutes before cutting and serving. This pairs well with ice cream.

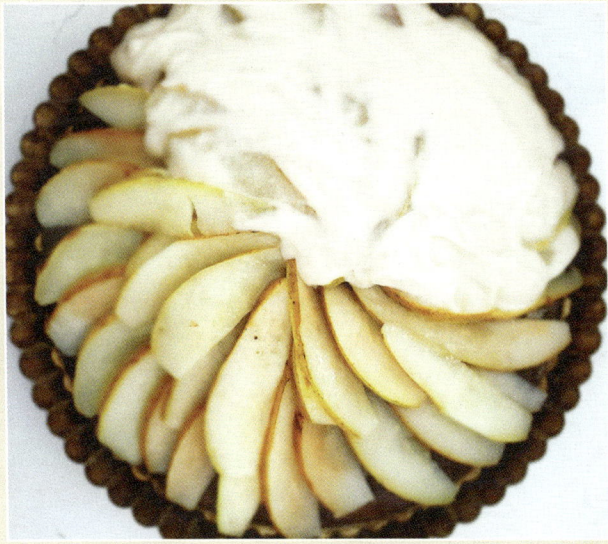

Above: *Adding the curd into the tart.*

Right: *Fully covered crumb topped "tatin."*

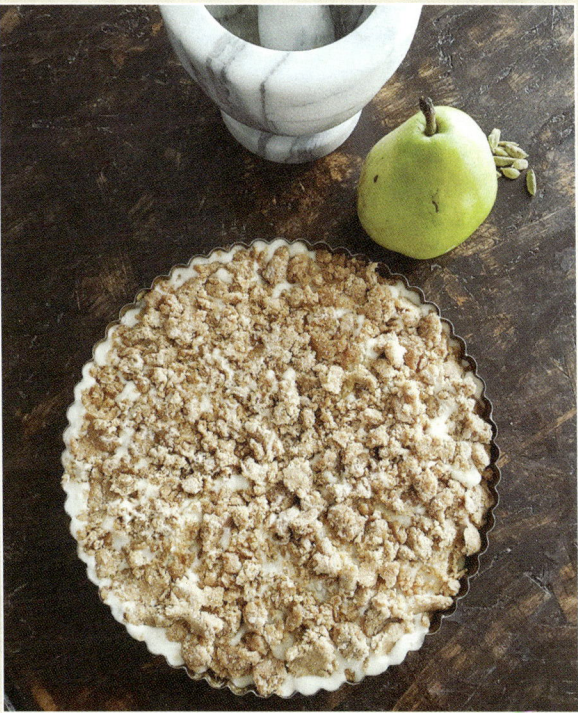

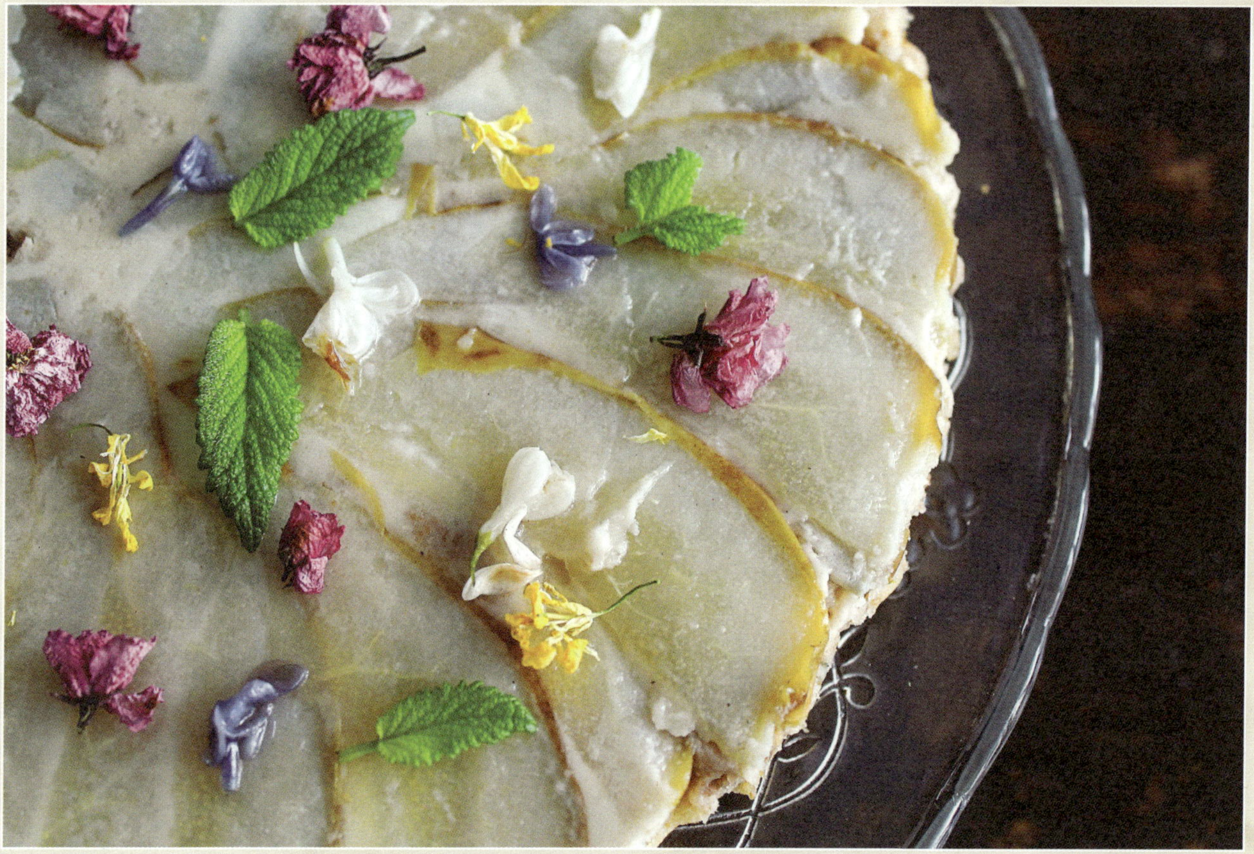

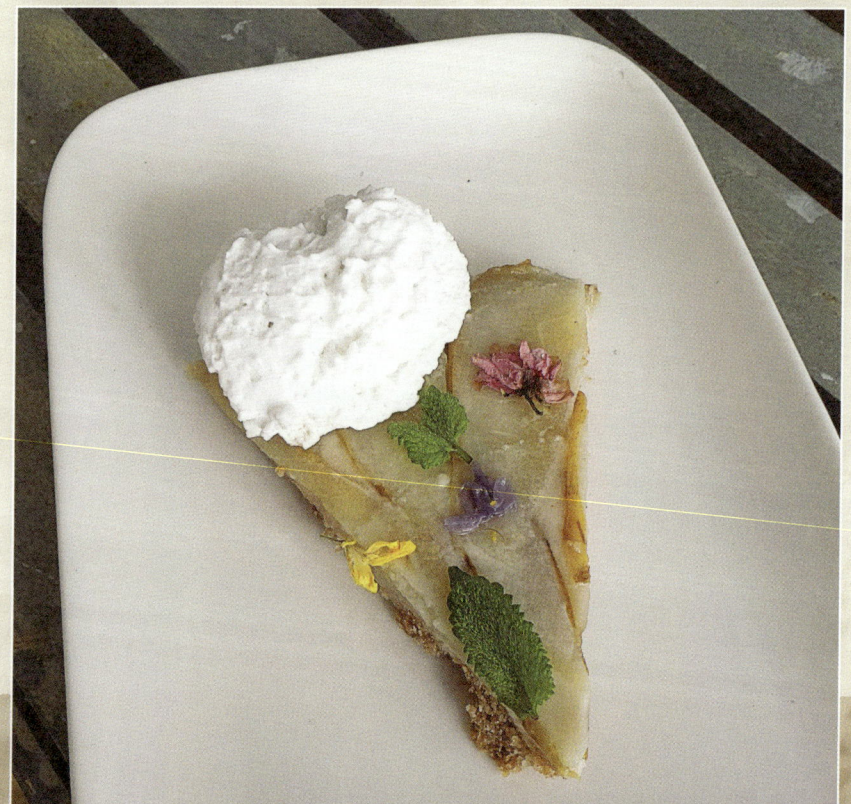

Above: Finished tarte tatin, garnished with salt cured sakura, dehydrated candied lilac, and fresh lemon balm.

Right: Serving the tarte tatin with a young blue cheese lightly sweetened curd.

## Something Savory

This section features several savory recipes using either by-products from cheesemaking or the cheeses themselves. As I feel that there are quite a lot of cheesy vegan recipes for mac 'n' cheese, caprese salad, grilled cheese sandwiches, and other such popular (for good reasons!) items, the recipes here will be a little different. Not to disparage those very popular items, but I think this is such an exciting time for vegan/plant-based cuisine that I think it is worth reaching outside the comfort food zone.

I am proud to highlight recipes from members of the Blue Heron team; Lucia Valenzuela (production supervisor), Jolene Vasallo (assistant operations manager), Karima Cellouf (production assistant and chef/nutrition educator), and Emily Davies, (sous chef and apprentice). Many of these recipes have been used in catering events we have done or at our short lived but well loved restaurant, SOIL. Recipes that do not have their names attached are mine.

# Jalapeño and Chive Biscuits with Cheesy Potato Chowder

**Tools and Equipment**

Thick cast stock pot or saucepan (medium to large)
Spatula
Knife, for chopping
Measuring spoons
Measuring cups
Wooden spoon
Cutting board

I made and served this chowder several times at SOIL and it was always surprisingly popular. I always like to garnish this with a spice infused oil or a chili sauce such as Pili Pili, a West African spicy pepper sauce that is a great condiment for so many dishes. We are fortunate in Vancouver to get ours from Kula Kitchen, a catering and products company focusing on Afrocentric plant-based foods. You can likely find Pili Pili in specialty food shops in your location.

## Cheesy Potato Chowder

### Ingredients

½ kg potatoes (German butter, Yukon gold, sieglinde, or similar variety), washed, skin left on, cubed
1 large carrot, washed, peeled if skin too thick, cubed or diced
2 ribs of celery cut into ½-inch slices
1 bay leaf
1 medium leek, washed well, white and light green sections only, sliced in rounds
2 cups corn niblets (omit if you wish)
2 cloves garlic, crushed, then minced
2 Tbsp grapeseed oil
3 Tbsp apple cider vinegar
1 round of 1–2 week aged cashew oat/white bean cheese broken into chunks or 2 cups cultured cashew curd
4 cups water
2 cups oat milk
½ cup nutritional yeast
2 tsp smoked paprika
1 tsp ancho chili powder
½ tsp cumin powder
salt and pepper to season (personal preference)
splash pickled jalapeño brine from 1 small can of pickled jalapeños (reserve jalapeños for biscuit recipe)
Spice infused oil or chili sauce

Optional: ½ cup tapioca starch stirred into 1½ cups water

## Method:

1. Wash and sanitize all work surfaces and tools you will use.
2. Wash and prepare all the vegetables ahead of time and set aside.
3. In a medium-large thick cast stock pot or saucepan, (heat the pot first for about 1 minute on low-medium heat), add the grapeseed oil and heat.
4. Add the garlic and leeks and sauté until they begin to soften.
5. Add the celery, carrot, and bay leaf and sauté over medium heat, allowing them to sweat for about 5 minutes. Then add the potatoes. Shake the pot or use a spatula or wooden spoon to move the potatoes and prevent them from sticking. After about 5 minutes, sprinkle a little salt, add the apple cider vinegar and a splash of jalapeño brine, then ½ of the water. This will slow the cooking down and allow the vegetables to sweat a bit longer, which will aid in flavor development. Allow the vegetables to cook on medium-high heat for about 30 minutes.
6. If you choose to add tapioca starch to make a thicker chowder, add it now so that the starch has enough time to cook into the chowder.

    Add the cheese, nutritional yeast, spices, salt and pepper, and stir into the mixture well. Add the remaining water and oat milk, and stir well for 1 to 2 minutes. Bring the mixture to a boil and cook for 5 minutes before reducing the heat to low-medium and allowing to slow cook for up to 1 hour. Add the corn (if you choose to use some) about halfway through this cooking period).
7. Garnish with spice infused oil or chili sauce and serve the chowder hot with the jalapeño and chive biscuits that follow.

## Jalapeño and Chive Biscuits
### (by Lucia Valenzuela, Blue Heron)

**Tools and Equipment**

Bowl
Cookie cutter
Food wrap
Fine mesh sieve
Rolling pin
Parchment or Silpat
Measuring cups
Measuring spoons
Spatula
Sheet tray

When we are about to release a new product we always test it in house. We are very fortunate at Blue Heron to have several chefs working with us. Our production supervisor and director of quality assurance, Lucia, is one of them and crafted this recipe while testing our cultured butter and our almond "buttermilk" (cultured by-product strained off from cultured almond ricotta).

### Ingredients

2 cups all-purpose flour (may substitute 1 cup of a whole grain flour like red fife or einkorn for 1 cup of all-purpose flour)
1 Tbsp baking powder
½ tsp baking soda
Pinch of salt
4 Tbsp cultured butter
1 small can pickled jalapeño, drained (fluid reserved for chowder above), finely diced
1 Tbsp dried chives (can be less if you want or substitute dried garlic)
1 cup almond "buttermilk" (the by-product of straining a fresh batch of cultured almond ricotta)

### Method

1. Wash and sanitize all work surfaces and tools that you will work with.
2. Preheat the oven to 425°F (approximately 220°C).
3. In a large bowl, sift together all of the dry ingredients, except chives.
4. With clean and sanitized hands, rub the cultured butter into the flour mixture until you have pea-sized lumps in the flour.
5. Add the chives and diced jalapeño and work through until evenly distributed.
6. Make a well in the mixture and add a little cold almond "buttermilk" at a time, working quickly but lightly with your hands to collect the mixture into a dough.
7. Once you have most of the mixture clumped into a dough, fold it repeatedly, kneading it and collecting the rest of the flour mixture in the bowl.
8. Turn the dough out onto a lightly floured surface and roll the dough out with a rolling pin until about 1 inch thick and in a rectangle. Fold this three times, and then roll again. Repeat this one more time. Wrap the dough and rest it in the refrigerator for 30 minutes.

9. After 30 minutes remove the dough from the refrigerator and repeat the folding steps one more time, and refrigerate to rest it for another 15 minutes. Then roll the dough out to about 1 inch thick and cut into rounds. Place on parchment- or silpat-lined sheet tray and bake at 425°F (220°C) for about 15 minutes or until golden brown.

### To serve

Top the chowder with a dollop of fresh cultured almond ricotta and a fresh herb garnish and serve with biscuits.

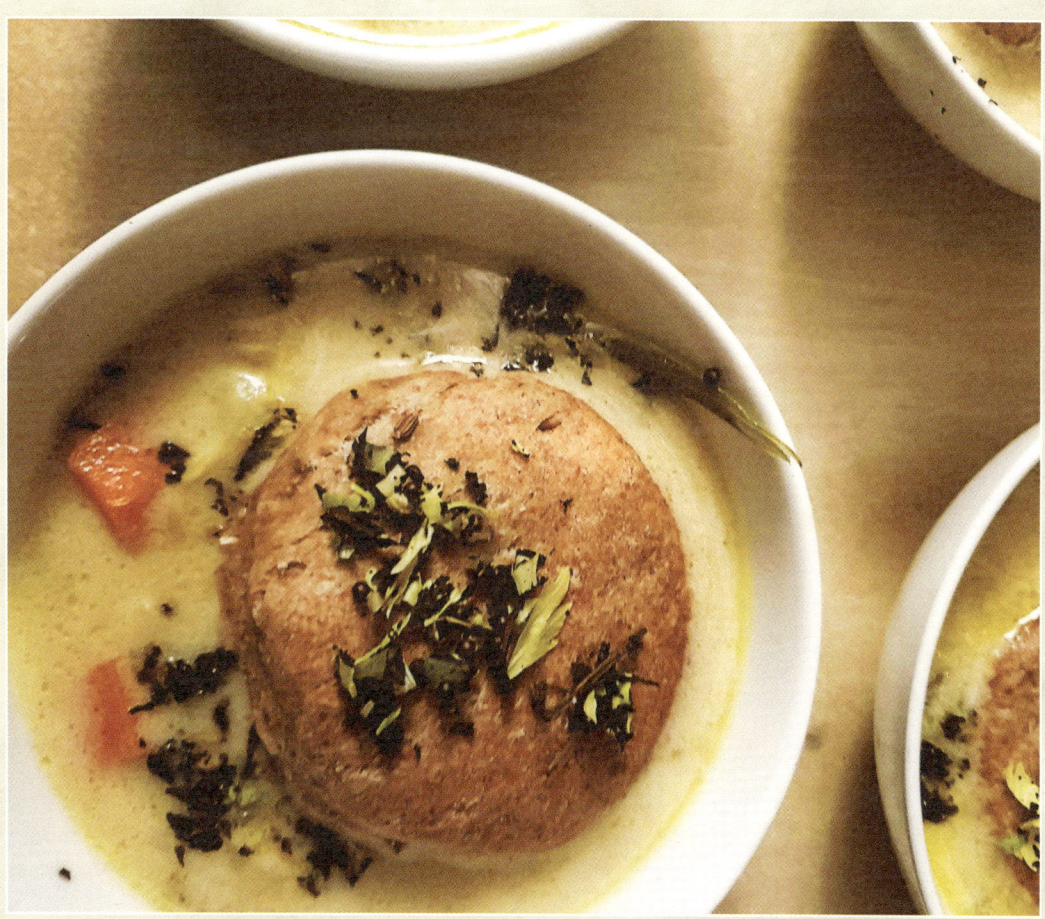

*Warm and comforting cheesy potato chowder with jalapeño and chive biscuits.*

# Millet Tabbouleh with Grilled Eggplant and Tzatziki

## Tools and Equipment

Thick cast saucepan
Baking sheet
Bowl
Knife
Fork
Spatula
Grater
Cutting board
Measuring cups
Measuring spoons
Fine mesh sieve
Cast iron grill pan or baking sheet

Our restaurant, SOIL, was not open for very long, (we needed to make a hard decision to close it in favor of pursuing the larger project of increasing Blue Heron's manufacturing capacity), but during that time Chef Emily Davies, who had worked very hard to become my apprentice and then sous chef, created some of our most popular recipes. This millet tabbouleh was part of an autumn dish served with glazed roasted carrots, but it can be adapted for use in many other ways. Here I have chosen to present it with grilled eggplant and a bright and fresh tzatziki recipe developed by Blue Heron's assistant operations manager, Jolene Vasallo.

---

## Ingredients

**Celery stock:**

grapeseed oil

3 tsp caraway seed

2 tsp fennel seed

4 ribs of celery, sliced

1 clove garlic, minced

6 cups water

**Tabbouleh:**

½ cup millet

1–1½ cups celery stock

2 bunches flat leaf parsley, washed, stems removed, chiffonade (chopped until very fine)

15 mint leaves (fewer if they are very large), stems removed, washed, and minced very fine

1–2 medium green onions, washed, chopped fine,

3–4 Tbsp lemon or lime juice (your preference)

½ cup fermented tofu feta (from this book, if you have made some)

olive oil, a drizzle

salt to season

1 large roma tomato diced,

1 small English cucumber sliced into thin rounds or diced

### Tzatziki:

250 mL cultured coconut yogurt (for a slightly thicker tzatziki you can substitute cultured cashew curd or blend some slightly aged cheese with a little coconut milk)

½ cucumber, washed, peel left on, grated. (English cucumbers are best for this.)

2 cloves garlic, crushed, then minced

2 Tbsp fresh squeezed lemon juice

¼ cup or more fresh dill, washed, dried, stems removed (If you love dill as much as I do and want a bit more layering of the dill flavor, add ½ Tbsp dried dill weed.)

### Eggplant:

1 medium long Japanese eggplant (my favorite type), or eggplant of your choosing

1 tsp salt

½ lemon

grapeseed oil for grilling

### Method: Celery stock

1. Wash and sanitize all work surfaces and tools that you will use.
2. Wash and cut the celery ribs.
3. Heat a splash of grapeseed oil in a thick cast saucepan, add the garlic, the caraway and fennel seeds, and sauté for 3 minutes. Add the sliced celery and sweat over medium heat for up to 10 minutes. Add the water, and bring to a boil. Cook at high heat for 5 minutes, then reduce to medium heat and allow the stock to reduce until there are about 4 cups of fluid remaining.

### Method: Tabbouleh

1. Wash and sanitize all work surfaces and tools that you will use.
2. Wash all vegetables that you will prepare.
3. Make the millet. Toast millet on a baking sheet in the oven at 375°F (190.5°C) for 5 minutes. Add to a thick cast pot, and then add the celery stock and a pinch of salt. Bring to a boil, allow to boil for a couple of minutes, and then reduce the heat and cover the pot. Allow the millet to cook for about 15 minutes. Remove from the heat, lightly fluff the millet with a fork, and pour onto a sheet tray to cool for 15 minutes. Optimal ratio for cooking millet is 1 part millet to 2 parts liquid.
4. In a large bowl place the millet, parsley, mint, lemon (or lime) juice, green onion, pinch of salt, and drizzle of olive oil. Rest in the refrigerator until serving, then add cucumber and tomato.

### Method: Tzatziki

1. Wash and sanitize all work surfaces and equipment that you will use.
2. Wash and set aside all vegetables you will prepare.
3. Place the coconut yogurt into a bowl, grate the cucumber over top, add the garlic, dill, and lemon juice. Fold in together until well combined.
4. If an especially thick tzatziki is desired, drain the tzatziki in a fine mesh sieve for about 15 minutes.

### Storage

Stored in a closed container in the refrigerator, this will keep for 1 week.

### Method: Grilled Eggplant

1. Wash and sanitize all work surfaces and tools that you will use.
2. Wash eggplant.
3. Slice eggplant into rounds or on the diagonal, rub the ½ lemon over the flesh of the eggplant, and then sprinkle with salt. Let rest for at least 15 minutes. This helps remove the bitterness that eggplant often has. Japanese eggplant is somewhat less bitter and becomes quite creamy when grilled, making it my favorite eggplant varietal to work with.
4. Heat a grill (a cast iron grill pan that sits on your stovetop will suffice). Brush the eggplant with grapeseed oil on both sides and grill until soft and browned.

### To serve

Place slices of warm, grilled eggplant on top of the tabbouleh, sprinkle a little cumin if desired, and top with tzatziki.

# Roasted Artichoke and Spinach Dip

I make this recipe frequently for catering services and use it in a number of ways. It can be a dip, cold or heated, served atop crostini as a canape with sliced olives; it can be used to stuff pasta (shells or cannelloni) or as a fun addition to a lasagne. This would also make a great crepe filling for a brunch dish, or baked with some chickpea flour into a 'frittata' of sorts. Be adventurous! A dip is never just a dip! Both the artichoke and spinach amounts can be adjusted to suit your preference.

**Tools and Equipment**

Baking sheet
Cutting board
Knife
Measuring spoons
High-speed blender
Cheesecloth

## Ingredients

1 can artichokes in brine (You may use fresh artichokes–the flavor is incredible and they are worth the work.) Reserve some of the brine for blending later.
1 bunch of fresh spinach (You can substitute frozen spinach.)
1 Tbsp grapeseed oil for roasting the artichokes
500 mL of cultured almond ricotta, drained (or macadamia ricotta or any of the young cultured curds)
3 cloves of garlic crushed, then minced, or add 4 cloves of roasted garlic
1 Tbsp lemon juice or preserved lemon
½ tsp salt
1 tsp black or white pepper
Optional: 2 Tbsp nutritional yeast

## Method

1. Wash and sanitize all work surfaces and tools that you will use.
2. Preheat the oven to 375°F (190.5°C). Roast drained artichokes with a drizzle of grapeseed oil and a sprinkle of salt for 20 to 25 minutes, or until they are lightly golden brown in color.
3. Remove the artichokes from the oven, and set aside to cool. While artichokes are cooling, saute garlic and spinach until softened.
4. In a high-speed blender, add a splash of artichoke brine, the spinach, garlic, lemon, and pulse a few times to break down the spinach. Add the artichokes, and pulse a few times before blending at low speed until mostly creamy but with some chunky texture remaining.
5. Add the cultured almond ricotta and pulse the mixture together; add the salt and pepper and pulse several more times.

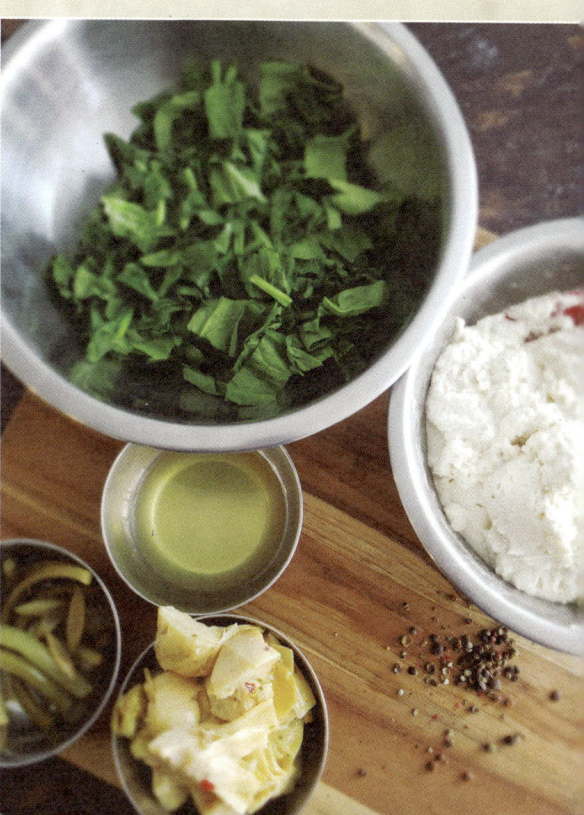

*The basic ingredients.*

6. For a thicker dip, strain the mixture in a fine mesh sieve for about 15 minutes to remove excess moisture. You can line the sieve with cheesecloth if you wish.

### Flavoring options

Baking the blended mixture will mildly caramelize the almond ricotta, adding depth of flavor and more creamy notes. If you choose to bake the dip, place the mixture in an ovenproof baking dish, and bake at 375°F (190.5°C) for 20 to 25 minutes, or until the top is golden brown.

Cold smoking the mixture will add a warm smoky flavor that amplifies the roasted notes of the artichoke. If you have a smoking gun this will be easy to do. I like to use dried sage leaves in the smoking chamber.

### Storage

Store in a covered container in the refrigerator. It keeps for up to 10 days.

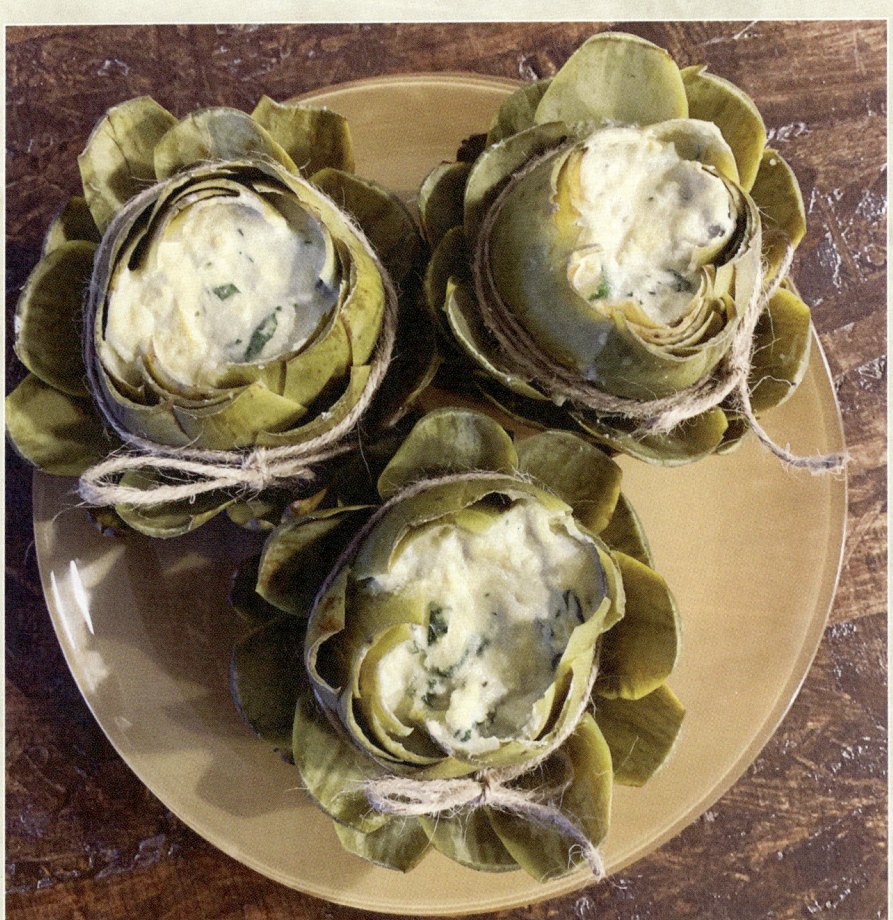

*Roasted artichoke and spinach dip served in artichokes.*
CREDIT: COLIN MEDHURST

# Potato and Celeriac Dauphinoise (gratin)

I have made several versions of this for weddings I have catered. This is adaptable to different root vegetables and each type changes the flavor profile. You may also play around with this recipe, using it to test the different types of cheeze or cheese. I adore tarragon, so I use that here, but you can change the herb to your preference. This makes a great side dish for family-style meals, and leftovers can be blended into a soup or sauce!

## Tools and Equipment

Vegetable peeler
Knife
Cutting board
Mandoline
Thick cast saucepan
Baking dish
Measuring cups
Measuring spoons
Spatula

## Ingredients

½ kg Yukon gold or similar style potato
½ kg celeriac
5 cups oat milk (or plant milk of your choice}
2 cloves garlic, crushed, then minced
1½ cups coconut cream
1½ cups of cheese you have made (can be cultured or non-cultured)
1 Tbsp fresh tarragon or a few rosemary leaves
1 tsp salt
¼ tsp black pepper
pinch of nutmeg
2 Tbsp cultured butter
½ cup blue cheese that you have made and set aside (or other cheese recipe that you have made from this book)

## Method

1. Wash and sanitize all work surfaces and tools that you will use.
2. Wash all vegetables very well. Peel celeriac. Use a mandoline to finely slice the potato and celeriac into approximately ¼-inch thick rounds. If the celeriac is large, you can cut it in half and then make half-moon shapes with the mandoline.
3. In a thick cast saucepan, add the vegetables, garlic, tarragon (or other herb choice) and oat milk and bring to a simmer. Simmer for 15 minutes. Be careful not to overcook. This is just to soften the celeriac and potato in advance of baking.
4. Preheat the oven to 350°F (176.6°C). Drain the infused milk off (reserve for use in other recipes), and then add the coconut cream, cheese, salt, pepper, and nutmeg. Return to a gentle simmer and allow to cook for another 10 to 15 minutes. Test the vegetables with a knife. Make sure to remove them from the heat before they are too soft.

5. Coat a baking dish with cultured butter or oil, and layer the potato and celeriac slices neatly and evenly. Pour the remaining pan cream overtop and top with your choice of cheese that you have made. My favorite is blue cheese mixed with some of the non-cultured mozzarella.
6. Bake in the oven at 350°F (176°C) for 35 minutes or until it is easy to slice a knife through the vegetables and the top is golden brown.

# Herb, Potato, Mushroom, and Asparagus Galette

Another one of my wedding catering go-tos is this herb and mushroom galette. Galettes are the name for a rustic folded tart, (no pie plate or tart pan necessary). In Italian they are referred to as crostatas. They can be sweet or savory. I often make these in miniature for canape/small bite service, but I have also served them larger as a primary meal served with the dauphinoise above and an arugula salad, or other such combination.

I love making this with golden foot chanterelles and lobster mushrooms during British Columbia's wild mushroom season, or less exciting but reliable mushrooms such as crimini during the spring when I can garnish the galettes with grilled British Columbia asparagus, but you can use whatever mushrooms are on hand in your region or ones bought at a grocery store or farmers' market.

## Ingredients

1 batch of your favorite pie crust recipe or use the pie crust recipe from the pear tarte tatin recipe and make it savory by adding black pepper and fresh herbs to the crust
½ kg mixed mushrooms (chanterelle, portobello, or your choice), sliced
1 large potato, peeled if skin is thick
½ bunch fresh asparagus
2 Tbsp cultured butter or grapeseed oil for sautéing
Garlic, 2 cloves, minced
a few fresh rosemary and tarragon leaves, chopped
1–2 sprigs fresh thyme, leaves stripped from the woody stems
1 fresh sage leaf, finely chopped
Pinch cinnamon
½ fresh lemon, juice and some zest
500g cheese or non-cultured cheeze of your choice made from this book (The mozzarella behaves well in this recipe as does the cultured almond ricotta, a 2–3 week aged cashew cheese, or almost any of the others. If you have camembert ready, it is a lovely fit for this recipe.)
salt and pepper to season

## Tools and Equipment

Rolling pin
Thick cast sauté pan
Spatula or wooden spoon
Knife or mandoline
Vegetable peeler
Measuring spoons
Measuring cups
Rolling pin
Baking sheet
Parchment or Silpat
Foil

*Core ingredients: cultured butter, cheese, sautéed mushrooms, herbs, pastry dough.*

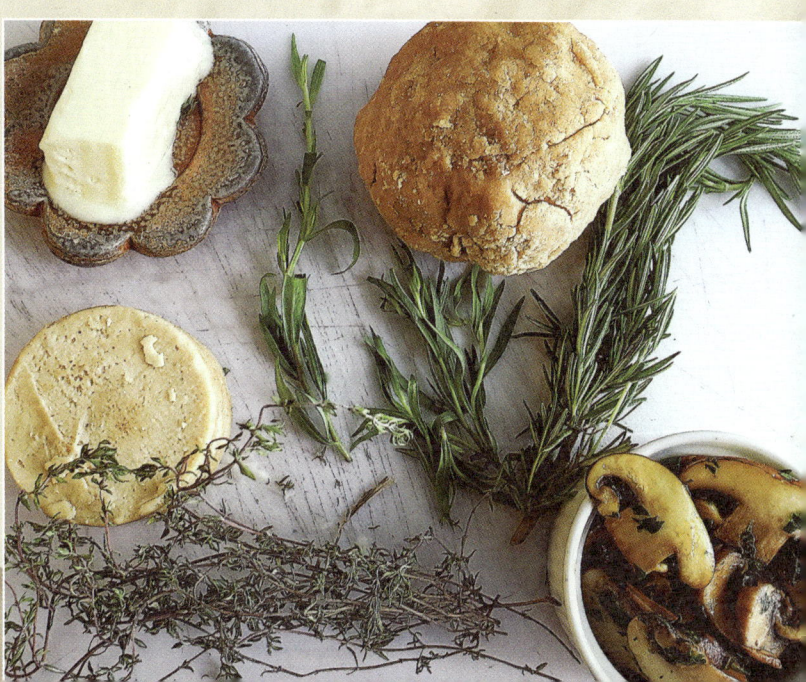

## Method

1. Wash and sanitize all work surfaces and tools that you will work with.
2. Wash/clean and slice the mushrooms and set aside.
3. Wash/clean the potatoes. If the skin is very thin, you do not need to remove it. Use a mandoline or a knife to make very thin round slices of potato. Set the slices aside.
4. Wash the asparagus, snap off the bottom ½ inch or so. Drizzle a little olive oil over them, and then grill them (if you have a grill) or par-cook in a thick cast pan with a small amount of water, just until the spears are brightened in color and lightly seared. This will prevent the asparagus from drying out during baking.
5. Roll out the pastry dough on a lightly floured surface into a circle about ¼ inch thick. Or make several smaller galette circles. Preheat the oven to 350°F (176°C).
6. In a thick cast sauté pan, heat the cultured butter or oil, add the garlic, and sauté until tender. Add the mushrooms and sprinkle with salt; allow them to sweat for about 2 minutes. Then add the fresh herbs, the fresh cinnamon, and allow to cook until mushrooms are quite soft, but not all the way cooked down. Be mindful here, mushrooms can cook down quite quickly, so be sure to keep your attention on them. You need them to retain some moisture and texture to withstand baking in the oven.
7. Just as the mushrooms are finishing, squeeze the lemon juice over them and zest a little fresh lemon zest in. Toss quickly. Remove the pan from heat and allow mushrooms to cool.
8. In the center of the galette circle break up the cheese you are using. Top the cheese with thin slices of potato, then sautéed mushrooms. Add a bit more cheese and potato if you wish. Then begin folding the edge of the dough around the filling, in overlapping layers that encircle the filling. Top each galette with asparagus spears. Sprinkle a little salt and cracked pepper over top, and, if you like, fresh herbs.
9. Place the galette or smaller galettes on a parchment- or Silpat-lined baking sheet and bake for 25 to 35 minutes at 350°F (176°C). Check at the halfway point to ensure that the crust is not overcooking. Place a layer of parchment or foil overtop if over-baking is a concern, or reduce the heat slightly.

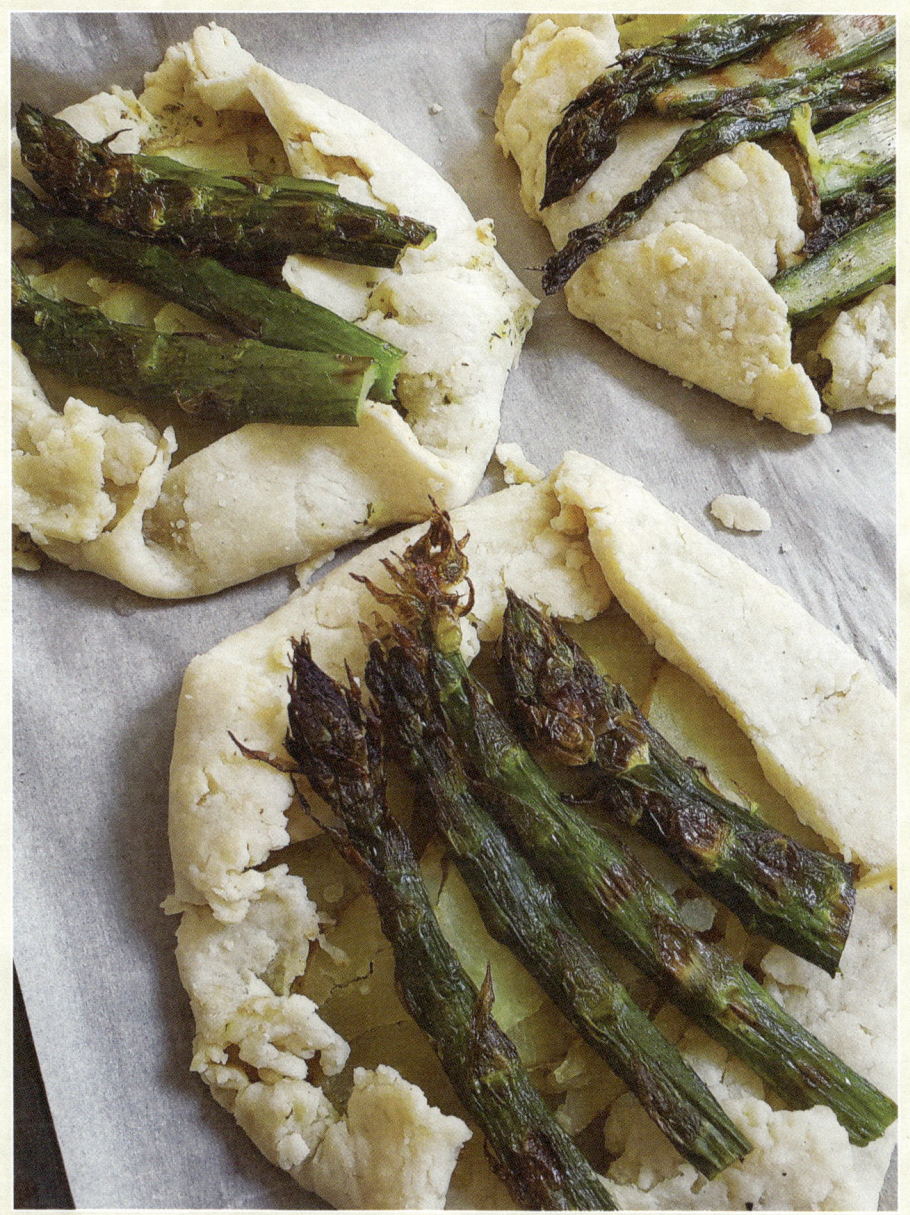

*Potato, mushroom and herb galettes topped with grilled asparagus, ready for the oven.*

# Camembert Stuffed Delicata Squash with Cranberries, Candied Pecan and Fried Sage

## Tools and Equipment

Knife

Cutting board

Baking sheet

Parchment or Silpat

Pie lifter (or other device to remove the squash rings from the baking sheet when done)

This little bite is another great side dish for late summer or throughout autumn and winter. It was created by accident when I was catering a vegan thanksgiving dinner with Chef KD Tighe and we cheekily made a little snack for the kitchen team while we were prepping. I had brought some of the Blue Heron test batch of oat/cashew camembert (white mold ripened cheese), and KD, Chef Tania, and another member of our team that night stuffed it into some scrapes of delicata squash and baked it. We ate it with remnants of cranberries, candied pecans, and fried sage that we had used for a salad. It was delicious.

## Ingredients

1 medium-sized delicata squash, also known as honeyboat squash (You may also use acorn squash or other squashes with edible skin.)

1 round of white mold ripened cheese that you have made

1 Tbsp grapeseed oil

pinch of salt

**Garnish:**

Dried cranberries, candied pecans, and fried sage leaves

## Method

1. Wash and sanitize all work surfaces and tools that you will use.
2. Preheat the oven to 350°F (176°C).
3. Wash the squash surface, but do not peel. Slice into 1-inch thick rounds, and scoop out the seeds. You can save the seeds, clean them off, and toast them as you would pumpkin seeds.
4. Place the squash rounds on a parchment-or Silpat-lined baking sheet. Break up the cheese and stuff the center of the squash with the cheese. Drizzle grapeseed oil and salt over the top. Bake at 350°F (176°C) until lightly golden on top and both the squash and cheese are very soft.
5. Remove from the oven, and garnish with dried cranberries, fried sage leaf, and candied pecans. Enjoy!

## Photosynthesis, a Smoothie

This is my favorite smoothie to date. It was designed by my sous chef/apprentice Emily Davies for the SOIL menu. We both like bananas, but we both were very tired of smoothies that rely on bananas for thickness. We also wanted to have a smoothie that combined ingredients (greens) that support the human gut biome and had a cultured element. This smoothie can be made to drink or as a smoothie bowl you dress up.

It requires a little advance preparation in that you need to keep the kale and orange frozen ahead of time and have a batch of coconut kefir or kefir-yogurt on hand, but once you have done it a few times, it is easy to keep doing. This recipe is for 1 smoothie.

**Tools and Equipment**
High-speed blender
Knife
Cutting board
Measuring cups
Measuring spoons

### Ingredients

80 g frozen kale (with stem), chopped up
130 g frozen orange (peeled)
1 tsp spirulina or E3 live blue-green algae
⅔ cup coconut or oat milk
pinch of salt
25 g dates, chopped
1 Tbsp (or more if you like) coconut kefir or kefir-yogurt
¼ tsp fresh grated ginger

### Method

1. Wash and sanitize all work surfaces and tools you will use.
2. Place the liquids into a high-speed blender, then the solids, and pulse a few times before moving to low speed continuous blending. Blend at low speed for 20 seconds before graduating to higher speed, ensuring the ingredients are emulsifying. Add a splash of water or lemon juice if you need more liquid.
3. Drink up!

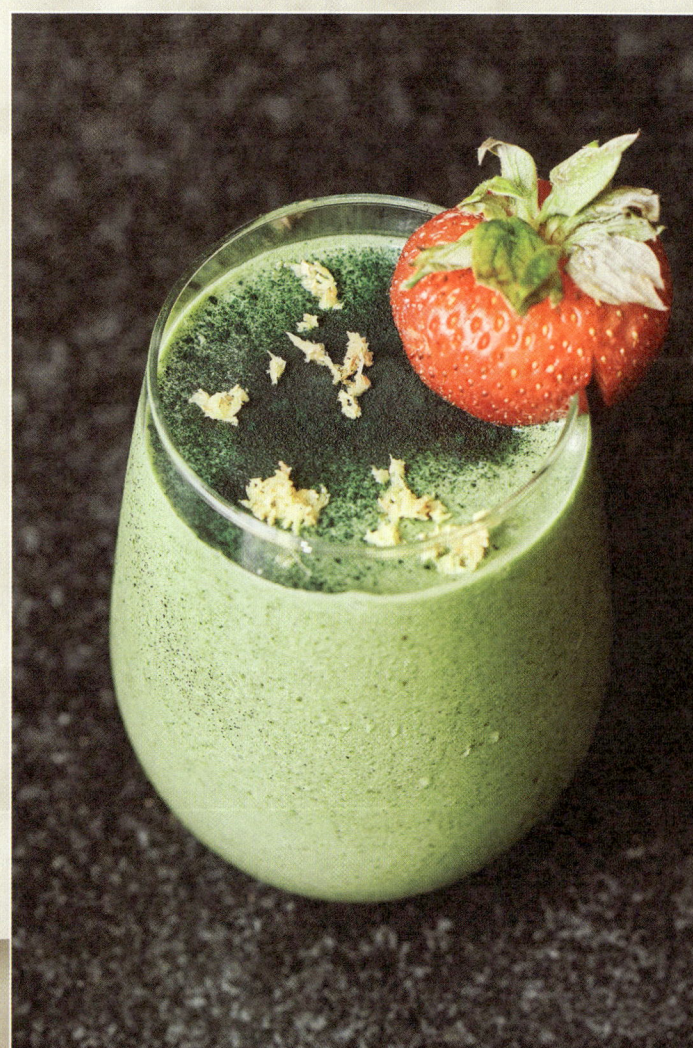

*The photosynthesis smoothie, anytime refreshment.* CREDIT: ANDRE SHEPPERD, DREMOND STUDIO

# Buttermilk Fried Tempeh

**Tools and Equipment**

Fork
Knife
2 x bowl
Thick cast sauté pan or small pot for deep frying
Probe thermometer
Plate
Cooling rack

This recipe comes from the talented Chef Karima Cellouf. Karima has been a production assistant with the Blue Heron team, but more significantly is an experienced chef in her own right, who is developing her nutrition/cooking consulting business. Karima, in addition to being a chef, is a certified nutritional practitioner. This recipe features buttermilk from drained almond ricotta, but you can also use loose coconut kefir, kefir-yogurt, or even blend up one of the cultured cheeses you make with a little plant milk to use in place of the buttermilk. As Karima says, this recipe makes one giant snack that may or may not be shared.

## Ingredients

**Marinated tempeh:**

1 x 200 g package of tempeh (fresh is preferred over frozen)*
3 large cloves garlic, finely grated
½ cup buttermilk from drained cultured almond ricotta (You may substitute coconut kefir, kefir-yogurt, or even one of the cultured cheeses you made, blended with a little water for the buttermilk.)
⅓ cup hot sauce (whichever your favorite is)
pinch of salt to taste

**Seasoned flour dredge:**

1 cup chickpea flour
1½ tsp garlic powder
1½ tsp onion powder
½ tsp cayenne
½ tsp cracked black pepper (or more if you like)
½ tsp salt

**Additional:**

sunflower or grapeseed oil for frying
salt to season
dipping sauce of your choice

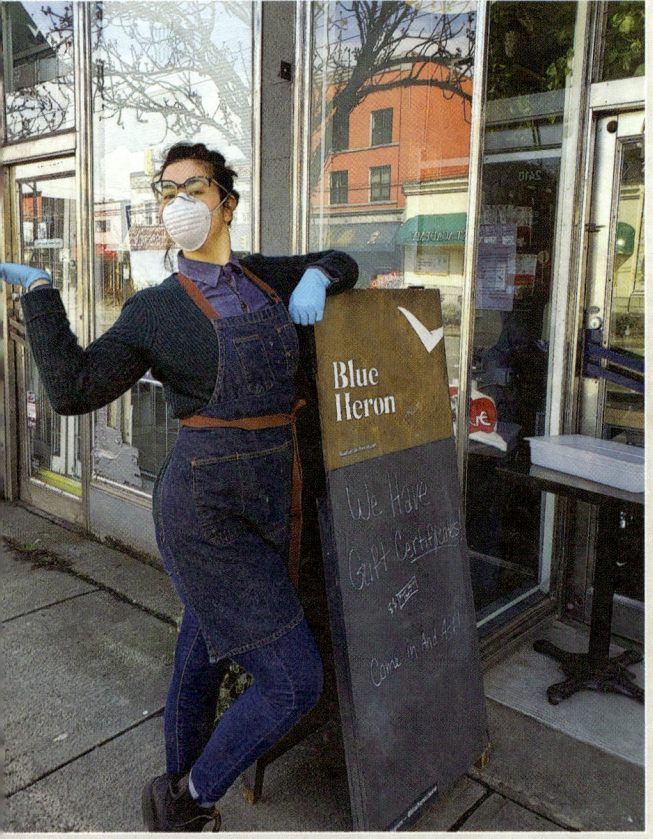

Chef Karima Cellouf, @heyhaveyoueatenyetx on Instagram and Blue Heron team member. Karima regularly highlights how to use Blue Heron cheeses and is a chef and certified nutritional practitioner.

*You may substitute extra firm tofu for the tempeh, but if you do, I suggest wrapping the tofu in cheesecloth, placing it on a perforated rack of some type, and pressing it with a heavy weight to remove excess moisture.

# Recipes: Putting Your Cheeses to Work

## Method

1. Wash and sanitize all work surfaces and all tools that you will use.
2. Prepare the marinade by combining the buttermilk, grated garlic, and hot sauce in a bowl and whisking together.
3. Using a fork, poke the tempeh several times in rows, on both sides, to allow the marinade to saturate. Tear (or cut) the tempeh into generous nugget-sized chunks. Add the tempeh to the marinade and ensure that it is well coated. Refrigerate for at least 12 hours, but if you can, overnight.
4. Remove the tempeh from the marinade and set on a plate to temper for 20 minutes and allow excess marinade to run off.
5. In a bowl, combine all the dry ingredients for the flour dredge.
6. Preheat a thick cast sauté pan, add the oil for frying. Use a probe thermometer to check the temperature. The temperature should be between 325°F and 350°F (163°C and 176°C).
7. Gently toss the tempeh in the dredge to ensure pieces are well coated, transfer to a plate, and tap off excess flour.
8. Fry the tempeh on both sides until crunchy and golden brown.
9. Transfer the pieces to a wire cooling rack, and immediately season with salt.

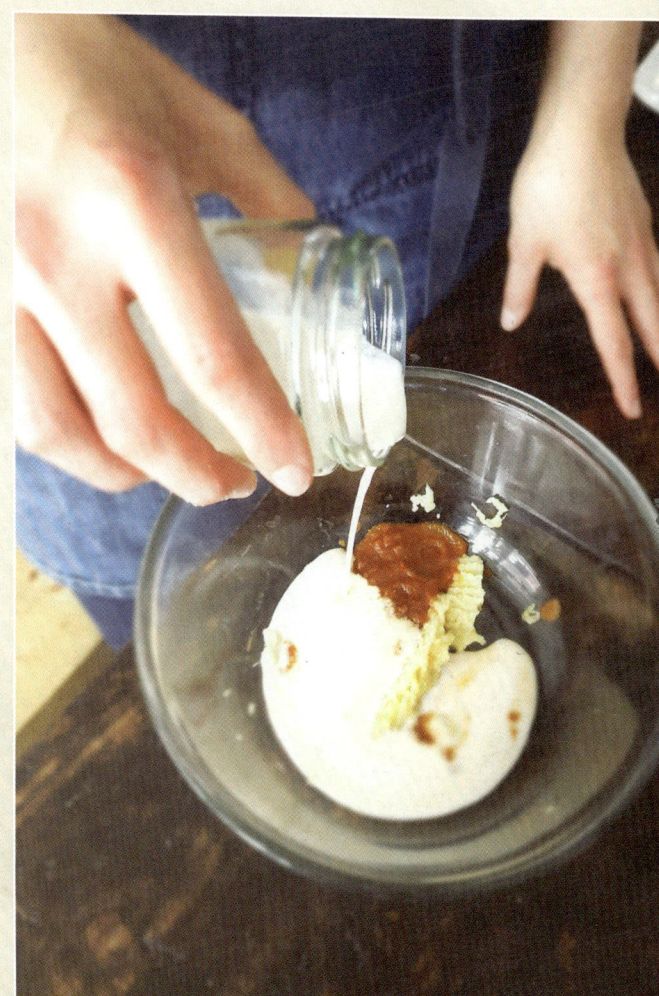

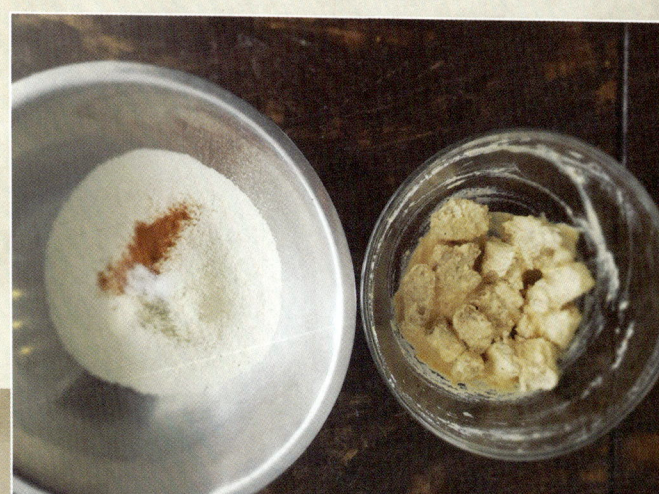

Top: *Making the marinade: adding the cultured buttermilk.*

Bottom: *Marinating the tempeh, with flour dredge at the ready.*

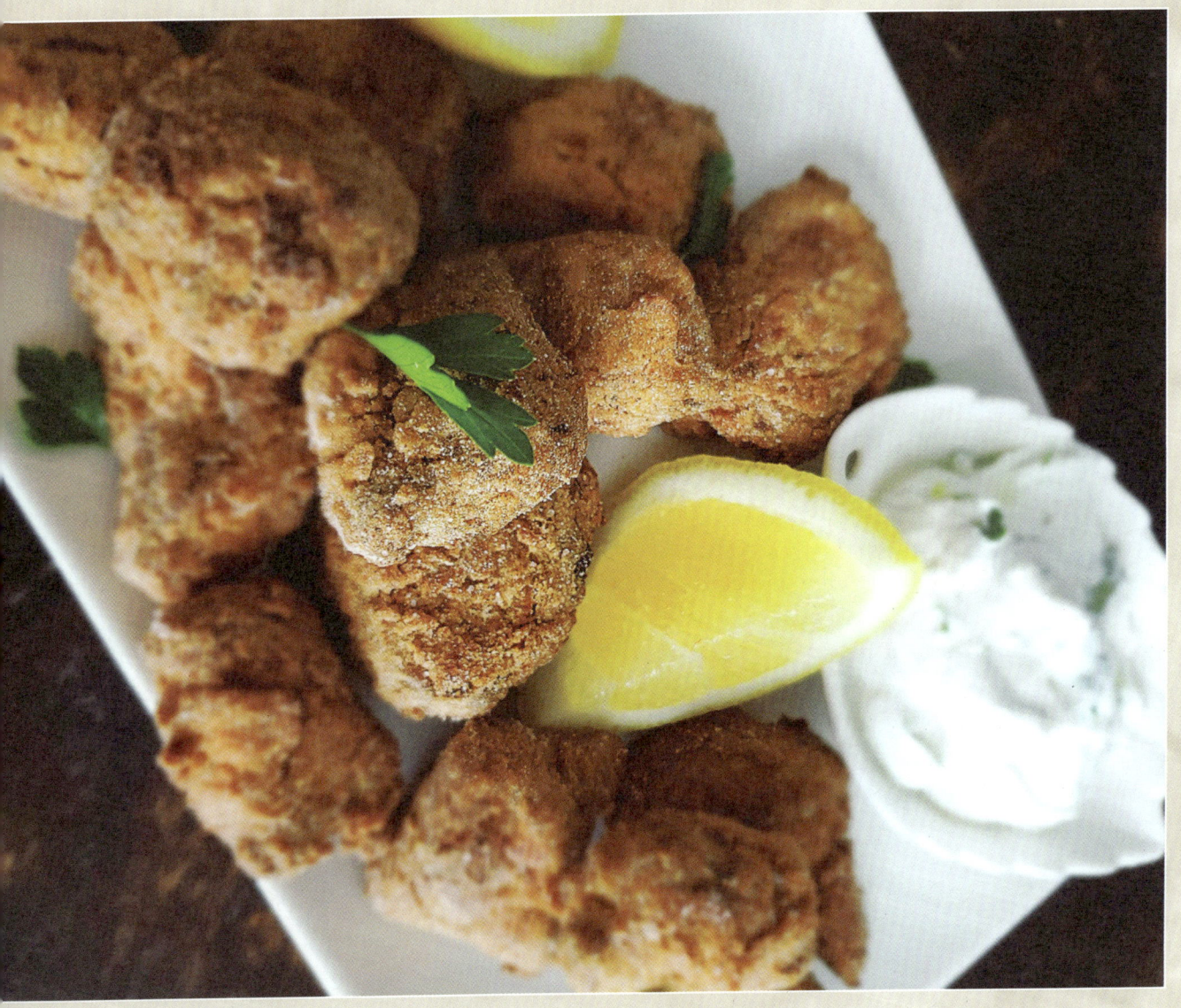

*Ready to eat! Serving up the buttermilk fried tempeh with some cooling tzatziki made with coconut milk cultured yogurt.*

# Appendix 1: Resources

How and where you source your ingredients for the recipes and processes in this book will depend to some degree on where you live. I based my recipes and processes on what is accessible to me locally, within my budget, and from online sources that sell to the public and not just to commercial producers.

In this section I outline some online sources for components like starter cultures and for specialty equipment, and I make suggestions regarding what to look for when shopping in your local area or when ordering online.

## Ingredients

A variety of ingredients can be used in making non-cultured and cultured cheeses. And a variety of ingredients can be added for flavor.

Whenever possible, seek fair trade and organic items and support locally owned businesses.

# Ingredients

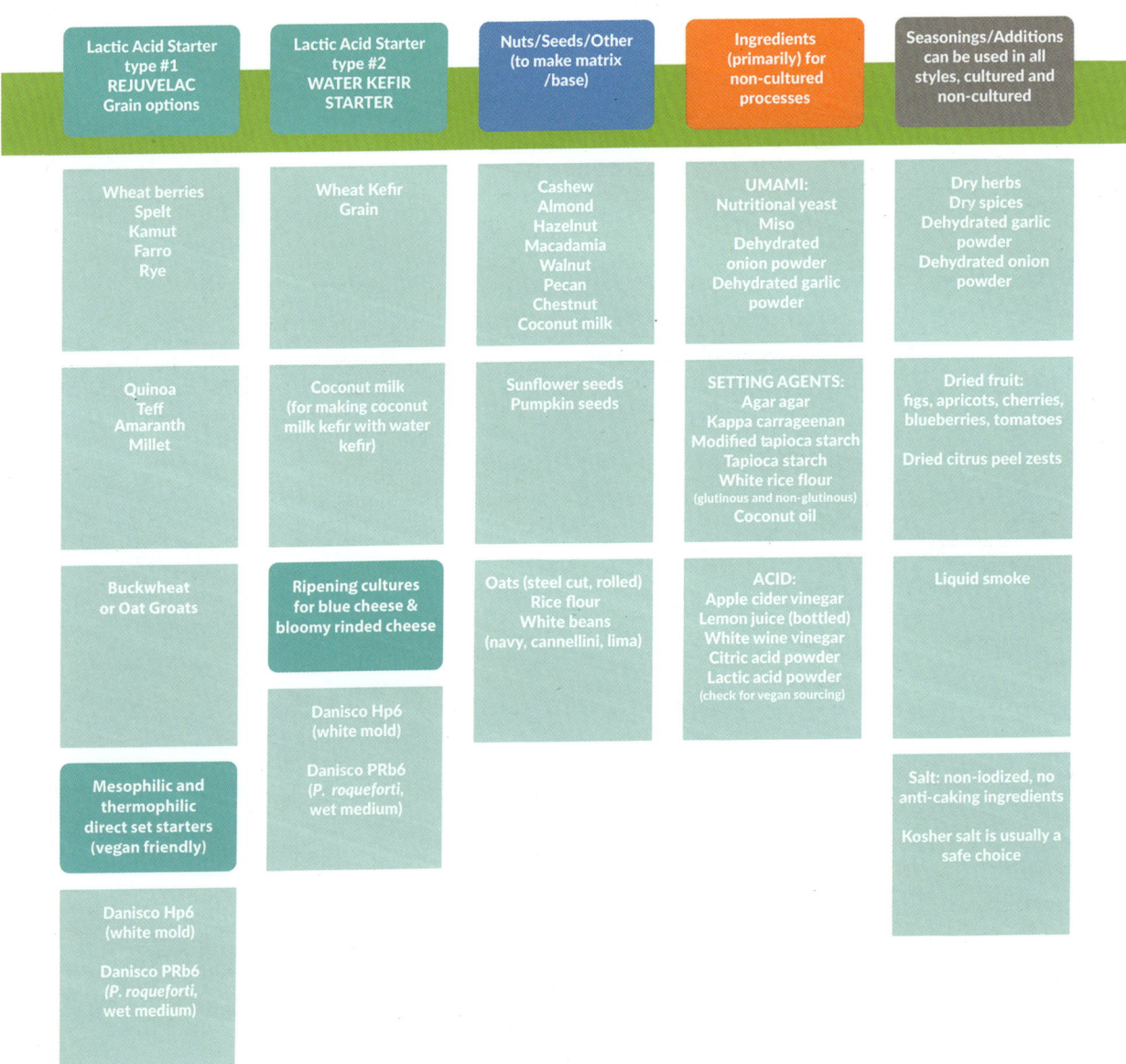

| Lactic Acid Starter type #1 REJUVELAC Grain options | Lactic Acid Starter type #2 WATER KEFIR STARTER | Nuts/Seeds/Other (to make matrix/base) | Ingredients (primarily) for non-cultured processes | Seasonings/Additions can be used in all styles, cultured and non-cultured |
|---|---|---|---|---|
| Wheat berries<br>Spelt<br>Kamut<br>Farro<br>Rye | Wheat Kefir Grain | Cashew<br>Almond<br>Hazelnut<br>Macadamia<br>Walnut<br>Pecan<br>Chestnut<br>Coconut milk | UMAMI:<br>Nutritional yeast<br>Miso<br>Dehydrated onion powder<br>Dehydrated garlic powder | Dry herbs<br>Dry spices<br>Dehydrated garlic powder<br>Dehydrated onion powder |
| Quinoa<br>Teff<br>Amaranth<br>Millet | Coconut milk (for making coconut milk kefir with water kefir) | Sunflower seeds<br>Pumpkin seeds | SETTING AGENTS:<br>Agar agar<br>Kappa carrageenan<br>Modified tapioca starch<br>Tapioca starch<br>White rice flour (glutinous and non-glutinous)<br>Coconut oil | Dried fruit:<br>figs, apricots, cherries, blueberries, tomatoes<br>Dried citrus peel zests |
| Buckwheat or Oat Groats | Ripening cultures for blue cheese & bloomy rinded cheese | Oats (steel cut, rolled)<br>Rice flour<br>White beans (navy, cannellini, lima) | ACID:<br>Apple cider vinegar<br>Lemon juice (bottled)<br>White wine vinegar<br>Citric acid powder<br>Lactic acid powder (check for vegan sourcing) | Liquid smoke |
| Mesophilic and thermophilic direct set starters (vegan friendly) | Danisco Hp6 (white mold)<br>Danisco PRb6 (P. roqueforti, wet medium) | | | Salt: non-iodized, no anti-caking ingredients<br>Kosher salt is usually a safe choice |
| Danisco Hp6 (white mold)<br>Danisco PRb6 (P. roqueforti, wet medium) | | | | |

# Sourcing Ingredients

| Item | Types of Shops | Online |
|---|---|---|
| nuts<br>seeds<br>oats<br>legumes<br>grains | • bulk/zero-waste shops<br>• health/natural food shops<br>• grocery store bulk sections | omfoods.com<br>nuthut.ca<br>ranchovignola.com<br>nuts.com<br>google: organic nuts/legumes/seeds near me |
| coconut milk | • grocery stores<br>• Asian grocers usually have some of the best quality coconut milk brands | |
| nutritional yeast | • most large grocery stores<br>• health food/natural grocers<br>• vegan/vegetarian specialty grocers | Easily found online at websites selling vegan ingredients |
| apple cider vinegar | • grocery stores<br>• health food/natural grocers<br>• supplement/nutrition shops (though generally more expensive in these) | |
| tapioca starch/modified tapioca starch | • grocery stores<br>• Asian grocers<br>• gourmet/specialty food shops | Expandex and Ultra-Tex 3 are both modified tapioca starch specialty products and most likely to be found online rather than in shops. |
| agar agar | • Asian grocers<br>• specialty food shops<br>• vegan/vegetarian grocers | easily found online |
| kappa carrageenan | • specialty food shops<br>• vegan specialty grocers | easily found online |
| salt, non-iodized | • grocery stores<br>• bulk/zero-waste stores<br>• readily available | |
| water kefir | • health food/natural food shops<br>• vegan grocers | culturesforhealth.com<br>upayanaturals.com |
| thermophilic lactic acid starters<br>Danisco CHOOZIT:<br>TA-061<br>TM-81<br><br>mold cultures<br>Danisco Choozit:<br>HP6 White mold (*P. candidum*)<br>PRB6 *P. roqueforti* | cheesemaking supply stores | Steve The Cheesemaker at thecheesemaker.com (see the "vegan" drop down menu) |

Nuts/seeds/legumes/grains: Bulk and zero-waste stores oriented toward healthy and organic choices will be more likely to have higher quality products. Make sure to smell and feel the nuts. Many nuts and seeds are not stored correctly and are already mildly rancid (that is, the oils have begun to leach from them). When shopping from bulk bins, make sure to dig the scoop deep to avoid the top layer which will be the most exposed to UV light and moisture loss.

Online ordering: Take some time to read the website and what the company stands for. Most should reveal where they obtain their nuts, seeds, legumes, and grains. If you want more detailed information about storage conditions or harvesting, send the company an email. My online suggestions above are in no way comprehensive. Google is your friend, and not all places ship to everywhere, so find places that suit your shopping requirements and that will ship to your location.

Coconut milk: Seek high fat coconut milk. Read the label and look for coconut milk fat percentage of 18–20%. Also look for the extraction percentage, which can vary from 50–85%. If you can find coconut milk in Tetra Paks (which will not be refrigerated as a rule), choose that over canned as the coconut fat quality seems to be better. Also, shake cans and Tetra Paks and assess how liquid it feels. If there is a lot of sloshing about, then even after refrigeration, there will be a lot of fluid content versus coconut milk fat content.

Other plant milks: If you use other plant milks in some of the recipes that call for the use of high fat coconut milk, it is generally preferable to make your own milks as you will obtain a higher fat, richer milk than the majority of store-bought ones. The store-bought plant milks are fine to use in the non-cultured agar agar/kappa carrageenan set cheeses but do not produce optimal results in the cultured recipes.

Apple cider vinegar: This can be found in virtually any grocery store these days. Brands to look for are Omega Nutrition, Braggs, and Spectrum. More importantly, look for "raw" apple cider vinegar. This is the vinegar that still has the mother in it, which has the bacteria and yeasts.

Nutritional yeast: Nutritional yeast is deactivated yeast that is produced by culturing live yeast on a medium (typically glucose derived from sugarcane or beet). It is deactivated with heat, harvested, washed, dried, and then packaged. This umami rich food supplement can be found in health food stores, shops focusing on vegan and vegetarian friendly products, and depending on the size of your city, likely even in some of the larger markets such as Whole Foods.

Soft wheat berries and other grains for making rejuvelac: Soft wheat berries and other grains such as spelt, teff, amaranth, millet, and quinoa can be found in a wide variety of grocery stores. Look for how grain is packaged or stored (if in bulk bins). If there are local grain producers that sell in your area at local farmers' markets, I suggest using their grains.

## Tools and Equipment

## Sourcing Tools and Equipment

| Equipment | Type of Stores | Online |
|---|---|---|
| bamboo sushi mats<br>mesh cheese aging mats | • cooking supply stores<br>• Asian grocers | readily available from several sources such as:<br>• New England Cheesemaking Supply Co. at cheesemaking.com<br>• Glengarry Cheesemaking at glengarrycheesemaking.on.ca<br>• Steve The Cheesemaker at thecheesemaker.com<br>Sometimes there are challenges with shipping cultures between countries. To avoid a problem with having equipment and cultures ship when ordered together at the same time, check out suppliers in your area or that ship within or to your country first. |
| wooden boards<br>Note: not all wood boards are suitable for use.<br>Pine is excellent, as well as bamboo boards, but boards that are made from multiple types of wood are generally glued together, and the glue could pose a risk. | You may need to do some work to find food grade/food safe wooden boards for the purposes of aging cheese.<br>• Start by checking with cheesemaking supply shops and some gourmet food stores.<br>• Avoid using construction materials as they are often sprayed with chemicals. | |
| probe thermometer (digital or otherwise) | • cooking supply stores<br>• well-appointed grocery stores/general goods stores | easy to find online |
| silicone spoons/spatulas/whisks | • cooking supply stores<br>• second-hand shops<br>• well-appointed grocery stores | easy to find online |
| thick cast pots/pans/saucepans | • cooking supply stores<br>• general goods stores<br>• second-hand shops | easy to find online |
| cold forms/ring molds/stainless steel hoops | • cooking supply stores<br>• general goods stores<br>• second-hand shops<br>• cheesemaking supply shops | • online cooking supply sites<br>• Steve The Cheesemaker at thecheesemaker.com |

## Sourcing Tools and Equipment cont.

| Equipment | Type of Stores | Online |
|---|---|---|
| cheese molds | • cheesemaking supply stores<br>• specialty/ gourmet cooking stores (especially those that teach cooking classes) | readily available from several sources such as<br>• Steve The Cheesemaker at thecheesmaker.com<br>• Glengarry Cheesemaking at glengarrycheesemaking.on.ca<br>• The New England Cheesemaking Supply Co. at cheesemaking.com |
| ripening boxes (large containers suitably sized for your project) | • Any shop that sells food grade containers of various sizes (e.g., Tupperware/Rubbermaid). | |
| pH meter | • cheesemaking supply stores | readily available from several sources such as<br>• Steve The Cheesemaker at thecheesmaker.com<br>• Glengarry Cheesemaking at glengarrycheesemaking.on.ca<br>• The New England Cheesemaking Supply Co. at cheesemaking.com |
| cheesecloth/butter muslin | • grocery stores<br>• cheesemaking supply stores<br>• specialty food stores<br>• homesteader/DIY stores<br>• fabric shops | Easy to find online |

# Appendix 2: Record-keeping

## Cheesemaking Culturing Log

This sample log can be adapted to create your own system for recording projects and tracking their development.

## Culturing Log

Cheese project: cultured cashew chèvre style cheese
Method: cultured (using lactic acid starter, water kefir)
Goal: semi-soft, chèvre style
Flavor: no added flavors

Date started:

| Action | Culturing | Notes on Culturing |
|---|---|---|
| **Date:** In this section include all the things you did. **Example:** <br>• soaked, rinsed, blended pistachio with cashew <br>• placed in container for culturing, added culture at 1300 hrs <br>• ambient temp 68.9°F (21°C) <br>• RH–could not measure <br>• container left on counter near kitchen stove | at 12 hours <br><br> pH: <br><br> aroma: <br><br> flavor: <br><br> texture: | Notes |
| | at 24 hours <br><br> pH: | Notes |

## Culturing Log cont.

| Action | Culturing | Notes on Culturing |
|---|---|---|
| | aroma:<br><br>flavor:<br><br>texture: | |
| | at 36 hours<br><br>pH:<br><br>aroma:<br><br>flavor:<br><br>texture: | Notes |
| | at 48 hours<br><br>pH:<br><br>aroma:<br><br>flavor:<br><br>texture: | Notes |
| **Post Culturing** | **Method** | **Notes** |
| Moisture loss/draining<br><br>Date Started:<br>Time started: | Example:<br><br>• placed curd in cheesecloth-lined sieve overtop a bowl<br>• sprinkled a pinch of salt over the top and gently pushed into the mixture<br>• allowed to rest at room temperature for 4 hours before returning to refrigerator to continuing losing more moisture | Here you can leave notes on taste:<br><br>aroma:<br><br>texture:<br><br>pH: |
| Shaping<br><br>Date started:<br>Time started: | Example:<br><br>• placed curd in cheesecloth-lined molds (on top of a bamboo mat). At this time I added a bit more salt, and decided not to add other flavors | Here you leave notes on taste:<br><br>aroma:<br><br>texture:<br><br>pH: |

## Culturing Log cont.

| Post Culturing | Method | Notes |
|---|---|---|
| Shaping cont. | • placed the filled molds on the bamboo mat inside a ripening box and returned to fridge<br>• left the lid askew but on top of the box, to allow airflow | You can also describe the changes you observe over days. |
| Aging<br><br>Date started:<br>Time started: | Example:<br><br>• curd in cheese molds still soft, but gently removed from molds and placed onto bamboo mat<br>• gently unfolded cheesecloth from sides and patted the sides with cheesecloth that had been soaked in a 10% brine solution<br>• returned cheese to ripening box and back to fridge<br>• will check daily | Here you record notes on<br>softness:<br><br>dampness:<br><br>aroma:<br><br>texture:<br><br>pH:<br><br>Be careful to observe and record changes especially with regard to how fast the cheese dries or if it starts to show cracks.<br><br>Record the brine solutions here and any other surface treatments you apply. |

## Cheesemaking Observation Log

This log is particularly useful for cultured or mixed method projects where you anticipate significant changes over time and where you need to monitor progress. It is based on a 7-day week and best used after you have finished the culturing time frame. Record all changes you observe. You can replicate this format for longer observation/aging periods.

## Observation Log

**Cheese project:** (insert your title here)
**Method:** (e.g. non-cultured, mixed method, cultured)
**Goal:** (e.g. soft, aged, etc.)
**Flavor:** (list any flavor/seasonings you are using here)
**Date started:**

| Observations | Day 1 Date: Time: | Day 2 Date: Time: | Day 3 Date: Time: | Day 4 Date: Time: | Day 5 Date: Time: | Day 6 Date: Time: | Day 7 Date: Time: |
|---|---|---|---|---|---|---|---|
| pH | | | | | | | |
| moisture | | | | | | | |
| texture | | | | | | | |
| flavor | | | | | | | |
| color | | | | | | | |
| issues | | | | | | | |

# Appendix 3: Common Issues for Starter Cultures

This is a quick guide for troubleshooting issues that frequently arise with starter cultures.

| Starter Culture | Problem | Cause | Solution Options |
|---|---|---|---|
| Water Kefir | Tight, small grain and poor or low rate of replication<br><br>Low level or non-existent tanginess (indicates poor metabolic activity) | Incorrect feed.<br><br>White sugar or evaporated cane juice offer little in the way of mineral content. Water Kefir grain will remain smallish and replicate slowly with this feed. | Option 1: Change the feeding solution. Move grain to new container, make a new feeding medium using a sugar with more mineral content such as raw cane sugar, coconut sugar, date sugar.<br><br>Option 2: Combining white sugar with mineral rich sugars is also an option. |
| Water Kefir | Sandy/gritty/detritus forming at bottom of container | Too much mineral content.<br><br>Coconut sugar, date sugar, or maple syrup when used alone can sometimes cause this issue. | Option 1: Change the feeding solution. Move grain to new container, make a new feeding medium using a sugar with less mineral content such as raw cane sugar.<br><br>Option 2: Combining a mineral rich sugar with a lower mineral content sugar is also an option. |

| Starter Culture | Problem | Cause | Solution Options |
|---|---|---|---|
| | | | Option 3: Strain water kefir grain and rinse gently under tepid water, then place into a new sanitized jar with a new feed. |
| Water Kefir | Complete disintegration of water kefir grain | This usually means something in the feeding environment killed the organisms.<br><br>This can be a result of big swings in temperature, sudden and frequent changes in environment, or too many changes to the feeding environment. | Sometimes a few grains can be salvaged, but it is best to start again with fresh grain. |
| Water Kefir | Growth on surface of solution which usually has a whitish, grayish, tan appearance but occasionally can appear orangish/pinkish | This usually indicates that wild yeast from the environment is present and growing.<br><br>This is particularly likely if there are other fermenting projects, such as kombucha, present. | Option 1: If caught early, you can usually slip the surface film off and monitor for its return.<br><br>Opton 2: You can also change the jar and feeding medium. Ensure that you use a clean, sanitized jar each time you change jars. |
| Water Kefir | Acidity develops too quickly, flavor becomes sour versus tangy | This usually indicates that the temperature is too high (24°C and higher). This will cause the microbes to metabolize the sugar too quickly, producing an uneven/undesired flavor. | Add more sugar (this will provide food for the microbes) and move to a cooler environment, even to the refrigerator during summer months. Refrigeration will slow the rate of metabolic activity, and this generally restores balance to the microbial community's activity. |
| Rejuvelac | Grain of choice not sprouting | This is a result of not enough moisture being applied consistently each day, so seeds are not staying damp enough.<br><br>If the seeds are very old, they may not sprout.<br><br>The temperature may be a bit too cool. | Option 1: Keep sprouting seeds damp by spritzing with water and rinsing daily (more than once a day).<br><br>Option 2: Get new seeds/grains.<br><br>Option: 3: Relocate the sprouting setup to an area |

Appendix 3: Common Issues for Starter Cultures  **223**

| Starter Culture | Problem | Cause | Solution Options |
|---|---|---|---|
| Rejuvelac cont. | | | that has a consistent warm temperature (inside oven with oven light on, if sprouting in a jar). |
| Rejuvelac | Sprouting grain has fuzzy growth | Invading mold spores have begun replicating before sprouting can begin. | Discard and start again. |
| Rejuvelac | Sprouting grain in a jar, but acidity is not developing | Something may be inhibiting proliferation of the lactic acid forming bacteria.<br><br>The grain in use may have been treated to prevent sprouting, which would render the seeds unusable for the purposes of making rejuvelac. | Option 1: Ensure jar has not previously contained chemicals.<br><br>Option 2: Move jar to warmer environment for up to 12 hours (oven with light on).<br><br>Option 3: Taste and smell every 12 hours to assess change in pH.<br><br>Option 4: If no change, discard and start again. |

# Appendix 4: Choosing a Base

This is a quick guide to selecting a base ingredient.

## Choosing a Base

| Nut/Seed/Groat | Component Balance (protein/fat/carbohydrate) | Notes | What you are looking for |
|---|---|---|---|
| Cashew | • Fat, protein and carbohydrate are well balanced.<br>• It produces a creamy texture.<br>• When cultured, it produces an even flavor. | • It can be blended with other nuts/groats to increase carbohydrates; a food source for bacteria. | • Plump, not shrivelled appearance; sweet not dusty or bitter flavor; color should be tan/beige, not gray.<br>• Avoid top layer in bulk bins. |
| Macadamia | • There is a bit more fat in relation to carbohydrate and protein than cashew has.<br>• This is a dense, firm nut, due to the high fat<br>• It has a mild flavor. | • It blends well with other nuts/seeds. | • Look for ones that do not feel too dry on the surface. Dryness could be a sign that some of the fat has leached out. |

## Choosing a Base cont.

| Nut/Seed/Groat | Component Balance (protein/fat/carbohydrate) | Notes | What you are looking for |
|---|---|---|---|
| Brazil | • This is high in fat and very dense. | • Culturing on its own is very difficult. A smooth texture is harder to achieve, and there is a tendency to rancidity because of the high fat content.<br>• This is high in selenium. Too much selenium can lead to toxicity. Selenium affects the thyroid gland.<br>• Use minimally and in combination with other nuts/seeds such as cashew or macadamia or even oat. | • Look for plump nuts that do not feel oily. An oily surface can indicate fat has leached out.<br>• Check smell. Brazil nuts have a distinctly sour aroma once they have gone rancid. |
| Almond | • This has higher protein in relation to carbohydrate and fat than cashew. (e.g., water kefir, coconut kefir, raw apple cider vinegar) produce rounder flavors.<br>• The risk of salmonella contamination on California almonds is minimized by observing sanitization protocols and overnight soaking in the refrigerator. Add a small amount of salt to the soaking solution to create a brine, which is a hostile environment for pathogenic bacteria. | • It has tannic acid as well as phytic acid in the skin.<br>• It has sulfur.<br>• It must be soaked for a minimum of 1 hour. Soaking overnight in a covered container in the refrigerator is recommended. Peel the skin before using.<br>• Optimal for a fresh/young cheese or in combination with other seeds/nuts.<br>• If cultured on its own, it is best for short, low acid cultures and fresh cheeses.<br>• Combine with more carbohydrate rich nuts for longer aging.<br>• Pay attention to sulfur and ammonia smells as cultured almond ages. Salt or citric acid can be used to control culture growth to inhibit these odors. The odors generally do off-gas.<br>• Fast culturing of almond can lead to bitterness, so yeast forward cultures | • Look for almonds that are plump, not shrivelled.<br>• They should be sweetish, not bitter. |

## Choosing a Base cont.

| Nut/Seed/Groat | Component Balance (protein/fat/carbohydrate) | Notes | What you are looking for |
|---|---|---|---|
| Walnuts, Hazelnuts, Pecans | • These nuts have skins that contain tannic acids.<br>• All have sensitive oils/fats that can run to rancidity during culturing because of the high fat content.<br>• Bitterness can be an issue because of the challenge of eliminating the tannic acid. | • These nuts are best used in combination with higher carbohydrate nuts/seeds.<br>• These need to be soaked for a minimum of 1 hour, but preferably overnight in the refrigerator.<br>• Add 1 tsp–2 tsp of baking soda to the soaking water depending on the volume of nuts and soaking water.<br>• Light toasting after soaking helps in removing skins. | • As with other nuts, look at how they are stored. If they are stored under bright store lights in bulk bins, be sure to scoop from the middle of the batch.<br>• Look for nuts that are not shrivelled or dried up looking, and are still plump.<br>• Walnuts, pecans and hazelnuts can all become rancid. Their oils are delicate and will break down if not stored properly. This will result in bitter flavor. |
| Pumpkin/Sunflower seeds | • These are lower in fat and carbohydrate than cashew or almond.<br>• They can become bitter after culturing because of the presence of sulfur and higher protein to fat and protein to carbohydrate ratios. | • Soaking in water to which 1 tsp–2 tsp baking soda has been added helps mitigate the bitterness. Rinse after soaking.<br>• These combine well with macadamia/cashew nuts.<br>• These work well for fresh cultured cream cheeses. | • Look for seeds that are plump, not shrivelled or soft. Shrivelling or softness indicates breakdown and poor storage conditions. |
| Oats | • A groat rather than a seed or nut, oats have low fat but high protein and long chain carbohydrate. | • They form a nice matrix for a cheese that will age.<br>• They are best in combination with nuts that have more fat, as fat is important in cheesemaking.<br>• They can be combined with plant-based liquids like coconut milk. | • Seek steel cut or rolled oats, but not oats that have been highly processed to become "quick oats."<br>• Whole oat groats do not work quite as well because of the presence of the oat germ. |

## Choosing a Base cont.

| Nut/Seed/Groat | Component Balance (protein/fat/carbohydrate) | Notes | What you are looking for |
|---|---|---|---|
| Rice | • Rice is a grass rather than a nut or seed.<br>• It is higher in carbohydrate and lower in fat and protein than nuts.<br>• It has potential as a base. | • On its own rice can have a tendency to produce ethanol (alcohol) during fermentation because of the high carbohydrate content, so it is best combined with another nut and/or coconut milk.<br>• The presence of long chain carbohydrate in non-white rices helps form a firmer matrix cheese. | • Look for sweet white rices.<br>• Red and black rice have anthocyanins, which are great antioxidants but can impart bitter flavor and sometimes can interfere with fermentation in cheese making.<br>• Look at how rice is stored, and like other bulk items, pull from the middle of the container and not the surface. |
| Legumes: lima, navy bean, great white northern, cannellini, butter beans | • Legumes/beans are high in protein, low in fat, and many have a good amount of carbohydrate. | • Due to a high protein content, legume only cheeses can be prone to drying too quickly.<br>• Canned beans do not require cooking. Dry beans require overnight soaking with baking soda and then cooking until soft.<br>• The white beans are a good place to start as they do not have other chemical compounds such as anthocyanins (from purple or red beans) that can produce bitter compounds when metabolized. | • You can use dry or canned beans.<br>• If selecting dry beans, make sure they are not shrivelled or dried out, or too old (storage age may be hard to find). |

# Appendix 5: Preparing Dry Beans

Dry beans need proper preparation for use in cheesemaking. The first and crucial step is soaking. Dry beans need to absorb water to become soft and to break down the starch that must be cooked in order to be digestible. Water is absorbed by the beans through a tiny opening called the micropyle, so the process of absorption is quite slow.

Soaking beans in water for many hours reduces the cooking time. However, in a pot of beans some beans may cook faster than others and become overcooked. This can lead to some beans bursting their skins while other beans don't cook enough to be soft and creamy inside. The natural pectin in beans strengthens the cell walls producing skins that are difficult to soften and expand, and this skin can burst when the inside of the bean becomes overcooked.

Soaking beans in a brine reduces the occurrence of skins bursting. Brine contains a low concentration of salt. During brining the sodium ions slowly weaken the pectin (through an ion exchange where sodium ions from the brine displace calcium ions in the pectin skin) so that the skins become more flexible and can expand without bursting as the interior cooks to a soft, creamy texture, which also makes the starch more bioavailable for the lactic acid forming bacteria to metabolize. Thus, brining accomplishes two things: it provides water to soften the beans, which reduces cooking time, and it produces beans that do not burst while cooking to the desired soft, creamy texture.

Baking soda has the same effect as salt on pectin, but it also reduces the amount of raffinose sugar in legumes and degasses the beans, so I recommend adding baking soda in addition to salt.

**Steps:**

1. Rinse the beans.
2. Place the beans in a container and fully cover with water. Add ½ tsp–1 tsp of baking soda or salt to the water (depending on the volume of water being used).
3. Soak for at least 24 hours in the refrigerator.
4. After the soaking period, drain the beans, and cook them until they are soft and are easy to mash.

# Index

Entries set in **bold** indicate a recipe. Page numbers set in *italics* indicate an illustration.

## A

absorption, 123, 160
 *See also affinaging; moisture removal*
acidification, 60–61
acidity/alkalinity, measuring, 137
acids
 acetic acid, 24–25
 used for non-cultured cheeses, 28, 61, *212*
 *See also lactic acid*
affinaging
 about, 159
 bandaging, 165
 brining, 160–162, *163*
 dry aging, 160–161
 dry salting, 160–161
 flavoring techniques during, 159, 161–162, *162, 163*
 leaf wrapping, *164*, 164–165
 moisture removal during, 123, 159
 oil curing, 164
 pH levels during, 159
 washing, 162, *163*
agar agar
 about, 41–42, *43*
 cultured curd with, *133*
 sources for, 213
 using, 4, 42–43, 45, 46–47, 126, 134, *212*
agarose agaropectin, 41
aged cheeses, longer
 cashew and coconut havarti/gouda-style, 123–128, *125, 127*
 cheddar-style, *104,* 129–134, *130, 133*
aged cheeses, short aged
 aging, *94,* 94–95, *95*
 **Coconut Kefir Cheese: Three Ways**, 97–104, *98, 99, 101, 102, 103, 104*
 shaping, *94,* 94–95, *95*
 **Soft, Short-aged Cultured Almond Cheese**, 110
aging
 about, 159
 boards, 2, 106, 160, 215
 coconut kefir cheese, *103*
 kefir/macadamia cheese, *106*
 longer aged cheeses, 123–128, *125, 127*
 mats, 26, *26, 27, 95, 101, 102, 103, 157,* 160, *179,* 215
 refrigeration requirements for, 120
 shorter aged cheeses, *94,* 94–95, *95, 103*
 time required for, 118
 *See also affinaging; aged cheeses, longer; aged cheeses, short aged*
alkalinity/acidity, measuring, 137
**Almond Curd Feta**, 114–115, *115*
**Almond Mocha Ricotta Mousse**, *181,* 181–182, *182*
almonds
 **Almond Curd Feta**, 114–115, *115*
 almond feta, 2
 **Almond Mocha Ricotta Mousse**, *181,* 181–182, *182*
 almond ricotta stuffed figs, *86*
 as a base, 226
 cultured almond curd, 107–109, *109*
 **Cultured Almond Ricotta, non-cooked**, *83,* 83–88, *84, 85, 86*
 culturing, 83, 107–109, *109*
 rejuvelac for almond paste, 63
 soaking, 32–33, *83*
 **Soft, Short-aged Cultured Almond Cheese**, 110
 sulfur in, 63, 69, 83, 107, 226
amaranth, *213,* 214–215
apple cider vinegar
 sources for, 213, *213,* 214
 using, 61, 83, *85*
Ardea Blue cheese, *149*
arrowroot, 40
artichokes, **Roasted Artichoke and Spinach Dip**, *199,* 199–200, *200*

**231**

Artisa, 11
*Artisan Vegan Cheese* (Schinner), 9, 19
*The Art of Fermentation* (Katz), 60
*The Art of Plant-based Cheesemaking*, 2nd ed. (McAthy)
  about, 12, 20
  changes re almond curd process, 107
  changes re miso, 78
  changes re non-heated coconut milk process, 97
  changes re probiotics, 77
  changes re tapioca starch, 40
Art of Plant-based Cheesemaking course, student cheeses, *15, 96*
*The Art of Plant-based Cheesemaking* (2017) (McAthy), xi, xii
asparagus, **Herb, Potato, Mushroom and Asparagus Galette**, 203, 203–205, *205*
*Aspergillus oryzae*, 78, 79

## B

*B. linens*, 58
back slopping, 77, 172
bacteria
  about, 1, 8, 22, 25
  *E. coli*, 22
  environment for, 23, 138, 160
  function of in cheesemaking, 18, 58, 59, 60, 61, 63
  lactic acid production by, 61, 62, 68, 70
  *Lactobacillus*, 68
  *Lactobacillus bulgaricus*, 171
  *Lactococcus*, 68
  *Leuconostoc*, 68
  *Listeria*, 22
  mesophilic, 79
  *Salmonella*, 22
  *Streptococcus*, 68
  *Streptococcus thermophilus*, 171
  thermophilic, 171, 174
  wild fermentation, 60
  *See also* LAB (lactic acid forming bacteria); microbes
bandaging, 165
bases, choices for, 27–28, 212, 226–228
Baudar, Pascal, 60, 78

bay leaf, **Blueberry Bay Compote**, 183, 186
BC Food Processors Awards, xii
beans
  dry, preparing, 229–230
  white, 37, 87, *212*, 228
biscuits, **Jalapeño and Chive Biscuits**, 194–195, *195*
bleach, as sanitizer, 24
Blöde Kuh, 11
bloomy rind. *See* white mold ripened cheese
blueberries, **Blueberry Bay Compote**, 183, 186
**Blueberry Bay Compote**, 183, 186
Blue Heron cheeses
  Ardea Blue, *149*
  Herbed Coconut Kefir cheese, *9*
  mold ripened cheeses, 136, *136*
  selection of, *xiii*, 13
  summer seasonal, *165*
  at Thrive dinner, *122*
  Wolf Flower, *118*
Blue Heron Cheese Shop
  author at, *xv*
  demand for products of, xi
  Jolene and Colin at, *xiv*
  opening of, xi
Blue Heron (company)
  awards for, xii
  complaint against, xiii–xiv, 10–11
  establishment of, 4
blue mold ripened cheeses
  about, 4, 20
  broken curd method, 154–159, *157, 158*
  creating veins in, 147, 149, *149*
  heat stimulated lactic-set curd method, 151–154, *153*
  mycelia on, 147, *147, 148*
  *P. roqueforti*, 4, 20, 58, 146, 150, *212*, 213
  salt for, 147
"bowls of food," 168
Brazil nuts, 2, 33, 83, 226
brine
  about, 160
  application techniques, 161, *162*

flavoring, 162–163
formulas for, 161–162
function of, 161
"butter," **Cultured "Butter,"** 170–171, *171*
**Buttermilk Fried Tempeh**, *208*, 208–210, *209, 210*
butter muslin, 26, 216

## C

Caldwell, Gianaclis, 8
camembert, macadamia, oat, cashew cheese, *139*
**Camembert Stuffed Delicata Squash with Cranberries, Candied Pecan and Fried Sage**, 206
camembert-style cheese
  about, 18, 20, 137
  camembert, macadamia, oat, cashew cheese, *139*
  **Camembert Stuffed Delicata Squash with Cranberries, Candied Pecan and Fried Sage**, 206
Canadian Food Inspection Agency (CFIA)
  complaint filed with, xiii–xiv, 10–11
*Candida*, 68
cannellini beans, 87
**Caramelized Pears**, 187, 188
carrageenan
  about, 43–44
  kappa carrageenan, 4, 44, 45, 134, 213
casein, 10, 12, 30, 58, 119, 143
**Cashew, Sunflower Seed or Macadamia Cream Cheeze**, 36–38
cashew and coconut havarti/gouda-style cheeses
  crossover method, *125*, 126–128, *127*
  culture and age method, 123–126
Cashewbert, 11, 19
cashews
  as a base, 27, *212*, 225
  **Cashew, Sunflower Seed or Macadamia Cream Cheeze**, 36–38
  cashew cheese on aging board, *2*
  and cheeze, 17
  macadamia, oat, cashew camembert, *139*

Oats, Cashew, and Coconut Yogurt, 174–175
  soaking, 32–33
  substituting macadamia nuts for, 87
casomorphins, 30
celeriac, **Potato and Celeriac Dauphinoise (gratin)**, 201–202
celery stock, 196, 197
Cellouf, Karima, 191, 208, *208*
CFIA (Canadian Food Inspection Agency)
  complaint filed with, xii–xiv, 10–11
chao, 116
Chao (commercial producer), 11
Chao (product), 116
cheddar-style cheese, *104*
  crossover method, 132–134, *133*
  culture and aged method, 129–132, *130*
cheddar-style cheeze
  about, 30, 39
  **Semi-Firm Cheddar-Style Cheeze Base**, 51–54
cheese
  about, 8
  defined by Codex Alimentarius, 10
  as a process, 3–4, 14, 62
  traditional definition of, xiv, 13–14
cheese analogs. *See* cheeze; cheeze styles
cheese boards
  for aging, 2, 106, 160, 215
  Blue Heron cheeses, *13*
  at wedding, *5*
cheesecake, **Unbaked Lemon Cheesecake with Blueberry Bay Compote**, 183–186, *184, 185, 186*
cheesecloth
  about, 26, *26, 101*
  aging in, *103*, 160
  bandaging cheese with, 164, 165
  as a liner, 48, 53, 56, *98, 102*
  shaping cheese with, 91, 94, *94, 95*
  sources for, 216
  using with sprouting jar, 65
  washing cheese with, 113, 161, 162
The Cheesemaker, 80
*The Cheesemaker's Apprentice* (Davies), 8

cheese molds, *26, 27*, 101, *102, 102, 157, 179*
cheese styles
  camembert, 18, 20, 137, *139*
  cheddar, *104*, 129–134, *130, 133*
  cream cheese, 100–104, *101, 102, 103, 104*
  feta, *2*, 112–113, *113*, 114–115, *115*, 116–117
  havarti/gouda-style, 123–128, *125, 127*
  ricotta, *83*, 83–88, *84, 85, 86, 181*, 181–182, *182*
**Cheesy Potato Chowder**, 192–193, *195*
cheeze
  about, 14, 16–18, 28, 30, 31, 33, 61
  soft cheeze process chart, *31*
Cheezehound, 11
cheeze styles
  cheddar, 30, 39, 51–54
  cream cheeze, 36–38
  feta, 31, 39
  havarti/gouda, 46–50, *50*
  mozzarella, 31, 39, 55–56, *56*
  ricotta, 34–35, *35*
chef, skills needed by, 30–31, 120, 168
cherries, **Syrah Infused Cherries**, 178, 180, *180*
**Chèvre-Style Cheese**, 90–93, *91, 96*
Choozit, 79, 141, 150
chowder, **Cheesy Potato Chowder**, 192–193, *195*
citric acid, 61
cleaning, 22–23
coconut kefir
  back slopping, 77
  **Coconut Kefir Cheese: Three Ways**, 97–104, *98, 98, 99, 99, 101, 102, 103, 104*
  **Coconut Kefir Curd Feta-Style Cheese (Macedonian-style Feta)**, 112–113, *113*
  draining, *98*
  **Lemon-Garlic-Herb Coconut Kefir with Macadamia**, 105–106, **106**
  process for making, *74*, 74–76, *75, 76*
**Coconut Kefir Cheese: Three Ways Labneh**, *99, 99*

Semi-Firm Cream Cheese, 100–104, *101, 102, 103, 104*
Soft Cream Cheese, 100
**Coconut Kefir Curd Feta-Style Cheese (Macedonian-style Feta)**, 112–113, *113*
coconut milk
  **Coconut Milk Yogurt**, *171*, 171–173, *173*
  culturing, *74*, 74–76, *75*
  **Oats, Cashew, and Coconut Yogurt**, 174–175
  qualities of, 74, 97
  sources for, 213, 214
**Coconut Milk Yogurt**, *171*, 171–173, *173*
Codex Alimentarius of the Food and Agriculture Organization of the United Nations, 10
**Coeur à la Crème with Syrah Infused Cherries**
  **Coeur à la Crème**, 178–179, *179, 180*
  **Syrah Infused Cherries**, 178, 180, *180*
cold smoking, 49, 166, 200
compote
  **Blueberry Bay Compote**, 183, 186
conidia, 147
Conscious Cultures, 11
contamination, preventing, 22, 59, 61, 64, 65, 138 *See also* sanitation
cream cheese/cheeze
  **Cashew, Sunflower Seed or Macadamia Cream Cheeze**, 36–38
  **Semi-firm Cream Cheese**, 100–104, *101, 102, 103, 104*
  **Soft Cream Cheese**, 100
crème fraîche, **Sour Cream/Crème Fraîche**, 176, *176*
crossover method
  cashew and coconut havarti/gouda-style cheeses, *125*, 126–128, *127*
  cheddar-style cheeses, 132–134, *133*
  elements of, 14–15, 17
  plant-based cheesemaking processes, 14–15, 17

culture and age method
  cheddar-style cheeses, 132–134, *133*
  havarti/gouda-style cheese, 123–126
**Cultured "Butter,"** 170–171, *171*
cultured cheese
  about, 14, 17, 18, 82
cultured cheese, soft
  process chart, *82*
cultured plant-based cheesemakers (commercial), 11
Cultures for Health, 70
culturing v. fermenting, 59–60
curd
  characteristics of, 123
  creating, 61, 138
  cultured almond curd, 107–109, *109*
  lactic acid curd, *89*, *91*
  testing at Graze, *3*

**D**
dairy cheese, about, 8, 30, 58
Daiya, 11
Danisco, 19, 59, 79, 80, 141, 150
Davies, Emily, *121*, 191, 196, 207
Davies, Sasha, 8
desserts
  **Almond Mocha Ricotta Mousse,** *181*, 181–182, *182*
  **Coeur à la Crème with Syrah Infused Cherries,** 178–180, *179*, *180*
  **Pear Tarte Tatin,** 187–190, *188*, *189*, *190*
  **Unbaked Lemon Cheesecake with Blueberry Bay Compote,** 183–186, *184*, *185*, *186*
dips, **Roasted Artichoke and Spinach Dip,** *199*, 199–200, *200*
direct set cultures, 79–80, *212*
dry aging, 160, 161
dry salting, 160
Dupont, 19, 59

**E**
*E. coli*, 22, 25
Earth Island, 11
eggplant, **Grilled Eggplant,** 197, *198*
emulsifiers, function of, 39
equipment, key, 26, *26*, *27*
evaporation, 123, 160
Expandex, 40

**F**
**Farm-Style Cheese,** *87*, 87–89, *88*, *89*
farro, 61, 63, *212*
fats
  in bases, 225–227
  effect of smoking on, 166
  function of, 28, 127
Feeding Change, 78
fermentation
  of grain, 66–67, *67*
  lactic acid, 59–60
  of water kefir grains, 72 –73, *73*
  wild, 60, 61
**Fermented Tofu Feta,** 116–117
fermenting v. culturing, 59–60
feta-style cheeses
  about, 31, 39
  **Almond Curd Feta,** 114–115, *115*
  almond feta, *2*
  **Coconut Kefir Curd Feta-Style Cheese (Macedonian-style Feta),** 112–113, *113*
  **Fermented Tofu Feta,** 116–117
  Macedonian v. Greek, 112
Field Roast, 116
figs, *86*, *164*
firmness, achieving, 39
flavoring
  during affinaging, 159, 161
  for brines, 162–163
  dried options, 37, 48, 49, 53, 92, 93, 103, *212*
  fresh options, 37, 51, 53, 92, 103
  preserved/pickled options, 49, 53–54, 92
  smoke options, 49, 53, 200
food addiction, 30
food borne illnesses, 22
*Full of Plants* (blog), 19

**G**
galettes, **Herb, Potato, Mushroom and Asparagus Galette,** *203*, 203–205, *205*
garlic, using fresh, 37, 51, 92
gelling agents
  agar agar, 41–43, 45, *212*
  carrageenan, 43–44, 45, *212*
  function of, 39
  pectin, 44–45
Gill, Alexandra, xii–xiv
*Globe and Mail,* xiii
GMP (guanosine monophosphate), 28
gouda-style cheese
  havarti/gouda-style cheeses, 123–128, *125*, *127*
gouda-style cheeze
  **Havarti/Gouda-Style Quick Vegan Cheeze,** 46–50, *50*
Gourmand World Cookbook Awards (2018), xii
grains
  fermenting, 66–67, *67*
  and making rejuvelac, 63–65, *65*, *212*
  sources for, 213, 214
Graze Vegetarian, 2, 2–3, *3*, 4
guanosine monophosphate (GMP), 28
*A Guide to Vegan Cheese* (Cashewbert), 19

**H**
hand-washing, 25–26
Happy Cheeze, xii, 11
hard cheeses
  Blue Heron products, 118, *118*
  cashew and coconut havarti/gouda-style, 123–128, *125*, *127*
  cheddar-style, 104, 129–134, *130*, *133*
  moisture removal for, 4, 118, 123
  refrigeration requirements for, 120
  time required for aging of, 118
havarti/gouda-style cheeses
  crossover method, *125*, 126–128, *127*
  culture and age method, 123–126
havarti/gouda-style cheeze
  **Havarti/Gouda-Style Quick Vegan Cheeze,** 46–50, *50*
**Havarti/Gouda-Style Quick Vegan Cheeze,** 46–50, *50*
hazelnuts
  as a base, *212*, 227
  soaking, 32–33
  sources for, 213
hemp seeds, 32–33, 213
**Herb, Potato, Mushroom and Asparagus Galette,** *203*, 203–205, *205*

herbs, using fresh, 37, 51, 92
heterofermentative bacteria, 59
heteropolysaccharides, 44
homofermentative bacteria, 59
HP6 direct set mold, 141, *212*, 213
hygiene, 22–26, *23*, 61

## I
Ikeda, Kikunae, 28
illnesses, food borne, 22
IMP (inosine monophosphate), 28
Impossible Foods, 12
inosine monophosphate (IMP), 28
Irish Moss. *See* carrageenan

## J
**Jalapeño and Chive Biscuits with Cheesy Potato Chowder**
  **Cheesy Potato Chowder**, 192–193, *195*
  **Jalapeño and Chive Biscuits**, 194–195, *195*

## K
kale
  **Photosynthesis, a Smoothie**, 207, *207*
Kanten, 41
kappa carrageenan
  about, 44
  effect of too much, 134
  sources for, 213
  using, 4, 44, 45, 46–47, *212*
*Kappaphycus alvarezii*, 44
Katz, Sandor, 60
kefir
  about, 68
  training to vegan medium, 68–69
  coconut kefir, *74*, 74–76, *75*, *76*, 77, *98*
  water kefir, 20, 68, 70–73, *73*, 79, *212*, 213, 221–222
Kinda Co., xiii
*Kloeckera*, 68
Kula Kitchen, 192

## L
LAB (lactic acid forming bacteria)
  in dairy cheesemaking, 18
  function of, 58, 60–61
**Labneh**, 99, *99*
lactic acid
  effect on blue mold, 147, 149
  function of, 61
  lactic acid cashew curd, *91*
  lactic acid cultured almond curd, 107–109, *109*
  lactic acid curd, 61, *89*
  lactic acid fermentation, 59–60
  lactic acid starters, *212*, 213
  production of, 58, 59, 62
lactic acid cultured almond curd, 107–109, *109*
lactic acid forming bacteria (LAB). *See* LAB (lactic acid forming bacteria)
*Lactobacillus*, 68
*Lactobacillus bulgaricus*, 171
*Lactococcus*, 68
lacto-fermentation, 59–60
La Fauxmagerie, xiii, 11
leaf wrapping, *164*, 164–165
lecithin, sunflower, 39
legumes
  as a base, 228
  preparing dry beans, 229–230
  soaking, 32–33
  sources for, 213, 214
  white beans, 37, 87, *212*, 228
**Lemon-Garlic-Herb Coconut Kefir with Macadamia**, 105–106, *106*
lemon juice, 61
*Leuconostoc*, 68
lima beans, 87
*Listeria*, 22
Living Food BCN, 11
log-rolling, 94, *94*
Luebke, Katie, 2, 68

## M
macadamia nuts
  as a base, *212*, 225
  **Cashew, Sunflower Seed or Macadamia Cream Cheeze**, 36–38
  **Lemon-Garlic-Herb Coconut Kefir with Macadamia**, 105–106, *106*
  macadamia, oat, cashew camembert, *139*
  soaking, 32–33
  substituting for cashews, 87
*Mastering Basic Cheesemaking* (Caldwell), 8

McAthy, Karen
  at Blue Heron Cheese Shop, xv
  experimentation by, 2–3, 19, 58, 68–69
  preference re sweetness, 177
  *See also The Art of Plant-based Cheesemaking, 2nd ed.* (McAthy); *The Art of Plant-based Cheesemaking (2017)* (McAthy)
Medhurst, Colin
  at Blue Heron Cheese Shop opening, xii
  and Blue Heron Cheese Shop plans, *4*
  business partner, xi, 4
  cheese board at wedding of, *5*
mediums, vegan status of, 79
mesophilic direct set cultures, 79, *212*, 213
microbes
  and aging, 118, 146, 161
  function of, 14, 15, 18, 58, 60, 63
  lab preparation of, 58–59
  native, 59, 60, 61
  pathogenic, 22, 23, 25, 64, 159, 160
  *See also* bacteria; LAB (lactic acid forming bacteria); molds; yeasts
millet
  **Millet Tabbouleh with Grilled Eggplant and Tzatziki**, 196–198
  sources for, *213*, 214–215
**Millet Tabbouleh with Grilled Eggplant and Tzatziki**
  **Grilled Eggplant**, 196, 197
  **Millet Tabbouleh**, 196, 197
  **Tzatziki**, 197, 198
miso, 51, 78
Miyoko's Creamery, 11
modified tapioca starch, 39, 40, *212*, 213
moisture removal
  absorption, 123, 160
  during affinaging, 123, 159
  evaporation, 123, 160
  with gelling agents, 39
  for hard cheeses, 4, 118, 123
mold ripened cheeses
  blue cheese, 146–158, *147*, *148*, *149*, *153*, *157*, *158*

commercial production of, 136
keeping separate during aging, 159, 160
preparation for making, 137
refrigeration requirements for, 137, 140–141
white mold ripened cheese, 137–145, *139, 140, 141, 145*
molds
blue mold appearing, 147, *147*, 148, *153*
conidia, 147
HP6 direct set, 141, *212*, 213
*P. candidum*, 58, 141, 213
*P. roqueforti*, 4, 20, 58, 146, *212*, 213
PRB6, 150, *212*, 213
role in cheesemaking, 18
sources for, 213
veins, creating, 147, 149, *149*
white mold appearing, *139, 140, 141, 145*
working with, 20
molds, cheese (equipment), *26, 27*, 101, *102, 102, 157, 179*
mousse, **Almond Mocha Ricotta Mousse**, *181*, 181–182, *182*
mozzarella-style cheeze
about, 31, 39
**Mozzarella-Style Cheeze**, 55–56, *56*
**Mozzarella-Style Cheeze**, 55–56, *56*
mushrooms, **Herb, Potato, Mushroom and Asparagus Galette**, *203*, 203–205, *205*
mycelia, 147, *147*, 148

## N
New England Cheesemaking Supply Co., 13
New Roots, xii, 11
*The New Wildcrafted Cuisine* (Baudar), 60
Noma, 60
*The Noma Guide to Fermentation* (Zilber and Redzepi), 60
nut cheeze, 17
nutritional yeast
about, 214
and cheeze, 1, 14, 17
sources for, 213

using, *31, 43, 212*
nuts
for bases, *212*
soaking, 32–33
sources for, 213, 214
Nuts For Cheese, xii, 11

## O
oats
as a base, *212*, 227
**Oats, Cashew, and Coconut Yogurt**, 174–175
sources for, 213, 214
**Oats, Cashew, and Coconut Yogurt**, 174–175
observation, 30–31, 120, 168
oil curing, 164
online, ordering, 213, 214

## P
*P. candidum*, 58, 141, 213
*See also* white mold ripened cheese; white molds
*P. roqueforti*, 4, 20, 58, 146, 150, *212*, 213
*See also* blue mold ripened cheeses
Palace Culture, xiii
papaya, 119
Parmela, 11
pathogens
about, 22
bandaging, 165
effect of lactic acid on, 59, 61
effect of salt on, 116, 125
and fresh herbs, 37, 51, 92
irradiation, 63
oil curing, 164
temperatures promoting, 32, 65
white mold cheeses and, 138
*See also* bacteria
pears
**Caramelized Pears**, 187, 188
**Pear Tarte Tatin**, 187–190, *188, 189, 190*
**Pear Tarte Tatin**, 187–190, *188, 189, 190*
pecans
as a base, *212*, 227
soaking, 32–33
sources for, 213, 214

pectin, 44–45
*Penicillium roqueforti* (*P. roqueforti*). *See P. roqueforti*
Perfect Day, 12
perseverance, 30, 31, 120, 168
pH levels
during affinaging, 159
for mold ripened cheese, 138, 139, 140
pH meters, 137
**Photosynthesis, a Smoothie**, 207, *207*
piercing, 147, 149, *149*
Pili Pili, 192
pistachio nuts, 32–33
plant-based cheesemaking
commercial producers, xii–xiii, 11, 19
common approaches to, 1–2
establishing language for, 96
evolution of, 16, 19
experimentation at Graze, 2–3
fermentation in, 1–2
opposition to, xiii–xiv, 10, 12
research and development, xiv, 96
standards for, 11
plant-based cheesemaking processes, 14–15, 16, 17
plant-based lifestyle, xiv, 8–9
plant milks, sources for, 213, 214
polysaccharides, 41, 45
**Potato and Celeriac Dauphinoise (gratin)**, 201–202
potatoes
**Cheesy Potato Chowder**, 192–193, *195*
**Herb, Potato, Mushroom and Asparagus Galette**, *203*, 203–205, *205*
**Potato and Celeriac Dauphinoise (gratin)**, 201–202
potato starch, 40
PRB6, 150
probiotics, 20, 77–78
proteins
in bases, 225–227
effect of microbes on, 13–14, 18, 123
function of, 17, 28, 44
sources for, 213, 214

pumpkin seeds
  as a base, *212*, 227
  soaking, 32–33
  sources for, 213, 214

## Q
quaternary ammonium chloride, 23–24
*Queen of Green* (website), 25
quinoa
  for rejuvelac, 63, *212*
  sources for, 213, 214–15

## R
Real Vegan Cheese, 79
Rebel Cheese, xiii, 11
record-keeping
  culturing log, 217–219
  observation log, 220
  usefulness of, 120, 122
Redzepi, René, 60
refrigeration, requirements, 120, 137, 140–141, 161
regulations, 10, 11
rehydration, of water kefir grains, 72, *73*
Reine, 11
rejuvelac
  about, 1, 19, 61
  chart of process for making, *62*
  choosing grain for, 63, *212*
  common problems with, 222–223
  and digestion, 62
  fermenting grain, 66–67, *67*
  sprouting grain, 63–65, *65*
  as starter culture, 62
  ways to use, 67
  and wild fermentation, 60
rennet, 10, 14, 18, 58, 119, 138
rhodophyta, 46
rice, 40, *212*, 228
ricotta
  **Almond Mocha Ricotta Mousse**, *181*, 181–182, *182*
  almond ricotta stuffed figs, *86*
  **Cultured Almond Ricotta, non-cooked**, *83*, 83–88, *84*, *85*, *86*
  **Walnut Ricotta**, 34–35, *35*
ring mold, 101, *101*, 102, *102*
ripening cultures

*P. roqueforti*, 4, 20, 58, 146, 150, *212*, 213
  white molds, 20, 141, *212*
  *See also* mold ripened cheeses
Riverdel, xiii
**Roasted Artichoke and Spinach Dip**, *199*, 199–200, *200*

## S
*Saccharomyces*, 68
*Salmonella*, 22, 25
salt
  dry salting, 160
  for mold ripened cheeses, 139–141, 147
  sources for non-iodized, 213
  using, 46, 116, 125
  *See also* brine
sanitation
  cleaning, 22–23
  hand washing, 25–26
  sanitizing, 23–25
  and starter cultures, 61
sanitizers
  acid based, 23, *23*, 24–25
  alkaline based, 23–24
Schinner, Miyoko, 9, 19
Schulte, Erica, 30
seaweed. *See* agar agar; carrageenan; kappa carrageenan
seeds
  soaking, 32–33
  sources for, 213, 214
semi-firm cheddar-style cheese, *104*
**Semi-Firm Cheddar-Style Cheeze Base**, 51–54
**Semi-firm Cream Cheese**, 100–104, *101*, *102*, *103*
shaping, 94, *94*, *95*, 101, *101*, 102, *102*
skills, development of
  observation, 30, 31, 120, 168
  perseverance, 30, 31, 120, 168
  record-keeping as tool for, 120, 122
slurry, 40, *41*
smoking, 49, 166, 200
smoothies
  **Photosynthesis, a Smoothie**, 207, *207*
  soaking, 31, 32–33

**Soft, Short-aged Cultured Almond Cheese**, 110
**Soft Cream Cheese**, 100
SOIL, 192, 196, 207
soups
  **Cheesy Potato Chowder**, 192–193, *195*
sour cream, **Sour Cream/Crème Fraîche**, 176, *176*
**Sour Cream/Crème Fraîche**, 176, *176*
soy
  about, 116
  chao, 116
  function of, 39
  tempeh, 79
  tofu, 39, 116–117
spelt
  and rejuvelac, *212*
  sources for, 213, 214–215
spinach, **Roasted Artichoke and Spinach Dip**, *199*, 199–200, *200*
sprouted grain
  contamination of, 64
  in making rejuvelac, 63–65, *65*
  uses for, 67
squash, **Camembert Stuffed Delicata Squash with Cranberries, Candied Pecan and Fried Sage**, 206
starches
  about, 39–40
  function of, 39
  sources for, 213
  using, 40–41, *41*
Star San, 23, *23*
starter cultures
  choosing grain for, 63
  coconut milk kefir, 74, *74*, *75*, 75–76, *76*, 77
  common problems with, 221–223
  mesophilic direct set culture, 79, *212*, 213
  probiotic capsules, 77–78
  rejuvelac, 19, 60, 61, 62, *62*, 63–65, *65*, 66–67, *67*, *212*
  role of, 61
  sauerkraut brine, 78–79
  thermophilic direct set culture, 79–80, *212*, 213

Index **237**

water kefir, 20, 68, 70–73, *73*, 79, *212*, 213, 221–222
stock, 196, 197
*Streptococcus*, 68
*Streptococcus thermophilus*, 171
sugar feeds, for water kefir, 70–71
sunflower seeds
   as a base, *212*, 227
   **Cashew, Sunflower Seed or Macadamia Cream Cheeze**, 36–38
   lethicin, 39
   soaking, 32–33
   sources for, 213
surface ripened cheese. *See white mold ripened cheese*
Syrah Infused Cherries, 178, 180, *180*

## T
tabbouleh
   **Millet Tabbouleh**, 196, 197
tapioca starch, 39, 40, *41*, 213
tempeh
   **Buttermilk Fried Tempeh**, *208*, 208–210, *209, 210*
   tempeh culture, 79
terminology, cheesemaking, 16–17
The Cultured Nut, xii, 11
thermophilic direct set culture
   about, 79–80, *212*
   and feeding mediums, 79–80
   sources for, 213
Thomas (blogger), 19
tibicos, 70
   *See also water kefir*
tofu
   about, 17, 39, 208
   **Fermented Tofu Feta**, 116–117
tools and equipment
   essential, 26, *26, 27*
   sources for, 215–216
Tzatziki, 197, 198

## U
umami, 28, 212
**Unbaked Lemon Cheesecake with Blueberry Bay Compote**, 183–186, *184, 185, 186*
   **Blueberry Bay Compote**, 183, 186, *186*
   **Unbaked Lemon Cheesecake**, 183–185, *184, 185, 186*

## V
Valenzuela, Lucia, 119, *119*, 191, 194
Vasallo, Jolene, *xiv, 119*, 191, 196
vegan cheesemaking. *See plant-based cheesemaking; plant-based cheesemaking processes*
vegan lifestyle, xiv, 8–9
VEGE, 59, 80
veins, creating, 147, 149, *149*
vinegar, as sanitizer, 24–25
Violife, 11

## W
**Walnut Ricotta**, 34–35, *35*
walnuts
   as a base, *212*, 227
   soaking, 32–33
   sources for, 213, 214
   **Walnut Ricotta**, 34–35, *35*
Wandering Deli, 11
washing, during aging, 162, *163*
water kefir
   about, 20, 68, 70, 79
   process for making, 72–73, *73*
   sources for, 213
   as starter, *212*, 221–222
   sugar feeds for, 70–71
wheat berries, 63, *65*, 213, 214–215
white beans, 37, 87, *212*, 228
   *See also beans: dry, preparing*
white mold ripened cheese
   about, 137–138
   about curd creation, 138–139
   about draining, 139
   about ripening, 139–141
   critical conditions for, 138
   macadamia, oat, cashew camembert, *139*
   lactic acid curd for, 138
   mold growth on surface, *140, 141*, 145
   pH levels in, 138, 139, 140
   process for making, 142–145, *145*
   refrigeration requirements for, 140–141
   salt for, 139–141
   susceptibility to pathogens, 138
white molds, 20, 141, *141, 212*, 213
*The Wildcrafting Brewer* (Baudar), 60
wild fermentation, 60, 61
*Wild Fermentation* (Katz), 60
Wolf Flower cheese, *118*

## Y
Yale Food Addiction Scale, 30
yeasts
   *B. linens*, 58
   *Candida*, 68
   *Kloeckera*, 68
   role in cheesemaking, 18
   *Saccharomyces*, 68
yogurt
   about, 171
   **Coconut Milk Yogurt**, *171*, 171–173, *173*
   **Oats, Cashew, and Coconut Yogurt**, 174–175

## Z
Zengarry, 11
Zilber, David, 60

## About the Author

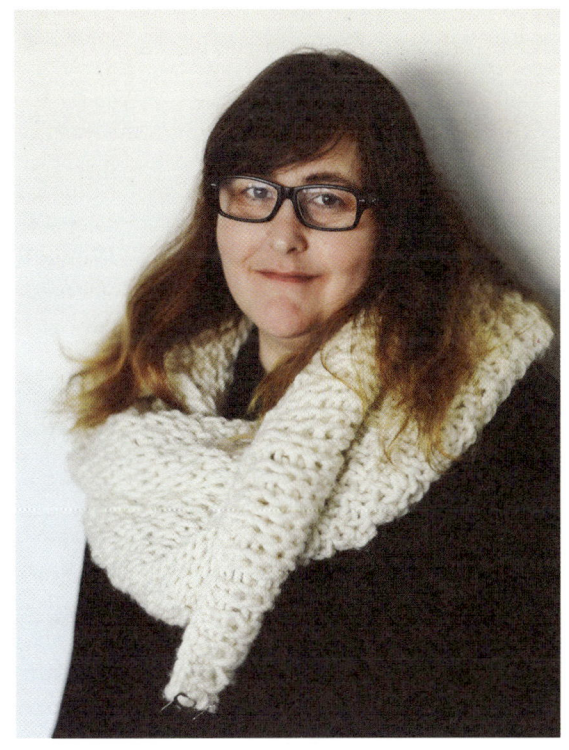

KAREN MCATHY is founder and co-owner of Blue Heron Creamery, a dairy-free, plant-based artisan cheese and vegan foods company in Vancouver, BC, which creates authentic and cultured non-dairy cheeses. McAthy is a sought-after educator in the world of plant-based food and award-winning author. www.blueheroncheese.com

## ABOUT NEW SOCIETY PUBLISHERS

New Society Publishers is an activist, solutions-oriented publisher focused on publishing books for a world of change. Our books offer tips, tools, and insights from leading experts in sustainable building, homesteading, climate change, environment, conscientious commerce, renewable energy, and more—positive solutions for troubled times.

We're proud to hold to the highest environmental and social standards of any publisher in North America. When you buy New Society books, you are part of the solution!

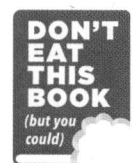

- We print all our books in North America, never overseas
- All our books are printed on **100% post-consumer recycled paper**, processed chlorine-free, with low-VOC vegetable-based inks (since 2002)
- Our corporate structure is an innovative employee shareholder agreement, so we're one-third employee-owned (since 2015)
- We're carbon-neutral (since 2006)
- We're certified as a B Corporation (since 2016)
- We're Signatories to the UN's Sustainable Development Goals (SDG) Publishers Compact (2020–2030, the Decade of Action)

At New Society Publishers, we care deeply about *what* we publish—but also about *how* we do business.

To download our full catalog, please visit newsociety.com/pages/nsp-catalogue.

Sign up for New Society Publishers' newsletter for information on upcoming titles, special offers, and author events (https://signup.e2ma.net/signup/1425175/42152/).

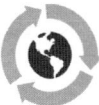

### ENVIRONMENTAL BENEFITS STATEMENT

**New Society Publishers** saved the following resources by printing the pages of this book on chlorine free paper made with 100% post-consumer waste.

| TREES | WATER | ENERGY | SOLID WASTE | GREENHOUSE GASES |
|---|---|---|---|---|
| 95 | 7,600 | 40 | 320 | 41,100 |
| FULLY GROWN | GALLONS | MILLION BTUs | POUNDS | POUNDS |

Environmental impact estimates were made using the Environmental Paper Network Paper Calculator 4.0. For more information visit www.papercalculator.org.

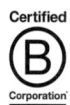
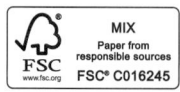
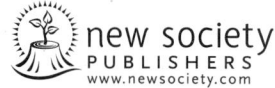